ENTER THE PHYSICIAN

History of American Science and Technology Series

General Editor, LESTER D. STEPHENS

ENTER THE PHYSICIAN

The Transformation of
Domestic Medicine
1760–1860

LAMAR RILEY MURPHY

The University of Alabama Press

Tuscaloosa and London

Library of Congress Cataloging-in-Publication Data

Murphy, Lamar Riley, 1953–
    Enter the physician: The transformation of domestic
medicine, 1760–1860 / Lamar Riley Murphy.
    p.   cm.—(History of American science and
technology series)
    Includes bibliographical references.
    ISBN 0-8173-0514-9 (alk. paper)
    1. Medicine, Popular—United States—History.
2. Self-care, Health—United States—History.
I. Title. II. Series. [DNLM: 1. Attitude to Health—
history—United States.   2. Delivery of Health Care—
trends—United States.   3. History of Medicine, 18th
Cent.—United States.   4. History of Medicine, 19th
Cent.—United States.   WZ 70 AA1 M97t]
    RC81.M965   1991
    613'.0973'09033—dc20
                                              90–10887

British Library Cataloguing-in-Publication Data available

For Bill

Contents

Illustrations

Preface

On 21 June 1741 Abigail Franks, daughter and wife of wealthy New York merchants, wrote her son Naphtali to thank him for sending her some medicine. Despite her gratitude, she thought his effort was pointless. Most illnesses in later years, Franks explained to her son, were simply to be endured. She scoffed at the idea of trying to cure them:

Its my Opinion as a person grows in Years they Contract Infirmitys that will hardly be removed. And as I have thank god Allways had a Great Share of health I must now begin to Expect those Little Ills humane Nature is Liable too And therefore Would not be Troublesome farther then there is a Necessity for to remove a preas[en]t pain nothing in Life should . . . ingage me to Confine my Self to any Rule by Way of Prevention people must be Very fond of Life to make it a trouble to them to prolong it My Physick is Temperence & Content wich I would Prescribe to all the world And would be the best Preventing dose they could Swallow.[1]

Abigail Franks's matter-of-fact passivity in the face of physical discomfort and illness was unusual. A more common series of events may be glimpsed in letters composed more than a decade later. On 8 February 1753 Aaron Burr sat down to write to Bostonian Sarah Prince, an intimate friend of his wife, Esther Edwards Burr. Burr said that Esther, daughter of Puritan theologian Jonathan Edwards and mother of the country's future second vice-president, had "been confind with a lingring Fever for about 2 Months—It intermits but seldom if ever goes clear off—We have been apprehensive of an Hectick—And am not yet without Fears it may issue in that." Though worried, the Burrs remained hopeful that she would recover. "We have of late," the letter continued, "taken

Encouragement from the Advice of a very skillful Phisician in these Parts—but have but just begun to use his Means."[2]

Six weeks later Esther Burr still lay ill. Her father, concerned about her "remaining great Weakness," sent advice on her spiritual and physical well-being. "As to means for your Health," Edwards penned, "we have procured one Rattle-snake, which is all we could get. It is," he reminded her, "a medicine that has been very serviceable to you heretofore, and I would have you trie it still. If your stomach is very weak and will bear but little, you must take it in smaller Quantities." He also sent ginseng, giving specific instructions about preparation and dosage: "trie stewing it in water, and take it in strength and Quantity as you find suits your stomach best." Another good method, he thought, would be to steep it "in wine, in good madera or Claret; or if these wines are too harsh, then in some good white wine." Whichever way she decided to prepare it, warned Edwards, she "had best to slice it very thin, or bruise it in an Iron mortar." The anxious father then suggested a cordial, recommending "spices steep'd in some generous Wine that suits your Taste, and stomach." The best strategy, however, would be to rely on medicine as little as possible. "And above all the Rest," advised Edwards, "use riding in pleasant weather; and when you can bear it, Riding on Horse-back; but never so as to fatigue you. And be very careful to avoid taking Cold." Edwards had one final word of counsel for his daughter: "And I should think it best pretty much to throw by doctors, and be your own Physician, [. . .] hearkening to them that are used to your Constitution." In a lengthy postscript, Edwards sent recipes and directions for remedies favored by his wife, one of which she had "found . . . very strengthening and comfortable to her in her weakness."[3]

We are not privy to more precise information about how Esther Burr managed her lengthy illness, but several things about the account strike the twentieth-century observer. First, the Burrs evidently did not call a physician until the sickness was already of long duration. Burr's letter, moreover, implies that seeking medical aid amounted to an admission of the seriousness of the illness, or at least the failure of domestic remedies. Indeed, one of the most noticeable features of Esther Burr's illness was its domestic management, from diagnosis to prescription and treatment. Esther's parents recommended remedies with obvious self-assurance, and they thought turning to a doctor would be almost certain folly. Thus while neither the Burrs nor the Edwardses responded passively to Esther's sickness, they did steer clear of professional advice. Instead—because they were more "used to [Esther's] Constitution" than any doctor could be—they took charge of the young woman's treatment, relying especially on "natural" therapies such as fresh air and exercise.

These were typical reactions to sickness, even in acute cases where disease progressed much more rapidly. On 1 January 1779 Grace Growden Galloway, left alone in Philadelphia after her prominent Loyalist husband fled, wrote in her diary: "Was taken so ill in the last Night that No Anodine wou'd ease Me. . . . [I]n the Morning I . . . sent for Dr Chevot Dr Cadwalader & Dr Redman but before they came I was taken with a pucking & found it was a True bilious Cholic & after the pucking stop'd I took a large Anodine & by the time the Drs Came I got ease but they all thought Me in a Dangerous Way but as I know how to conduct Myself I think Next to providence the Anodine saved My life."[4]

Like Esther Burr and Grace Galloway, other citizens two hundred years ago fully expected to diagnose and treat a host of diseases, certainly at their onset and often until their resolution. Many of the illnesses—for instance, fevers, cancer, smallpox, and gout—were maladies for which most twentieth-century Americans automatically visit a doctor. Our forebears not only treated these illnesses themselves, but most of them firmly believed that experienced lay healers were better prepared to diagnose and treat sick people than were learned physicians. Today only minor ailments and first aid remain within the nonprofessional's diagnostic and therapeutic purview. Present-day Americans rely on doctors not only in acute and chronic illness but for preventive advice as well.

Traditionally, historians have focused on the activities of doctors to explain changes in medicine.[5] Until recently they have ignored or only tangentially addressed the experiences of the other actors in medical history: patients, caregivers, and nonprofessional healers.[6] Nor have they given much attention to exploring the importance of the domestic setting and its implications for health-care roles and responsibilities. Thanks especially to the scholarship of the past twenty years, we now understand more about both professional and nonprofessional dimensions of medical practice, but there is still a great deal to be learned.[7] How were literate Americans equipped to make decisions about matters pertaining to medicine, health, and disease? To whom or what did they look as authority?[8] How and why did this change over time? How and why have professional and nonprofessional responsibilities in health and medicine shifted over time?

To answer some of these questions, I have juxtaposed a number of different kinds of historical sources. In order to assess the nature of the health and medical information available to the literate citizen, I have examined domestic health guides, popular magazines, and textbooks.[9] Popular literature has been supplemented by professional writings— journal articles, learned essays, and handbooks of medical practice. Advice and professional literature, however, primarily allow us to reconstruct prescriptive values. To gauge the extent to which they reflected and influenced actual behavior, these public documents have been enhanced by material drawn from private sources: letters, diaries, and autobiographies. Each of these sources is more fully described in the bibliographic essay following chapter 6.

Though my survey has not been exhaustive, I believe that it has been representative, at least for a certain broadly defined group of Americans: literate, middle- to upper-class, white Protestants. My focal point should not be interpreted as denigrating the health-care experiences of other American groups, for they have certainly been important and should be closely examined as well. Nor do I wish to slight the importance of the vast amount of medical information conveyed by word of mouth and through ephemeral media. In many times and for many people, this kind of information was probably more accessible than any other, and it deserves serious scholarly attention.

To interpret the material used in this study, I have drawn on a number of different historical fields. Medical history is, of course, indispensable. It introduces the principal figures, documents powerful reasons for action, and shapes the chronology. But medical developments do not take place in a vacuum, and by itself medical history cannot fully explain changes in medical care.[10] Several other fields are crucial to the story, and they overlap considerably: the history of women, sexuality, the family, childhood, and education. Publishing history is also pertinent. Broader questions of social and cultural history—reform, religion, politics— provide essential context.

Recent research suggests some of the interconnections among these fields. Used together, they enhance each other, enriching our understanding of the past.[11] Popular health literature has most commonly been used to help explain the triumph of orthodox medicine over its sectarian challengers.[12] Though it is plausible to assume that changing popular attitudes were a key factor in this victory, no one has adequately documented the extent to which this was true. Moreover, this assumption distorts the reality of the nineteenth-century medical world by pitting orthodox physicians against challenging practitioners of every hue. If we *begin* with the literature and its writers, we find that conventional questions yield novel answers and that new dimensions appear. It is my contention that health writers—men and women from every medical perspective and the lay world—played a pivotal role in reshaping the accepted boundaries of lay and professional medical responsibilities. They had an important concomitant and interrelated role as well, for they popularized and reinforced age-old ideas about the individual's responsibility for disease prevention through healthy living.[13]

This book is organized topically and in rough chronological order. The first chapter stresses the eighteenth-century coexistence of domestic, lay, and professional spheres of medical practice. It argues that scholars have overlooked or minimized the crucial distinction between orthodox reaction to *domestic* as opposed to substandard or sectarian practice. During the colonial period, the boundaries between professional and nonprofessional medical responsibilities were not rigidly, clearly, or permanently defined. Contemporary evidence suggests that medical self-help was not the overriding issue for learned doctors before the 1830s. Rather, post-Revolutionary elite physicians, imbued with republican ideas, sought to induct the population into a learned medical ethos in which self-help occupied an integral but newly auxiliary role.

But boundary issues did begin to assume greater importance, as two different conceptions of medical legitimacy and authority increasingly collided. One conception, generally associated with nonprofessionals and rooted in tradition, vested healing authority in those demonstrating practical experience reinforced by folk teachings. The other, more characteristic of professionals, derived healing authority from formal training supplemented by bedside lessons. The two conceptions grew more and more incompatible as formally educated American physicians in the post-Revolutionary decades sought to establish and uphold European standards of learned medical practice. It was in this context that health publicists initiated a multifaceted campaign to educate Americans about medical matters. Though their efforts predated sectarianism, they eventually embraced that battle as well.

This pedagogical crusade, visible in and shaped by advice literature, blurred sectarian lines. Sectarian identification remained important in therapeutic and affiliational terms but became more fuzzy in light of other, larger concerns. Advice literature points to two areas of overarching importance during the century prior to the Civil War: first, establishing the characteristics and qualifications of the medical healer; and second, defining the nature and scope of the responsibilities of all health-care participants: healer, patient, and caregivers. The earliest writers—all orthodox practitioners—published "family physicians," encyclopedic volumes designed to educate the population about the proper management of disease. Their goal was not to destroy domestic practice, but was to improve and restrict it to more sharply defined tasks and situations.

The nature of health popularization, however, began slowly but perceptibly to change during the first third of the nineteenth century.[14] This was due in large part to the coincidental conjunction of two broad trends. The first, as examined in chapter 2, dovetailed with growing cultural investment in the concept and duties of motherhood. As orthodox doctors sought to claim healing authority superior to that traditionally exercised by women, they placed a premium on the woman's role in preventing disease and rearing healthy children, thereby seeking to assure the future of the republic. In the process, a campaign in which questions of gender were subsumed in issues of expertise evolved into one for which gender became central. An unanticipated but far-reaching consequence was to justify the exclusion of women from formal medical training, a powerful legacy for generations to come.[15]

Changes in health popularization also resulted from the deepening realization that the quest to enlighten Americans was in many ways counterproductive to the interests of established medicine. Chapter 3 examines the regulars' mounting alarm as herbalist Samuel Thomson glorified self-help, perverting the Revolutionary heritage by wresting domestic practice from its essential but ancillary role within the learned medical tradition. Few of Thomson's followers were as radical as he, and most challenged the dominant therapeutic system rather than the structure of the healing relationship. Most Thomsonians agreed that both an educated citizenry and a medical profession were indispensable, and they shared the emphasis on disease prevention that was increasingly visible among orthodox practitioners. The regulars' experiences with Thomsonianism underscored the inadequacy of legislation in fighting sectarianism as it highlighted the hazards of focusing popular educational efforts on treatment.

Accordingly, beginning in the middle third of the nineteenth century, regular physicians turned to another type of popular education, downplaying information about disease *treatment* and stressing facts about disease *prevention*. In this crusade they were joined by a disparate group of people: health reformers; sectarians, including Thomsonians, homeopaths, and hydropaths; and quasi-professional women. From the physicians' perspective, this was a precarious alliance; they were constantly on guard to detect and discredit popularizers of Thomson's ilk, who they felt did not observe the fine line between instructing the population on health matters and invading the physician's realm. Chapter 4 presents the ideas of popular crusaders for healthy living, spotlighting Sylvester Graham

and William A. Alcott, and documents their fortunes in winning orthodox support. Increasingly, however, professionals and nonprofessionals
alike realized that general behavioral guidelines alone could not adequately or appropriately prepare individuals—even the most dedicated—
to meet the challenges of attaining and maintaining health.

Starting in the 1830s, orthodox physicians thus promoted a new type
of popular health literature as a necessary and ideal complement to existing sources of written advice: textbooks in anatomy, physiology, and
hygiene. Chapter 5 analyzes this pioneering educational effort, which
minimized or completely omitted information about disease treatment
and instead explained how people could prevent illness and be healthy.
Imbued with the perfectionism and pietism prevalent in mid-nineteenth-
century America, textbook authors—physicians and nonprofessionals,
men and women—defined their crusade as much in terms of moral as
physical redemption. In more concrete terms than ever before, nineteenth-century citizens learned about how to discharge their obligations
to themselves, their families, and their country. For the first time, then,
on the eve of the Civil War, there existed for popular consumption written behavioral guidelines based on increasingly systematic scientific arguments. As textbook authors sought to enlighten the population about the
physiological underpinnings of good living, they also helped to redefine
professional and nonprofessional roles in health and medicine.

During the same mid-nineteenth-century decades, as chapter 6 ex-
plores, there were many other advocates of healthy living. Among the
most prolific were hydropathists, homeopathists, and female practitioners. Though each in varying ways posed a threat to the medical establishment, there were significant areas of tacit or explicit consensus among
orthodox physicians and their rivals. Crucial issues about how to cope
with disease and promote health transcended acrimonious rhetoric and
boundary disputes: most notably, that physicians should supervise disease treatment; that lay people should assume responsibility for preventing illness; that patients and their caregivers should adhere to certain
physician-defined rules in caring for the sick; and that all Americans
should be properly educated about health and disease.

Inherent in this ongoing educational process was the ever sharper re-
allocation of treatment responsibility. Health popularizers more and more
strenuously insisted that disease management lay within the physician's
rightful and exclusive purview. Nonprofessionals, even those with healing skills honed through extensive practical experience, lacked medical
training and the superior expertise thereby conferred. Their participation

in disease treatment should therefore be confined to nursing and emergency care.

Underway for more than a century by the time of the Civil War, this process of boundary redefinition, though discernible and increasingly authoritative, should not be imagined as constituting a straightforward progression from one arbitrarily chosen point in time to another. At the mid-eighteenth-century inception of the health popularization campaign, like-minded physicians articulated a common vision of the individual and societal rewards to be reaped by diffusing medical knowledge. The loosely defined homogeneity of the trailblazers, however, disappeared within a generation, as a wide range of professional and nonprofessional people adopted the educational crusade. Antebellum health popularizers, often representing antagonistic therapeutic positions, were united by their mutual interest in defining appropriate lay and professional health-care responsibilities.

Change was gradual and uneven but *real*. Though established medicine remained on precarious footing on the eve of the Civil War, a doctor practicing in 1860 enjoyed greater authority in the sickroom than had his colleagues fifty or a hundred years earlier. Much of this change came from the work of three generations of health publicists. As popular medical writers helped oust the lay person from accustomed roles, they assigned each individual responsibility for prevention, which they deemed crucial to the nation's ability to survive. The broad diffusion of preventive knowledge would take on new importance with the postbellum discovery of the germ theory. Bacteriology revolutionized health care in the five decades following the Civil War, but the groundwork had been laid by doctors and reform-minded writers in the preceding century.

Acknowledgments

I have accumulated many debts since beginning this study, and they are a pleasure to acknowledge. Kathleen Neils Conzen, who chaired my dissertation committee at the University of Chicago, read and reread every chapter, and I have profited from her advice. Neil Harris taught me that clear writing and aggressive editing are inseparable, and Jan Goldstein offered constructive criticism and solid support at several crucial moments. During my undergraduate years at Tulane University, Sylvia Frey set an inspiring example of rigorous scholarship and precise exposition.

Many people read and commented on early versions of the first chapter. I would particularly like to thank Julia Antelman, Eileen Brewer, Jeffrey Brooks, Karen Brooks, Stephen Freedman, Alexa Hand, Stewart Herman, Sarah Kilpatrick, Stephen Lestition, and Kathleen McCarthy. Ann Durkin Keating, James Lewis, and Anthea Waleson tackled every word of my dissertation draft, and I count myself lucky to have had their pointed criticisms and their sustaining friendships. On many occasions Kenneth Cmiel gave as much thought to this study as to his own, and his suggestions have been invaluable. For years Kathleen Schwartzmann strayed from her work in sociology to serve as my behind-the-scenes adviser; had I not had the benefit of her good-humored prodding and practical suggestions, I am certain this project would have lasted several more years.

This study simply could not have been done without extensive use of the University of Chicago Library's Interlibrary Loan office. I am deeply grateful to Janet Fox, Sandra Applegate, and other staff members for their good-natured, creative, and rapid processing of a flood of requests over many years. My former colleagues in the University of Chicago Library's Department of Special Collections provided a stimulating and friendly work environment that helped immeasurably. Special thanks go to Michael Ryan and especially Daniel Meyer, whose support and feedback eased the path more than he imagines. Robert Rosenthal shared my love of popular medical books, and he created a remarkable collection that has served as the backbone of this project. Because of his untimely death, he will not see the completion of the project he so enthusiastically nurtured. Jean Block's wisdom and wit helped me through countless rough spots, and I wish the current manuscript had had the benefit of her review. All of the illustrations in this book come from material in the University of Chicago Library, and I am delighted to have received permission to use its rare, science, and general collections in this way.

Julia Antelman, Paul Carnahan, Therese Chappell, Kimberly Shively, Katherine Uradnick, and especially Bruce Peterson readily supplied essential computer assistance. Nearly a decade ago Susan Kerr decided to educate me about computers, and she has responded cheerfully and speedily to every ensuing plea for help. Steadfast support from Carol Eck and especially from Patricia Prieto has helped me weather the ups and downs of getting this project done.

Thanks to excellent support from The University of Alabama Press, the process of preparing the manuscript for publication has been surprisingly smooth. Jean Tyrone's copyediting helped immensely, as did the editorial suggestions made by Ellen Stein and the staff of The University of Alabama Press. Malcolm MacDonald and Lester Stephens have offered consistent support and guidance, and I have very much appreciated their confidence in this project. I am also grateful to David Pofelski, who created an excellent index in a short period of time.

I grew up in Greenville, Alabama, a town that is attuned to its history and the history of its inhabitants. I am certain that my parents, Mary and James Riley, never imagined that the stories they told me from a young age would have such a great influence. I have also relished the link to the past through my grandparents: Lois Boggan Riley, Fred H. Riley, Sr., Marguerite Cureton Riley, Ethel Jackson Williamson, and Edward Lamar Williamson, whom I never met but for whom I was named. I very much appreciate their nurturing my inquiring spirit and encouraging my endeavors for so many years. Long before I began this study, my brother, James Riley, stood firmly behind me, and his unwavering faith has fortified me.

Since my marriage I have been blessed with the companionship of another family for whom historical matters are important. Professor Edna

McGlynn, Priscilla McGlynn Murphy, and Philip Murphy responded to this project with special enthusiasm, and I have appreciated their confidence.

A latecomer to this project, my husband, Bill Murphy, brought with him extraordinary good humor, historical sensitivity, and editorial expertise. For his generous help with this project and so many other things, I thank him.

ENTER THE PHYSICIAN

The Family Physician

"All the nation are already physicians," observed Nicholas Culpeper about England in his 1649 *Physicall Directory.* "If you ail anything, every one you meet, whether a man or woman, will prescribe you a medicine for it."[1] Culpeper's remark acknowledged the plethora of practitioners in mid-seventeenth-century Britain. As Culpeper implied, not all healers were licensed or professional physicians, but he did not comment on the nature of the relationship between the licensed and the unlicensed healers. Had he done so, he would have described a culture in which the boundaries between and within the two groups were fluid and often blurred. In fact, even separating them into two groups confers a bipolarity that is somewhat artificial. To echo several recent scholars, the most realistic way to view healers of this period would be to imagine them "shad[ing] into each other along a continuum" that was elastic, multidimensional, and dynamic. Today, on the other hand, we take for granted the existence of clear distinctions between doctors and the lay public, between professional and lay knowledge, and between professional and lay areas of expertise. In Culpeper's time, both licensed healers and the population at large viewed unlicensed healers as a necessary and legitimate part of the medical fraternity.[2]

But there were differences among Old World healers during this period, the most discernible stemming from the sources of their authority and legitimacy. All licensed healers belonged either to a trade or a profession and therefore had to meet certain qualifications in terms of knowledge. Unlicensed healers did not have to satisfy legal standards of knowledge because they were not members of a trade or profession.

However, they derived comparable legitimacy from their experience in healing, which in many cases was far greater than that of more learned practitioners.[3]

Licensed healers were either physicians, apothecaries, or surgeons. In earlier days, law had classified them as separate orders, but by the time of Culpeper's writing they overlapped considerably in terms of function and knowledge. Only physicians were considered to be members of a profession, while apothecaries and surgeons, who worked with their hands, belonged to the trades. All three groups diagnosed and prescribed, but physicians preferred that apothecaries compound medicines and that surgeons perform operations. Physicians usually did receive more formal training than apothecaries or surgeons, but the lengthy and theoretical nature of that training—traditionally, a liberal British university education—left them less well equipped to treat disease than were many other healers, licensed and unlicensed. To gain more practical experience, physicians increasingly were to supplement their schooling with apprenticeships and study abroad at more clinically oriented universities. Physicians overlapped in other ways with their lay counterparts. For instance, they familiarized themselves with subjects like alchemy and astrology, and they incorporated folk cures into their materia medica.[4]

Unlicensed healers ran the gamut from domestic and lay practitioners to quacks. Quacks, often called "empirics" because of their reliance on experience over theory, existed on the fringes of medical respectability. Some, like oculist and former tailor William Read, won royal favor. Others, such as Bishop George Berkeley, proponent of tar water, sparked widespread literary debate over the merits of their nostrums. James Graham was typical of many. As the creator of the Temple of Health, featuring a Celestial or Magnetico-Electrical Bed, Graham achieved brief notoriety before returning to obscurity. In short, the term *quack* embraced a variety of individuals united by their self-proclaimed but often pretended medical knowledge and their entrepreneurial zeal.[5]

Unlike quacks, domestic and lay practitioners occupied a legitimate position in the medical world. Except among the advantaged, they rarely had even a smattering of learned medical knowledge. Instead, they used folk remedies and understanding acquired by experience to minister to their own families and often to neighbors as well. Neither physicians nor quacks, domestic practitioners were defined by one 1542 British statute as "divers honest persons, as well men as women, whom God hath endowed with the knowledge of the nature, kind and operation of certain herbs, roots and water and the using and administering of them to such as be pained with customable disease." These were the healers consulted by most people, who were confined by income, residence, learning, or preference to this sphere. Only the wealthiest sought the services of the elite, learned practitioner.[6]

Not only were few seventeenth-century English citizens directly exposed to learned medicine, but many well-educated lay people dismissed orthodox medicine and praised folk remedies and practitioners. King James I, for instance, ridiculed academic medicine as mere conjecture and therefore useless. Francis Bacon insisted that "empirics and old women" were "more happy many times in their cures than learned physicians," and many of his contemporaries agreed. Among them was Thomas Hobbes, who stated that he would "rather have the advice or take physic from an experienced old woman that had been at many sick people's bedsides, than from the learnedst but unexperienced physician."[7]

There was no certain litmus for distinguishing between scientific and empirical practice. In fact, to most people such a distinction would have seemed irrelevant. What mattered most was proven ability to cure diseases. In the absence of generally accepted professional and societal standards, each individual had to decide whom to trust. "Prestige and confidence," as Joseph Kett has summarized, "not formal qualification, became the touchstones of success."[8]

A large part of the reason for these attitudes was that learned physicians in the seventeenth and eighteenth centuries had very little diagnostic or therapeutic advantage over their unlearned counterparts. For over two thousand years physicians had relied on the same three basic tools to determine the nature of a person's illness: listening to the patient's own description of the situation; observing the patient's appearance, behavior, and wastes; and examining the patient's body, which was usually fully or partly clothed. Some diseases could be fairly easily recognized by the presence of telltale rashes or lesions that accompanied them, and there was rarely any doubt about the primary injury caused by obvious trauma, such as broken bones or sprained joints. In many other cases, however, the principal symptom was something less specific, such as fever, aches, or fatigue. Given the resources available, the people who were most successful at diagnosis were those who had had considerable medical experience—whether physicians or lay healers—and could recognize a wide range of diseases. Formal education could be helpful, but familiarity with the patient's constitution and history was usually more pertinent. As a result, in many cases patients trusted their own instincts or the judgment of family members over the advice of a physician.[9]

Just as the means of diagnosis had remained largely unchanged for centuries, so too had the means of treatment and the understanding of the treatment context. Until well into the nineteenth century, medical theory and therapeutics were strongly influenced by humoralism, formalized by Galen in the second century A.D. According to this tradition, health resulted from a natural balance of four bodily humors (yellow bile, blood, phlegm, and black bile) and their manifested qualities (cold, heat, moistness, and dryness). Furthermore, every part of the body was inextricably related to every other part, so that an imbalance in any one part resulted in illness for the whole. This meant that the body had to achieve and maintain equilibrium both with itself and with its environment. The need to pay attention to bodily functions *and* environmental conditions spawned advice literature on how to attain internal and external balance through proper ventilation, diet, clothing, excretion, perspiration, and so forth.

The humoral framework also had repercussions for treatment. Healers and patients believed that treatment was most effective when it seemed to correct imbalances and restore equilibrium. Feverish patients, for example, would be advised to follow a cooling regimen; they might also be bled to help lower high temperatures produced by too much blood. Those suffering from chills and a runny nose would take preparations that warmed and dried. If a patient's stool was abnormally dark, the doctor might prescribe an enema or oral laxative to eliminate excess black bile. What was important to both healer and patient, as Charles Rosenberg has pointed out, was that the therapies "worked"—that is, that they "provid[ed] visible and predictable physiological effects." Not only did a drug's activity indicate to both healer and patient that it was effective, but the results also provided valuable insights into prognosis. Healers, caregivers, and patients carefully monitored the patient's responses and examined all physical signs and products to evaluate how the body was doing and what should be done next. These assumptions encouraged healers and their patients to adopt a very active role in disease management.

Even if a physician were called in to direct treatment, his authority and the efficacy of his prescriptions were inevitably affected by a number of factors. To begin with, the patient would almost certainly have already undergone numerous treatments, whether self-administered or supervised by family and friends. The fact that a physician had been asked to consult usually signaled that the patient's condition had deteriorated or failed to improve. In order to diagnose and treat effectively, the physician was completely dependent on the memory and truthfulness of the patient and his attendants. Even if they faithfully revealed every symptom, medication, and response since the onset of the illness, the physician still had to exercise sensitivity and ingenuity in understanding the information being imparted. The doctor's book learning gave him a different, though not necessarily better, perspective on health and illness from that of the lay person. As a result, there was always the danger that, without being aware of it, doctors and lay people would attach different meanings to the same words, thereby inadvertently increasing the gulf between professional and nonprofessional. Whether their patients cooperated or not, all doctors obviously would have had great difficulty in predicting what effects previous actions might have on their own therapies.[10]

The physician's authority and the utility of his advice were also undermined by the fact that treatment took place in a domestic setting, typically with the active participation of family, relatives, friends, and local healers.[11] Here the doctor was at a significant disadvantage: he was rarely present all day and night to ensure that his instructions were being followed, or to see the results of his treatment unfolding. The domestic context of illness forced the physician—and any other healer—to forge an alliance with the people in the home. Without their reports on the patient's condition and their cooperation in treatment, the healer's ability to practice was seriously handicapped or even nullified.[12]

There were virtually no trained doctors among the early immigrants to the New World, and colonial domestic and lay practice flourished, encouraged rather than contested by lawmakers. Status distinctions were blurred, and even quackery was more or less tolerated. By the eighteenth century, however, the situation had begun to change, as an incipient medical elite appeared.[13] To explain the consequences, Paul Starr has rightly stressed the eighteenth-century American coexistence of domestic, lay, and professional spheres of medical practice. In the democratic fervor of the post-Revolutionary period, Starr says, nonprofessional medicine had heightened appeal, exacerbating the latent tension between professional ideals and a democratic culture. By the first decade of the nineteenth century, learned physicians were acutely conscious of their precarious cultural authority. They blamed lay healers, principally those affiliated with mushrooming medical sects—first Thomsonianism and eventually hydropathy, homeopathy, and many others. Sectarians rejected learned medicine in favor of their own treatment regimens, and learned doctors thought sectarian tenets also reinforced the self-help tradition. Elite physicians tried to assert authority, Starr argues, in part by publishing domestic health guides to spread *regular* medical knowledge. Starr sees the results as paradoxical. In the long term, domestic manuals did extend learned medical authority, for they reached a broad and unenlightened spectrum of the population. In the shorter term, however, Starr agrees with other students of American medicine: domestic manuals *undermined* professional authority by providing the endorsement and knowledge conducive to medical self-reliance.[14]

Certainly the struggle for cultural authority was central to post-Revolutionary medical developments, and, over the long term, nonsectarian health guides indeed enhanced the legitimacy of established medicine. To understand the shorter-term reality, however, it is essential to differentiate more carefully learned medical reaction to *domestic* or *lay,* as opposed to *substandard* or *sectarian,* practice. Contemporary evidence suggests that medical self-help was not the overriding issue for learned physicians before the 1830s. Rather, beginning in the 1770s, they sought to induct the population into a learned medical ethos in which self-help occupied an integral but newly auxiliary role. Two factors made this undertaking imperative: first, the determination of elite physicians to raise professional standards and restrict medical practice to men accredited by formal medical schooling; and second, the republicanism of the Revolutionary era, which mandated a well-educated citizenry to ensure social health and national survival. During these years of the new republic, ideas about lay and professional responsibilities—as defined by doctors *and* by lay people—remained fluid and mutually tutorial.[15] Learned physicians made progress, slow and erratic but real, toward establishing a new definition of legitimate medical credentials, a definition in which experience was necessarily supplemented by formal medical training.

A New Genre Emerges

What the eighteenth-century citizen did when taken sick of course depended on many things, but the most important determinants were the apparent severity of the illness, ease of access to medical care, and social and economic position. In the truncated version of the British guild system that developed in the colonies, there existed no recognized body of physicians whose authority rested on formal medical schooling, nor were there adequate and enforceable legal or professional barriers to medical practice. In this situation well-educated men, usually learned but rarely formally trained in medicine, constituted the medical elite. Benjamin Franklin was a notable exemplar of this group, but less renowned gentlemen in every colony—ministers, politicians, plantation owners, merchants—shared Franklin's fascination with medicine. Many, such as William Byrd and George Logan, assembled fine libraries with sizable medical holdings, and some developed reputations as skilled healers.[16] Most colonists, however, had little or no acquaintance with the learned medical tradition. Except in alarming cases, the average citizen relied on treasured family recipes or chose from an array of folk practitioners: bonesetters, cancer doctors, herbalists, nostrum dealers, apothecaries, midwives, and neighborhood women. Diaries, letters, cookbooks, almanacs, and newspapers were sprinkled with traditional wisdom pertaining to health, disease, and medicine.[17] Canons of learned medicine sporadically intruded, particularly in controversy when doctors used newspapers and pamphlets to compete for the approbation of their medical colleagues and the reading public.[18]

Colonists also could turn to domestic health manuals, many of which were longevity texts, such as Luigi Cornaro's *Discourses on a Sober and Temperate Life*. A sixteenth-century tract on physical salvation through temperate living, the Italian nobleman's testimonial was a perennial British favorite after its 1704 London publication. Reprinted in America by Benjamin Franklin in 1793, Cornaro's book was reissued three years later by Parson Weems in combination with Franklin's *Immortal Mentor, or Man's Unerring Guide to a Healthy, Wealthy, and Happy Life*. The message still had wide appeal, for as book agent Weems wrote to Philadelphia publisher Mathew Carey in October 1796, "My subscribers are numberless and very impatient for their books."[19] London physician George Cheyne's writings also found a large audience, especially his 1724 *An Essay on Health and Long Life,* of which six English-language editions appeared the next year and ten before 1745.[20] These volumes conveyed age-old, common-sense advice for healthy living and provided only limited information about specific diseases and therapies.

Citizens who wanted to know more about therapeutics consulted curatives, a genre that had existed in some form at least since the Middle Ages. Herbals predominated, their British popularity boosted by the 1652 appearance of Nicholas Culpeper's *The English Physitian* and the 1747 publication of John Wesley's *Primitive Physick*. Though Culpeper was ambivalent toward learned medicine, the Methodist theologian violently opposed it. Both generally followed the cookbook pattern, organizing their handbooks according to names of diseases, symptoms, remedies, and injuries, and then giving appropriate information under each heading. Occasionally they added a line or two of description derived from learned authorities, but more often—like other contemporary sources of lay medical information—they transmitted folk traditions.[21]

The 1769 Edinburgh publication of William Buchan's *Domestic Medicine* marks a turning point in the type of medical information available to the average citizen. A medical graduate of the University of Edinburgh and a Fellow of the Royal College of Physicians of Edinburgh, Buchan was squarely within the learned medical tradition. He denied that his goal was to teach nonprofessionals to be their own doctors, but he argued that

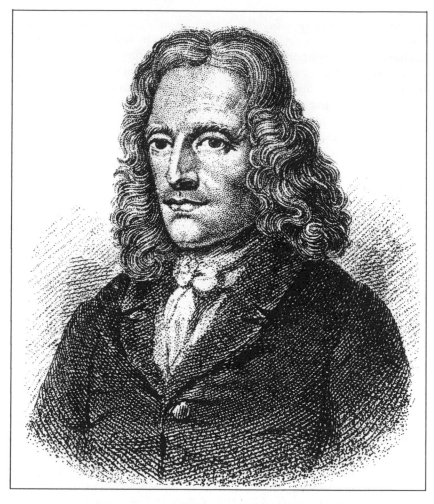

Portrait of William Buchan, author of the path-breaking *Domestic Medicine* (Edinburgh, 1769), from the frontispiece of his *Advice to Mothers* (Philadelphia, 1804).

it was the physician's duty to instruct the public about "the importance of due *care* for the preservation of health, and of the proper *regimen* in diseases." There were situations, he recognized, "where something must be done, and no medical assistance can be had, [and] it is certainly better to direct people what they ought to do than to leave them to blunder on in the dark." By educating the benevolent, Buchan also hoped to encourage their efforts to reduce the poor's reliance on "quacks and conjurers, and the folly of their own superstitious notions."[22]

Buchan fused the two older traditions, and his creation differed strikingly from those of his predecessors within either genre. The first third of his book, devoted to health and its maintenance, resembles longevity texts in its organization according to the ancient doctrine of the nonnaturals, those "factors external to man which inevitably and continuously influenced his physical well-being." The six elements included air, food and drink, motion and rest, sleep and wakefulness, evacuation and retention, and the passions of the soul. Though these subjects harkened back to ancient interests, providing information on these topics meshed well with contemporary ideas about how to avoid and treat disease. Furthermore, Buchan sounded a more activist and secular tone compared to most earlier advice books.[23]

The remainder of Buchan's book broke new ground. Instead of printing lists of cures as did existing curatives, Buchan gave detailed information about diseases, including for each one a discussion of causation, symptoms, regimen, treatment, and prevention. Rather than following the alphabetical structure used in most curatives, Buchan arranged his *Domestic Medicine* according to nosological principles. In short, Buchan's book, as Charles Rosenberg has pointed out, differed importantly from its forerunners in that it was meant to be *read* as well as *used*. By Rosenberg's count, *Domestic Medicine* appeared in at least one hundred fortytwo separate English-language editions between its original publication and the 1871 Philadelphia version.[24] Not surprisingly, it was widely cited, imitated, debated, and plagiarized, particularly during the first half-century after publication.

Domestic Practice and Practitioners

Abigail Adams, wife of Massachusetts patriot and future president John Adams, noted in her diary in 1784 that she was reading "Buchan Domestick Medicine. He appears a sensible, judicious and rational writer."[25] It is tempting to assume that the appearance and popularity of a domestic manual offering such detailed disease and treatment information indicated the existing or incipient decline of established medicine. Some people did voice dismay. Vicesimus Knox, a popular British essayist, summarized the major reservations in a 1788 essay "On the Rashness of Young and Adventurous Writers in Medicine." Problems arose, Knox explained, when those "totally ignorant of medicine, both practical and theoretic," decided that their symptoms matched those described in a book and "[took] the medicine, just as it is prescribed, without regard to the difference of age, seasons, or symptoms." This was exactly the wrong sort of behavior, said Knox, who advised readers to "abstain . . . from medical books; and apply, in sickness, to the best physician or apothecary within reach of your situation." Licensed healers, Knox argued, had two important advantages: they had "speculative and practical skill" and they operated "with a cooler and more deliberate judgment" than a person dosing himself or his loved ones could possibly possess.[26]

Despite Knox's words, it must be remembered that learned practitioners of this time not only tolerated home health care but *expected* it; for them, the domestic or lay role was complementary, not threatening, to that of the professional. Benjamin Rush, the most eminent American physician of the latter half of the eighteenth century, exemplifies this stance. As Rush cautioned a group of 1789 medical graduates, medical improvements did not come exclusively from colleges and universities. "Systems of physic are the productions of men of genius and learning[,]" he clarified, "but those facts which constitute real knowledge are to be met with in every walk of life." Rush urged his listeners to look everywhere for insight into disease management. Discussions with quacks would be profitable, he explained, partly because they would highlight the "ignorance and temerity" of many learned practices. The fledgling doctors should also "converse with nurses and old women" and "even Negroes and Indians," because they often knew facts that had "escaped the most sagacious observers of nature." Nor, Rush concluded, should the students neglect "persons who have recovered from indispositions without the aid of physicians," being certain to "mark the plain and home-made remedy to which they ascribe their recovery." Rush himself kept his so-called "Quack Recipe Book" in his coat pocket so that he could scribble home remedies in it as he discovered them.[27]

A dozen years later Rush was still giving the same advice. He warned that, because "disease is a lawless evil," it could be understood only if it were "inspected every hour of the day and night." This meant that the novice practitioners could learn a great deal "from sitting up with sick people," as would be obvious "from conversing with sensible nurses." Once again, Rush advised that those who wanted to be successful would have to "inquire after, and record cures which have been performed by time, by accident, or by medicines, administered by quacks, or by the friends of sick people."[28]

Rush followed his own advice and sought counsel from lay people. As Elizabeth Drinker, wife of a respected Philadelphia merchant, wrote in her diary on 5 September 1807: "Dr Rush came he ask'd me what I thought of my husband loosing 6 ounces more blood, he was sure it was necessary, I told him from the appearance of his blood that was taken, and from his pulse, as far as I could judge, it was what I expected—he orderd 6 or 8 ounces more taken, which was accordingly done—and it appears worse than any yet taken from him—."[29] This passage also demonstrates Elizabeth Drinker's expertise and stature in disease treatment, which was based on long experience, folk wisdom, and medical literature, including Buchan's *Domestic Medicine*. Drinker did not always wait to be queried; on 24 December 1794, she resolved to challenge a diagnosis made months earlier:

I have been led to think, I may say to conclude, on reading Docr Rush's acct of the Yallow fever, that my daughr Nancy had it towards the later end of October last, at Clearfield—and do suppose that Docr Kuhn, who attended her, knowing that we would steadily attend her, be it what it would, kindly endeavord to conceal it from us—he say'd it was the Jaundice and some thing of the fall fever—it is possible it may be so,—but as it has pleas'd kind providence to restore her, I intend at a sutable oppertunity to tell the Doctor of my opinion of the matter, and I have no doubt of his candour on the occasion,—I suspected it while nurseing her by many of the symptoms, and finding many others in Dr Rs book, seems a confirmation.[30]

Like Elizabeth Drinker, most domestic practitioners were not passive recipients of medical knowledge. The elderly Reverend Devereux Jarratt, telling his life's story in letters to a Maryland minister friend, mentioned a facial tumor in January 1795. By April he was complaining about a copious and aggravating discharge. Reasoning that the discharge was "an effort of nature to relieve itself," Jarratt "for the first time, applied a small plaister of salve to the orifice to keep it open and afford vent to let out the water." However, he still had "not applied to any of the faculty to have their opinion," and on the basis of Buchan's handbook he felt optimistic about his condition: "At present, I cannot think there are any symptoms of a cancer, according to *Buchan's* description of a cancer." By 1796, however, the tumor had grown much worse, and he had consulted medical personnel: "Neither doctors nor surgeons know what it is."[31] In this case it is not clear that learned physicians offered any advantages over domestic practitioners.

Another who could not muster total faith in the power of learned medicine was Fisher Ames. An eminent Federalist and the son and brother of doctors, Ames registered his skepticism in a letter to Thomas Dwight on 22 September 1795. "I am told," he wrote, "my case is nervous, bilious, a disease of the liver, atrophy, etc., as different oracles are consulted. I am forbidden and enjoined to take almost every thing." Consequently, he trusted himself far more than he did physicians: "*I* prescribe, and take meat, some cider, a trotting horse, keep as warm as I can, abstain from excess of every kind, and I have still faith I may recruit."[32] As in Jarratt's case, Ames had no evidence that following his own instincts was detrimental to his well-being, and he suspected that it would be more beneficial.

Unlike Elizabeth Drinker, neither Jarratt nor Ames was well known for his healing skill. Virginian Landon Carter, on the other hand, could note that "the whole neighbourhood are almost every day sending to me. I serve them all." His diary is an absorbing account of how one planter met incessant medical challenges, and it illuminates the dynamic interplay between theory and experience that characterized his approach to sickness. Carter's social position and his familiarity with learned medical doctrines distinguished him from much of society, but his pragmatic approach to sickness mirrored the best domestic and learned practices of the times.[33]

Carter displayed an impressive command of contemporary medical literature, frequently ruminating on works by Boerhaave, Cullen, Arbuthnot, Huxham, and other eminent physicians. Like a growing number of elite doctors, Carter contended that theoretical knowledge by itself could not provide an adequate preparation for practice because it was merely "the Grammar to Experience"; evidence abounded "that from the Imperfectness of theory, there was still room for experience to improve it." He was equally "positive" that experience had to be informed by theory: "there must be experience Joined with reading to produce Success in Practice."[34] Carter took this formula seriously. He conscientiously updated his library with standard texts and journals, and preserved excerpts and self-assured evaluations in his diary for future reference and experimentation. There he also scrupulously transcribed treatments administered to himself, his dependents, and his neighbors. The planter compared anticipated with actual results, which he painstakingly monitored. Learned provenance usually did guarantee a treatment's trial, but only successful results determined whether the treatment would be rejected or used again.

Carter's typical approach can be seen in the case of an aged and faithful slave who had a relapse in June 1774 of "a Stoppage in his urine besides a costiveness."[35] Despite submission to "every endeavour" conceivable, he lay dying. As a last resort Carter applied a large blister to his back, borrowing from the *London Medical Essay* a method he had "tried . . . once before in a dropsical Youth with vast success." Dissatisfied with the results, he switched a day later to a treatment recommended by David McBride, a British medical writer, chemist, and physician. When Carter next mentions the slave on 25 August it is to lament his death, though he still insisted that "if that man had not been so vastly old, I should have cured him."

Carter's expertise was not confined to general medicine, for his diary also documents theoretical and practical knowledge in midwifery.[36] On 7 July 1766 he rushed to his parturient daughter-in-law, "almost in dispair," with "every body about her in a great fright." He judged that her condition was favorable, though "the child was dead and the womb was fallen down and what not." Carter superintended delivery of the stillborn child and afterbirth, but "another prodigeous alarm" arose when there was no lochial discharge. Tempering his anxiety, the landowner "reasoned from the dead state of the fetus the possibility of such a circumstance though I never read of it in any Author." He further reassured himself by observing other signs which "all authors do say" mitigated against the importance of the lochial discharge. Nonetheless, Carter administered some medicine and was delighted that it produced a lochial discharge. Despite his success, Carter did not relax until the doctor arrived and pronounced nothing amiss. On the eighth and ninth he rejoiced over his daughter-in-law's health, concluding on the latter day that if she continued to recuperate, "books and experience have not yet amounted to all the particular cases in Midwifery." Her experience "of hardly any Lochial discharge" proved to Carter that there were "such cases not dangerous, although every author says it is."

Carter usually did seek professional medical attendance except for minor problems, but the self-confidence derived from reading and experience made him a far from docile onlooker. His conduct during his daughter Judy's month-long illness in the summer of 1766 reveals a great deal about the tensions inherent in the relationship between physicians and domestic practitioners.[37] Stricken on 17 July, she first received professional care in an overnight visit from Dr. Mortimer on the twenty-fifth. During the physician's brief consultation on the twenty-seventh, Carter "advised a Plaister to her Stomach," but "the Dr. was angry and for a while rejected it." When "her pulse continued very low and a dead sickness [was] even felt outwardly," Mortimer changed his mind. He "put on the plaister which in two hours by the help of clysters eased and her pulse rose." The planter does not comment on how Mortimer reacted to the efficacy of the treatment that Carter had suggested and he had originally opposed. Since the patient seemed to be improving, the doctor left.

Mortimer was unavailable when next summoned on the twenty-ninth, so Carter reluctantly took charge of his daughter's treatment. Judy Carter rallied under her father's care, as Mortimer observed when he returned on August second. She grew worse during the night, however, so Carter wrote to the doctor "to tell him of her purging 18 or 19 times since he left her yesterday." The landowner also implored the physician "to make her a visit so that he might see her period of remission or intermission which I was perswaded if ever it did happen was only in the night." Mortimer responded with "a second very severe letter treating me extremely rude ridiculous and scandalous," but he did appear for another overnight stay. After the doctor's early morning departure, Carter penned another missive "in which I put forth the Parent's right to object to harsh medicines such as were condemned by the best of men and especially such as he had experienced before in a fatal manner." Though Carter did not spell out the exact nature of the conflict between his daughter's physician and himself, it is quite obvious that there *was* a conflict and that it arose primarily because of Carter's repeated challenges to the doctor's treatment advice.

Judy Carter's condition continued to vacillate, and on the ninth the landowner recorded Mortimer's written advice that she be purged as soon as her father judged appropriate. The final entry about this illness appears on 20 August; the prognosis must by this time have been favorable, because Carter mentioned the length of her indisposition only as a convenient measurement of "roguery" in dairy production figures. Whatever the patient's precise condition, the entries about Judy Carter's illness illustrate the fact that the doctor and landowner had different ideas about treatment roles and prerogatives. In several instances Carter invited the doctor's help and deferred to his experience and knowledge, and some passages convey the relief Carter felt when the doctor's advice matched his own. But Carter also believed that there were times when the doctor should defer to the landowner's judgment, honed through extensive practice and wide reading. There is no evidence that Carter intended to be disrespectful; his actions instead seem guided by the conviction that he and the doctor were partners in health care and should behave in a suitably collegial manner. The doctor's reactions reveal a different understanding of the relationship. From the physician's perspective, Carter's presumption of equality challenged the doctor's authority and violated protocol.

More than a decade later, Carter and local doctors were still struggling to define the nature and scope of their respective health-care duties and privileges. Now toward the end of his life, Carter recorded a painful bout of the colic that had plagued him since childhood. Though the diary provides exhaustive evidence of the remedies he had used over the years, in this case he eventually consulted a physician.[38] Soon displeased with the doctor's remedies, he "left them off" and began taking a nostrum that had relieved him during an earlier attack. Carter's actions annoyed his doctor. As the planter penned, "my Physician it seems grew affronted with me for it; and first from one occasion and then another, showing his unwillingness to attend me."[39] When the doctor withdrew from the case, Carter expressed sorrow rather than anger. He implied that an older and therefore wiser doctor would not have interpreted Carter's actions as those of a recalcitrant patient determined to interfere with medical authority. Instead, he would have graciously acquiesced to the planter's unmatched understanding of his own system. Carter could see no reason why he should automatically defer to trained doctors, for his reading and experience gave him a poise and expertise in medical matters that he felt approximated and sometimes surpassed theirs. As these episodes suggest, there was a great deal of tension inherent in the relationship between domestic and professional spheres of practice; while the proper boundaries between the two were sometimes questioned, their coexistence was not. It was this literate, middling-to-elite group of Americans—like Carter, Jarratt, and Drinker—that early writers of health guides especially addressed.

Educating Lay People

Because Buchan's book appeared at a time when domestic involvement in disease management was accorded an active and respected role, learned physicians in America were not hostile to his *Domestic Medicine*. On the contrary, they immediately began issuing new editions, some, like a 1795 printing, "revised and adapted to the diseases and climate of the United States of America." The editor of that 1795 version was Samuel Powel Griffitts, then professor of materia medica at the University of Pennsylvania, but formerly a pupil of Adam Kuhn and student in Edinburgh, Paris, and London.[40] A Quaker, Griffitts was known for his humanitarianism and philanthropy, particularly his role in the 1786 founding of the Philadelphia Dispensary. He also crusaded on behalf of abolitionism, the Vaccine Society, and a National Pharmacopoeia. "Doctor Buchan's *Domestic Medicine* has long since had a place in most families," Griffitts wrote, but he aimed to "[make] this valuable and popular work more intelligible, and consequently more useful." Rather than tampering seriously with Buchan's text, Griffitts used footnotes to modify, contradict, or support the author's advice. Probably because of his own absorbing interest, Griffitts appended to Buchan's discussion of smallpox a ten-page essay, "Of Vaccine Inoculation." Also new to this edition was a section on yellow fever, a subject of pressing concern to ravaged Philadelphians of the period.[41]

Reissued two years later by the same Philadelphia publisher, the Griffitts edition met competition from Isaac Cathrall's 1797 version, "adapted to the climate and diseases of America."[42] Cathrall's medical lineage was equally distinguished, for he had supplemented his study under physician John Redman with instruction in the same three European cities as Griffitts. Also a Quaker, Cathrall channeled his humanitarian impulses more narrowly, serving at the city almshouse for a decade. His book is evidently based on a different edition of Buchan than that used by his colleague, but he too relied primarily on footnotes to endorse or amend Buchan's views. Like Griffitts, Cathrall added a discussion of yellow fever.[43]

Learned medical men did not limit their support of health manuals to Buchan's. When the first American edition of Robert Wallace Johnson's *Friendly Cautions to the Heads of Families* appeared in 1804, a reviewer in the *Philadelphia Medical Museum* expressed "sincere pleasure" that "so many works of merit" were being reprinted from European editions.[44] The New York *Medical Repository* echoed this opinion, its writer pointing out that the work covered areas "which nurses are apt to neglect, and physicians too frequently disdain to superintend." There was also praise for "Mr. Humphreys, the publisher, for the zeal he exhibits in the republication of practical and well-selected books."[45] These favorable notices were doubtless encouraged by the thrust of the book: Johnson did not discuss specific remedies or disease characteristics, but instead gave general instructions to nurses on how to cooperate with physicians in caring for sick people.

Humphreys had introduced another book of British origin the year before, *The Town and Country Friend and Physician*. Published anonymously, its author was British physician James Parkinson, better remembered for his 1817 *An Essay on the Shaking Palsy,* or Parkinson's Disease.[46] Though this manual contained more treatment information, the *Medical Repository*'s critic reassured his professional brethren that the author had not been "so indiscreet as to betray mysteries of the craft, and instruct the people in the art of living without their services."[47] The situation, he conceded, did seem alarming given the abundance of books with titles such as *Family Physician, Guide to Health, Hygeia Herself, Villager's Friend,* and *Every Man His Own Doctor.* Despite appearances, the reviewer found no real cause for concern, because "the greater part of the faculty . . . generally continue . . . wisely observing the distinction between the *preventing a man from getting sick,* and *curing him after he is sick.*"

Promoting prevention won commendation for New York physician Shadrach Ricketson's 1806 *Means of Preserving Health, and Preventing Dis-*

eases.[48] Ricketson, explained the notice in the *Medical Repository*, neither offered new ideas nor challenged current medical thinking. This lack of originality was a strength, since the work transmitted to the public "a body of sound precepts for the preservation of health, and the avoidance of diseases."[49] By excluding treatment guidelines and concentrating on hygienic living, Ricketson's volume remained faithful to the old tradition of the non-naturals, as summarized in his title: "Founded principally on an attention to AIR AND CLIMATE, DRINK, FOOD, SLEEP, EXERCISE, CLOTHING, PASSIONS OF THE MIND, AND RETENTIONS AND EXCRETIONS." The volume was to be distributed in New York, Philadelphia, Baltimore, Boston, Hartford, New Bedford, Albany, and Troy. There must not have been great demand for it, however, since it appears that it was never reprinted.[50]

Curative information was also available, as shown by Henry Wilkins's *Family Adviser*, printed first in Philadelphia in 1793. The Baltimore author, another medical graduate of the University of Pennsylvania, belonged to the state's Medical and Chirurgical Faculty and advocated a National Pharmacopocia.[51] In his book Wilkins adhered to the format reminiscent of pre-Buchan works, offering limited discussion of diseases keyed to a numbered list of remedies in the appendix. Bound with most of the seven editions of Wilkins's volume was John Wesley's *Primitive Physick*, which heightened the association with the earlier form.[52]

More typical of the new genre was James Ewell's *The Planter's and Mariner's Medical Companion*, originally published in Philadelphia in 1807.[53] From a prominent Virginia family, Ewell settled in Pennsylvania after studying with respected physicians in Alexandria and Baltimore. Before 1805 he had moved to Savannah, where he is said to have been the first to vaccinate there for smallpox. Ewell's medical guide followed Buchan's model in that it covered both the prevention and the treatment of disease. The 1816 edition retained endorsements by many highly respected American physicians, including Shippen, Chapman, Barton, Caldwell, Woodhouse, and Ramsay. Each praised Ewell for having provided a non-European domestic manual for those, as Caldwell and Ramsay phrased it, "remote from medical aid."[54]

Yet the *Philadelphia Medical Museum*'s reviewer had no praise for Ewell's book. "The venerable Buchan's work" was sufficient alone, he argued, and there was no reason to add to it unless there were some "new and important discoveries" to communicate to readers. Not only did Ewell have nothing new to offer, but the reviewer thought that his solicitation of recommendations was "disgraceful for a professional man" because it gave the appearance of trying to influence what people thought of

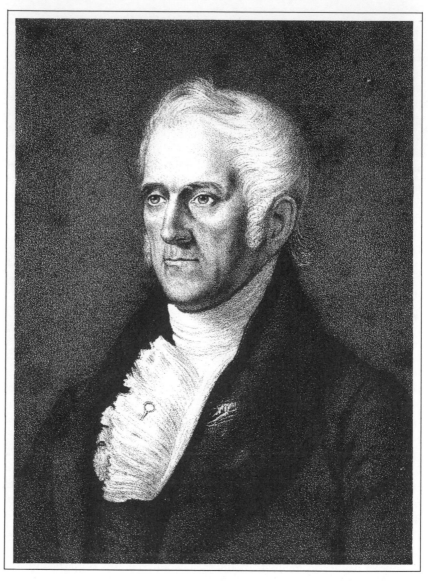

Portrait of James Ewell, author of *The Planter's and Mariner's Medical Companion* (Philadelphia, 1807), from the frontispiece of a later edition, *The Medical Companion* (Philadelphia, 1847).

his work. On top of all of this, the reviewer used roughly half of his essay to list specific instances in which he felt that Ewell had chosen inappropriate therapies, which he thought was unforgivable "in a work expressly intended to be the *vade mecum,* or medical *fac totum* of the secluded planter." The reviewer in the *Medical Repository* took the opposite view and defended the publication of health manuals, including Ewell's. "We are not attached to monopolies of any kind," read the notice, especially any that would suppress "the information which will teach man how to prevent sickness and pain, and to remove these ills when they invade."[55]

None of these handbooks advocated medical self-sufficiency, which James Parkinson labeled "domestic quackery" in the 1803 New Hampshire edition of *Medical Admonitions to Families.*[56] Nor did they share the irascible and learned physician Thomas Cooper's stance. Half of his 1824 *Treatise on Domestic Medicine* was devoted to cookery, and his disease advice frequently consisted of terse suggestions to "Apply to a physician" or "Send for a surgeon."[57] Most writers agreed with naval surgeon Thomas Ewell, brother of James and also a graduate of the University of Pennsylvania. He maintained in his 1824 *American Family Physician* that medical knowledge would predispose a person to consult a doctor promptly when sick and then obey his instructions.[58] But because these guides were designed for people in sparsely populated areas or faced with emergencies, they did discuss routine surgical procedures, first-aid techniques, pregnancy, childbirth, and specific remedies for diseases.[59] Many also gave catalogues of the medicines and supplies that should be kept on hand, for, as James Ewell argued, it was "a god-like act" for knowledgeable citizens to be well supplied with remedies. In fact, Ewell, like many apothecaries and practitioners, sold medicine chests in conjunction with his *Medical Companion*. The chests were not only for home use but were also meant to benefit "sick and indigent neighbours, who often suffer, and sometimes perish" due to lack of proper medication.[60] Contrary to their stated intentions, then, authors of these "family physicians" *did* facilitate domestic practice, although for the first time they provided a learned framework for home health care.

If learned medical men were not using health guides to contest domestic medical practice in this period, what were they trying to accomplish? Post-Revolutionary manuals varied in tone and method, from the self-consciously learned and expostulatory to the more anecdotal and moralistic. Horatio Gates Jameson, a respected Baltimore surgeon trained at the University of Maryland, wrote portions of his 1817 *American Domestick Medicine* in a technical style that was probably more accessible to his medical colleagues than to a nonprofessional audience.[61] James Ewell, on

Recipe 25.

MERCURIAL PILLS.

Take of
　　Calomel, one drachm
　　Opium and
　　Tartar emetic, each ten grains
　　Crumb of bread a small quantity
　　Sirup, or mucilage of gum Arabic, sufficient to
form a mass.
　　Divide into forty parts. One pill to be taken night
and morning by an adult.

Recipe 26.

MERCURIAL SOLUTION.

Take of
　　Corrosive sublimate, twenty-four grains
　　Laudanum, half an ounce
　　Spirits, one pint and a half.
　　Mix. Dose for an adult, from three to six drachms,
twice a day.

Recipe 27.

SATURATED SOLUTION OF ARSENIC.

Take of
　　Arsenic in powder, about one drachm
　　Water, half a pint.
　　Boil it for half an hour in a Florence flask, or in a
tin sauce-pan; let it stand to subside, and when cold,
filter it through paper. To two ounces of this solution,
add half an ounce of spirit of lavender. A dose to be
taken twice or thrice a day.

Dispensatory recipes from James Ewell's *The Medical Companion*
(Philadelphia, 1816), p. 614. Although Ewell was an orthodox
physician, he did not confine himself to heroic remedies such as
these but also recommended botanic and folk cures.

the other hand, freely used verse and anecdotes to vitalize and reinforce his message. Ewell even added to his third edition an eyewitness account of the capture of Washington, D.C. during the War of 1812.[62]

Regardless of such differences, authors of these guides had the same approach to establishing authority. To justify their didactic roles, writers depicted healing skill as derived from experience and regular medical training assisted by Divine favor. Though the elements of the equation remained familiar, their relative weights slowly changed as authors increasingly stressed the necessity of formal medical training. Most copiously cited illustrative passages from established medical texts and contemporary journals, relying on Boerhaave, Sydenham, Cullen, Brown, Rush, Barton, and other eminent Europeans and Americans. Horatio Jameson, like the others, usually adorned these names with adjectives such as *great, illustrious, excellent, learned,* and *celebrated.*[63]

Buchan's *Domestic Medicine* also found a place on the list of authoritative works invoked by many of the authors. A few of Buchan's disciples were more selective in their allegiance than others. Jameson, for example, enthusiastically endorsed some of Buchan's therapies but found several others to be "extremely dangerous."[64] Anthony A. Benezet, on the other hand, had nothing but praise for Buchan, the man who, standing "almost alone," had "triumphed over the test of opposition in Europe." Benezet, who claimed a learned pedigree, documented his reliance on Buchan in many cases, such as his discussion of bodily elimination, where he "borrow[ed] very freely from Dr. Buchan." But he readily admitted that his debt to Buchan was much greater, and Benezet did incorporate without attribution numerous passages from Buchan's opus into his own work. In fact, as with his discussion of scrofula, Benezet lifted many sections verbatim from Buchan's work and then abridged, omitted, or added paragraphs. In many other sections, such as the one on fevers, the words are different from those Buchan used, but the meaning remains the same.[65]

By thus educating the public about the sources of medical authority, writers hoped to enable citizens to make wise health-care choices. They believed that this educational process, if undertaken and directed by learned physicians, would guarantee the diffusion and perpetuation of a medical ethos based on received medical authority. This task assumed particular urgency beginning in the mid-eighteenth century, not at first because quackery was new or necessarily spreading, but because a "new breed" of European-trained doctors had appeared in the colonies.[66] Joining the handful of older colleagues who had supplemented their apprenticeships with study abroad, these physicians articulated different ideas about the sources and nature of medical legitimation and authority. Like their older colleagues, they believed practical experience and familiarity with ancient authorities were essential for good medical practice. What distinguished this emerging group was a growing agreement that formal medical schooling in both clinical and theoretical subjects should be made the mandatory prerequisite for entry into the medical profession.[67]

Pennsylvanians were at the forefront of medical reform efforts, since many of them had benefited from European opportunities, particularly in London and Edinburgh. Clinical instruction formed the backbone of a London medical education, and the city was widely regarded, as Samuel Powel Griffitts said, as "the Metropolis of the whole World for practical Medicine."[68] In addition to four teaching hospitals where students could "walk the wards" with a physician or surgeon, there were private schools of anatomy, surgery, and midwifery. During the mid-eighteenth century, London boasted John Fothergill and John Coakley Lettsom, highly respected Quaker physicians and philanthropists; William Hunter and his brother John, the foremost anatomists of the day; Colin McKenzie, famed for his skill in midwifery; and John Pringle, acclaimed for his work in military hygiene. London preparation, nonetheless, did have one shortcoming: its neglect of theory. As Robert Whytt warned, "Many of the English Physicians run down all Theory in Physic so much, that either they, or the Successors, if they tread their steps, will soon become mere Empiricks."[69]

Edinburgh courses, on the other hand, were renowned for their theoretical bent, slighting or omitting clinical training altogether. By the 1730s Edinburgh had surpassed Leyden as the preeminent center of medical experimentation and training. The "efflorescence of genius" extended far beyond medicine, for mid-eighteenth-century Scotland was blessed with exceptional thinkers in science, philosophy, and law.[70] It was exhilarating, as Benjamin Franklin buoyantly wrote Jonathan Potts and Benjamin Rush. "You have great Advantages," penned the eminent American, "in going there to study at this Time, where there happens to be collected a Set of truely great men, Professors of the Several Branches of Knowledge, as have never appeared in any age or country."[71] Rush's own evaluation coincided, and he rejoiced to Jonathan Bayard Smith, a former Princeton classmate, on 30 April 1767: "'Tis now in the zenith of its glory. The whole world I believe does not afford a set of greater men than are at present united in the College of Edinburgh."[72] Seven years later when Griffitts was a student, he exposed the heart of the matter in a letter to Rush: "It would have been a great mortification to me not to have passed a winter at Edinburgh."[73]

Edinburgh medical professors included Joseph Black in chemistry, John Hope in materia medica, Alexander Monro *secundus* in surgery and anatomy, William Cullen in the institutes of medicine (physiology and pathology), James Gregory in the practice of medicine, and Thomas Young in midwifery. Demonstrations sometimes supplemented lectures, as young Samuel Bard explained to his physician father in 1762: "As [Cullen] goes along he explains his Theory by a variety of experiments."[74] Bard, however, had already studied in London, but, for Quaker George Logan and others whose clinical knowledge was weak, the emphasis on theory could pose problems. John Fothergill recognized this and recommended to William Shippen, Jr., as he normally did to his American protégés, that he "lay a foundation in practice [before entering] upon theory."[75] Shippen followed his advice, but Benjamin Rush adopted the opposite course. London, he arrogantly predicted to John Morgan on the eve of departure, would probably offer him little in the wake of his Edinburgh preparation. "After attending the lectures and practice of the great Dr. Cullen for two years," concluded Rush, "I am sure little knowledge can be acquired from the random prescriptions of the London hospital physicians."[76] Yet he was resigned to spending some time there, because he was afraid that failure to do so would damage his reputation. As Rush had anticipated, he found that few of them practiced medicine "upon philosophical principles," but after several months he had to concede that "they have enriched the science with a number of very useful facts."[77]

It would be hard to overrate the impact of European training, especially that at Edinburgh under Cullen, on mid- and late-eighteenth-century American medicine. The entire faculty of the nation's first medical school at the University of Pennsylvania—John Morgan, William Shippen, Jr., Adam Kuhn, and Benjamin Rush—had been Cullen's students, and Thomas Bond, though his degree was from Leyden, had studied in Edinburgh as well. The curriculum and many of the lectures followed the Edinburgh course, as did those of the second medical school, King's College in New York.[78] The Pennsylvanians made one major change and stressed practical medicine as well. As Pennsylvania Hospital physician Thomas Bond said in 1766, theoretical expertise should always be united with practical knowledge "for Language and Books alone, can never give . . . Adequate Ideas of Diseases, and the best methods of Treating them. For which reasons, Infirmaries are Justly reputed the Grand Theaters of Medical Knowledge."[79]

Edinburgh graduates—of whom there were more than a hundred Americans between 1760 and 1800—were inclined to define professional status in terms of medical school education, including possession of the medical degree. Together with other medical graduates, they began in the 1760s to take steps, as Dedham, Massachusetts, practitioner Nathaniel Ames, Jr., explained it, "to prevent the intrusion of every ignorant drone that assume[d] the title of doctor" into their ranks.[80] With varying degrees of success, physicians promoted licensing laws and sought to establish medical schools, hospitals, and medical societies. John Morgan, recently home from studying abroad, spelled out with greatest clarity the rationale for formal medical education in his 1765 *Discourse on the Institution of Medical Schools.*[81]

The practitioner trained by the apprenticeship system, Morgan maintained, regardless of his intelligence and hard work, would never have more than superficial knowledge. Without systematic study of the different branches of medicine, Morgan said, "all our ideas are but crude conceptions, a rope of sand, without any firm connection." It would be both foolish and presumptuous to embark on medical practice without proper exposure to scientific experimentation and observation. Those who practiced without the necessary qualifications were doomed to be plagued by "continual perplexities." Morgan graphically portrayed this type of practitioner as operating "at random and in the dark; not knowing whether his prescription might prove a wholesome remedy, or a destructive poison." Without adequate knowledge, how would the practitioner know when to begin or end a particular treatment or for what effects to watch? The consequences, argued Morgan, could be fatal: "He may thus interrupt the salutary attempts of nature, or, not knowing how to second them, tamper with the life of his patient, and idly waiting to see what nature herself is capable of doing, neglect to succour her, till it is too late, and the fatal hand of death is just closing the gloomy scene."

Implicit in Morgan's vision was the assumption that the properly qualified practitioner would be male. Though Morgan did not dwell on this facet of his plan, its centrality should be underscored, particularly since it created formidable practical and conceptual problems: the vast majority of the healers in the latter half of the eighteenth century not only lacked formal schooling but also were women. In addition, elite practitioners recognized that many of their lay counterparts had greater experience—and often greater success—in diagnosing and treating illnesses than they did. As physicians of this and later generations grappled to redefine legitimate medical practice, they also eventually transformed the relationship between domestic and professional medicine. In the process, a campaign in which questions of gender had been subsumed in issues of expertise evolved into one for which gender became central. One unanticipated but far-reaching consequence, which we will explore more fully in the next chapter, was to justify the exclusion of women from formal medical training, a powerful legacy for generations to come.[82]

Medicine in the New Republic

The timing of this move to raise standards and therefore restrict practice was a logical outgrowth of the European training that larger numbers of Americans were receiving. From another perspective, however, it seems contradictory, since ideals of republicanism and independence increasingly prevailed after mid-century. Recent research has emphasized the extent to which republicanism had different meanings for Americans of different social ranks and regions, but few educated citizens of any region would have equated republicanism with the leveling of all distinctions. They thought distinctions should still exist but that they should be based on merit rather than heredity, wealth, or power. Yet the position of this "natural aristocracy" seemed very insecure in the face of an eroding deferential social order.[83]

For these Americans the political revolution was "an act of faith." Convinced that the survival of republics depended on a virtuous citizenry, Revolutionary leaders believed they had to preserve or instill the proper moral character in both their contemporaries and their descendants. Essential qualities included frugality, temperance, industry, self-reliance, intelligence, good judgment, and competence. A nation inhabited by people lacking these qualities would face catastrophic consequences: individual corruption, familial degeneration, and ultimately societal decay. Thus republican government necessarily entailed vigorous promotion of public and private virtue, internal unity, and social solidarity. This, Jeffersonians and Federalists agreed, could be achieved only with an educated and politically sophisticated citizenry.[84] Though not everyone would have been comfortable with his rhetoric, Benjamin Rush gave voice to a widely held view when he spoke of "convert[ing] men into republican machines. This must be done," he explained, "if we expect them to perform their parts properly in the great machine of the government of the state."[85]

Spreading knowledge in all fields thus became extremely important. This generation's understanding of the concept of knowledge owed much to the Scottish Enlightenment, particularly to the philosophy of common sense, whose central thinker was Thomas Reid. Reid's influence is usually discussed in terms of his later essays, but Garry Wills has elucidated Reid's ideas as earlier presented and disseminated.[86] In his 1764

Inquiry, says Wills, Reid describes knowledge as having three main parts: root, trunk, and branches. The root is simple perception, exercised by men, women, children, brutes, and even lunatics. This is the realm of experience and has no foundation in anything prior to itself. Next is the trunk, or the sphere of common sense and rational experiment, with immediate conclusions drawn from self-evident propositions. All rational adults share in the ability to use common sense, but, unlike simple perception, it is fallible. The final part, the branches, is the realm of argument and reflection about the remote and less-certain consequences drawn from self-evident propositions. This last kind of knowledge, that of the sciences, is the highest but most vulnerable achievement of the human mind. These "branches" are sound only when still connected with the "roots" of simple perception and the "trunk" of common sense.

For leaders of the Revolutionary era, this conception constituted a mandate to seek knowledge everywhere in an effort to retrieve facts, which illuminated the fixed and absolute external reality. "Facts," said Rush, "are the morality of medicine. They are the same in all ages and in all countries." Man's knowledge of facts, however, could be perverted. Not only did superstition and ignorance interfere with true understanding, but theorizing and systematizing could be equally corrupting. In his eulogy on Cullen, Rush warned his audience of this danger. "To believe in great men," he stated plainly, "is often as great an obstacle to the progress of knowledge, as to believe in witches and conjurers."[87] Common sense alone was not a reliable guide, regardless of its being "the perception of things as they appear to the *greatest* part of mankind." Rush hammered home his central point: no matter how widely held, beliefs based solely on common sense had "no relation to their being *true* or *false, right* or *wrong, proper* or *improper.*" This had enormous social repercussions: "In the uncultivated state of reason, the opinions and feelings of a majority of mankind will be *wrong,* and, of course, their common or universal sense will partake of their errors. In the cultivated state of reason, *just* opinions and feelings will become general, and the common sense of the majority will be in unison with truth."[88]

Thus only citizens armed with cultivated knowledge—and therefore reason—could make responsible decisions. Physician and author Elihu Hubbard Smith stressed the importance of the universal diffusion of knowledge: "The ignorant are ever the slaves of passion; easily swayed by accidents; readily improved upon; & at the command of every intriguer." The "well-informed," he continued, "hear, attend, read, reflect, investigate." Samuel Stanhope Smith captured the essence of the issue in a 1783 letter to Rush: "The diffusion of knowledge is the diffusion of virtue and freedom."[89]

This belief fueled a great post-Revolutionary expansion in educational opportunities. Leaders looked not only to schools but to churches and families to inculcate and sustain civic virtue. George Washington spoke for many Americans in his 1796 farewell address when he said that "virtue or morality is a necessary spring of popular government." Spreading knowledge was therefore of the utmost importance. "In proportion," he concluded, "as the structure of a government gives force to public opinion, it is essential that public opinion should be enlightened."[90]

The legacy of the Revolution was tangible and compelling for this generation of learned doctors. Rush again phrased it well, writing to a nonprofessional audience in the *American Museum*. "The American war is over[,]" he explained, "but this is far from being the case with the American revolution. On the contrary, nothing but the first act of the great drama is closed." What remained, continued the doctor, was the great work of bringing "the principles, morals, and manners of our citizens" into conformity with republican institutions.[91] Rush in fact wanted to incorporate medical study into academic education; this in his eyes would entail not the abolition of the medical profession, but the inclusion of more of the population within that ethos.[92]

But how was this to be done? Learned medical men purported to be able to identify quacks by their empiricism, but this yardstick was in reality completely inadequate and often totally irrelevant. For instance, the Reverend William Bentley recounted in his diary Captain Chever's treatment in April 1790 by "A Mr Newman . . . , who is celebrated for his success in Cancers." At the beginning, "the Physicians encourage[d] his experiments," commented the Salem minister; nine months later, however, an elite physician amputated the limb, since Chever's "cancerous humour . . . had resisted every method of cure." Bentley, however, mentioned no conflict between the lay and professional healers.[93]

Physician Alexander Hamilton's experiences during his travels provide additional evidence of the problems inherent in using empiricism as a gauge of medical competence. Accustomed to a world in which professional gradations were immediately recognizable by cultivation and social position, Edinburgh-born Hamilton was repeatedly forced to reevaluate practitioners he met. The doctor was continually surprised when a person's outward characteristics belied his actual skill as a practitioner. In Wrentham, Massachusetts, for instance, "the learnedest physician" wore odd clothes that Hamilton thought incongruous with his stature. He was more discomfited by the eminent practitioner, William Douglass.

Douglass, he wrote, was "a man of good learning but mischievously given to criticism and the most compleat snarler I ever knew. He is loath," Hamilton continued, "to allow learning, merit, or a character to any body." Hamilton had no trouble pinpointing the source of his disquiet: "He is of the clinical class of physicians and laughs att all theory and practise founded upon it, looking upon empyricism or bare experience as the the the only firm basis on which practise ought to be founded." Worse still, maintained Hamilton, Douglass had surrounded himself with "a set of disciples who greedily draw in his doctrines and, being but half learned themselves, have not wit enough to discover the foibles and mistakes of their preceptor." Douglass, he concluded, was "a notorious physicall heretick, capable to corrupt and vitiate the practise of the place by spreading his erroneous doctrines among his shallow brethren."[94]

The situation was complicated further by the fact that there was no clearly superior therapeutic system. Horatio Jameson bluntly acknowledged this in his 1817 *American Domestick Medicine.* "It still remains," he wrote, "for some future genius, to unfold and explain the laws by which disease, in its varied forms, can be properly and safely distinguished; and, until that happy epocha, the practice of medicine must be difficult, and clouded with uncertainty."[95] If such knowledgeable physicians as Hamilton and Jameson had difficulty assessing medical legitimacy, how was the average citizen to cope?

Beginning in the 1770s the issue of medical legitimacy assumed greater and greater importance for learned physicians. It was at this point that they began to use health guides to establish criteria for professional evaluation and to define the legitimate parameters of professional behavior. Writers started to outline the sources and limits of the doctor's authority with respect to his colleagues as well as to the patient and his or her entourage; the patient's responsibilities and behavior; and the duties of nurses, friends, and relatives. These books were peppered with admonitions to the patient to trust the doctor; to obey his instructions fully and exactly; to divulge all symptoms to facilitate accurate diagnosis and correct prescription; and to forbid interference from well-meaning friends, family, and lay healers. There were equally numerous comments directed to friends and relatives about proper conduct in a sickroom and around a sick person, and nearly all of these books included strenuous remarks about the selection, behavior, and character of children's nurses.

These concerns were clearly expressed in James Parkinson's 1804 *Medical Admonitions to Families.* Parkinson wanted to give his readers enough information so that they could determine when it would be safe to forgo medical advice or when they might risk "sacrificing a friend, or perhaps a beloved child, by delay or improper interference, in some insidious disease." He also wanted to teach sickroom attendants about how to help physicians and to spell out what might happen if they neglected or contradicted doctors' directions. Aware that "a weak mind" might not discriminate but might "fly with confidence to their oracles" in every disorder, Parkinson vowed to restrict his directions for cure "to those [diseases] in which no risque can be incurred, by trusting them to the management of a domestic practitioner." He intended to pinpoint the symptoms that signaled the need for professional attendance as well as "the mischiefs [that were] likely to arise from improper interference."[96]

Parkinson's book opened with a table of symptoms, which he hoped would help domestic practitioners identify the disease at hand and determine whether its treatment should be directed by a physician. His resolution to limit treatment details was undermined somewhat by the necessity of educating people who were in situations where medical aid was not available. But Parkinson did withhold specific treatment guidelines for some afflictions. It would be "fruitless" to include such advice for the slow nervous fever, he maintained, "since it would be certainly safer, to omit medicine entirely . . . in so dangerous a malady" rather than entrust its management to anyone other than a trained doctor. In fact, in any case requiring a doctor's care, it was imperative that the patient and caregivers place total confidence in the physician and carefully follow all instructions, "since the most trifling omission may occasion the death of the patient."[97] Writing in the same year, Robert Wallace Johnson endorsed these views in equally strong language. "It behoves the patient . . . ," said Johnson, "to regard [the physician's] rules, the nurse to see them punctually observed, and both, to be cautious how they deviate from them; as fatal consequences may sometimes arise, from what may seem to have been but a trifling variation."[98]

But, as James Parkinson bemoaned, patients and caregivers frequently violated the physician's rules without compunction and then blamed the doctor for what was in reality their own fault: "The patient, soured by the long continuance of his disease; angry with the physician, for having pointed him out, as the cause of his own sufferings; and vexed with himself, for his weakness, and want of resolution; will rail at the inefficacy of the art, and perhaps at the ignorance of its professors; asserting, that the admonitions he has received, are such lessons of austerity, as his monitor himself, has neither the power, nor the inclination to follow."[99] Caregivers were just as bad as patients, Anthony Benezet concurred, primarily because they stubbornly used their own judgment based on inherited wisdom instead of listening to "such instruction as would, perhaps, induce them to forsake practices which they have been taught to believe correct, or to which they adhere merely because they are accustomed to walk in the tracks of their predecessors." It was crucial for nurses to be trained properly, Benezet argued, because especially in remote areas "those deemed experienced nurses, have great control over the management of the sick in every respect."[100] The consequences of presumptuous behavior could be dire, concluded Robert Wallace Johnson, since such actions had been known to "aggravate" a disease so greatly that it was "diverted from its natural course . . . ; so that new symptoms have arisen, and very often a new disease, which adding force to the former, the power of medicine hath been resisted, nature has been overcome, and death has ensued."[101]

In order to promote proper medical behavior, American authors also began to instruct the population about body structure and functions. Deviating from Buchan's example, many included brief sections on anatomy and physiology in their household health guides. As James Ewell explained, there is no rational way to take care of one's body without understanding something about its parts and operation. Benezet agreed, pointing out that "the whole human frame is an exquisitely constructed laboratory, where thousands of unnoticed operations are ceaselessly progressing." Since "the disturbance of some apparently unimportant function [was] often followed by disease and death," it was critical to know something about anatomy and physiology.[102]

This knowledge, argued Jameson, was especially important for preventing chronic diseases, such as consumption, gout, and scrofula. It was not the fault of physicians that those sorts of diseases were increasingly prevalent, but, wrote Jameson, "the fault lies wholly in the people, who by enervating habits, carry about a chronick debility, which occasions those new disorders: and for which there is no remedy, in the *Materia Medica*."[103] This perception of the necessity of educating the population about anatomy and physiology, novel and faintly articulated in these works of the early national period, was to be promoted increasingly in the middle third of the nineteenth century.

Reallocating Health-Care Responsibilities

By arming citizens with nonsectarian health manuals, learned doctors sought to equip them to make responsible health-care decisions. The object, as the anonymous physician-author of *The Manual for Invalids* so succinctly phrased it in 1829, was to instruct each individual so that he or she would know what to do when disease struck: *"Thus far should I go, and no farther: here I can assist my health, and here should consult my physician.*"[104] Writers of manuals encouraged rather than challenged domestic medical practice as they pursued their overarching goal of fighting quackery. Again Benjamin Rush's perspective is instructive. In 1809 he compared current medical practice with that characteristic of the early 1760s, pinpointing one major change in these words: "From the diffusion of medical knowledge among all classes of our citizens, by means of medical publications, and controversies, many people have been taught so much of the principles and practice of physic, as to be able to prescribe for themselves in the forming state of acute diseases, and thereby to prevent their fatal termination. It is to this self-acquired knowledge among the citizens of Philadelphia that physicians are in part indebted."[105]

Over the course of the new century, health writers would exhibit growing concern over demarcating appropriate spheres of lay and professional medical practice. As the guides increasingly stressed the promotion of health over the treatment of disease, authors defined the doctor-patient relationship more and more sharply by selectively circumscribing and enlarging the lay person's areas of health-care responsibility. Writers had no doubt which audience was most critical to their success: the female domestic practitioner, especially the mother. The crusade to reach that audience, which overlapped in time with the effort described here, is the subject to which we now turn.

2

The Maternal Physician

For centuries one province had been beyond the purview of physicians and indeed of men: female complaints, including pregnancy and childbirth, and by extension children's diseases. Here women, especially midwives and mothers, were the reigning figures, but in the mid-eighteenth century this sphere too attracted the attention of learned doctors. Orthodox practitioners criticized midwives as ignorant, meddlesome, and harmful, and at first they envisioned improving women's care by formally educating midwives rather than by excluding them from practice. But at the same time, learned doctors advocated a new and central role for themselves in women's health care. Led by European-trained William Shippen, colonial physicians joined their overseas counterparts in proclaiming a "new obstetrics," touted as more scientific, rational, and safe. Judith Walzer Leavitt has described the New World response: "Women overturned millenia of all-female tradition and invited men into their birthing rooms because they believed that men offered additional security against the potential dangers of childbirth. By their acknowledgement of physician superiority, women changed the fashions of childbearing and made it desirable to be attended by physicians." As Walzer warns, however, these statements are seriously misleading unless placed within the proper historical context.[1] Male physician-accoucheurs did make rapid gains among advantaged urban women, but attendance was sporadic, control was tenuous, and influence was uneven. It is more accurate to view the post-Revolutionary decades in terms of transition, as a time of flux and sorting out, one in which doctors, educators, and lay people were actively involved in trying to set parameters and differentiate prerogatives.

As historians have chronicled this shift in authority, some have equated it with medical and male usurpation of control.[2] More frequently, scholars have identified this shift with the birth of modern, improved obstetrics and gynecology.[3] Few, however, have recognized anything positive for women about the concomitant redefinition of women's medical and health responsibilities. In fact, as Leavitt has argued, historical evidence suggests that women remained powerful—and in many cases primary—actors in the birthing process until early in the twentieth century, when childbirth increasingly moved to hospitals. Male physicians were indeed asserting authority and gaining entry into birthing chambers, but that did not mean that they were trying to strip women of all responsibility for family medical care. On the contrary, an integral part of the physicians' enterprise was to *enhance* woman's familial health-care role. As most of these doctors first envisioned it, they would educate women about health matters and join them in creating a health-care partnership characterized by mutual cooperation and deference.[4] As part of the scenario, they advocated that women assume responsibility for preventive living. Advice literature was a potent weapon in their campaign arsenal.

Women as Healers

Childbirth, as many historians have documented, was traditionally a social event in which all the participants were women.[5] Normally the parturient woman "called her women together," and the midwife superintended delivery and immediate postpartum care.[6] Especially after the first third of the eighteenth century, doctors were summoned in cases of protracted or complicated labor or when the baby threatened to arrive before the midwife. Inevitably there were times when doctors and midwives attended the same delivery, but such situations did not automatically breed conflict. Rather, the experiences of Martha Moore Ballard suggest that there existed a tacitly accepted protocol. A respected midwife in the Augusta, Maine, vicinity, Ballard left a careful record of nearly one thousand deliveries between 1778 and her death in 1812. In troubling cases she sent for a doctor, and sometimes she divulged the division of responsibilities between them. On 17 November 1793, for instance, she extracted the child, while the physician "chose to close the loin."[7]

The interactions between Ballard and area doctors, however, should be viewed within a larger context. Like many midwives, Ballard was also a locally renowned nurse and lay practitioner, so she encountered doctors in many medical situations outside the birthing room. For example, she regularly collected herbs and made medicines, which she administered herself or dispensed to neighbors. The Ballard home often sheltered patients, many of them brought by doctors appreciative of her expert care. Occasionally she noted the praise her actions had won from a physician. On 5 December 1798, for instance, after an exhausting day and night with a very sick woman, she was delighted that "[Dr. Cony] approved of what I had done."

Often Ballard worked in tandem with medical practitioners. Many such cases ended in death, suggesting that professional aid was requested when illness became undeniably serious. Part of the physician's responsibility may have been to predict impending death, as happened with Mrs. Cragg's sickness. Ballard began treating the woman in late March of 1790, but within two weeks that patient was "exceeding ill." When Cony was called in, the diarist stated simply that he "plainly told the family that Mrs. Cragg must die." His prognosis was correct.[8]

Just as Ballard sought professional aid when cases under her direction worsened, she referred supplicants to doctors when she judged necessary. After examining a young boy's swollen thigh on 13 February 1791, she "recommended their apply to some person of skill for the safety of the child." Ballard also consulted physicians when serious illness struck her or other family members. Thus after trying frantically to revive her grandson, apparently dead after having "drank spirrit," she sent for Cony, who "used some means and he recovered through the goodness of God."[9]

Of course doctors could not always cure. Yet once a physician had been consulted, protocol dictated that he had supervisory authority over the case. Even if his treatment proved to be unsuccessful, the diarist was evidently not expected to intervene after having surrendered control of the case. On the first day of March in 1800, Ballard began treating another grandson, her dismay deepening as he continued to decline. Within two days she had sent for Cony, but in his absence asked a different physician to prescribe. That evening Cony endorsed the course set out by his colleague, but the child remained sick throughout the night. Though more medicines were prescribed, Ballard's frustration mounted; she "used according to his directions to a punctilio, but to no effect; the illness still increases." Additional medication came the next day, but the family feared the child was dying even though, as the diarist moaned, "we followed his directions." When Cony then suggested a blister, no objection was recorded, but one wonders what lay beneath Ballard's notation that "he cast very hard reflections on me without grounds, as I think."

Perhaps in her despair she had somehow overstepped her bounds, as she had been charged with doing the previous autumn. On 24 October 1799 Cony, called to visit Ballard's husband, took the opportunity to air some grievances. Cony, she wrote, "accused me with going to Mr. Dingley's in his sickness and objecting to his prescriptions and prescribing some of my own and seting Mrs. Dingley crying by giving my opinion of the disease, and said this was one of many instances I had done so." Two days later Dingley himself was at the Ballard house, and the lay healer told him what had happened. Ballard recorded her neighbor's response: "He declares no such thing mentioned by him or his wife as the doctor represented to me." Whatever the truth in this anecdote, it highlights the tensions inherent in a sphere where there were potentially colliding views of authority. Physicians increasingly displayed credentials derived from formal education and accreditation, whereas domestic practitioners still traced their healing expertise to practical experience and custom.[10]

As Ballard's diary documents, this problem of overlapping jurisdiction was not confined to childbirth and midwifery. Nor were midwives and doctors the only participants in disease management. Rather, all wives and mothers traditionally had the prerogative within the domestic arena. The experiences of widow Margaret Morris offer another fascinating glimpse of the dynamics of domestic medicine. Daughter and sister-in-law of doctors, this Philadelphia matron assumed many medical duties, though sometimes reluctantly. In a letter of 7 January 1794 to her sister and brother-in-law, she told of the illness of another sister, "confined to her bed . . . with what I take to be a general rheumatism, flying pains all over, from her head to her shoulder, and yesterday very bad in her left side. At first," she continued, "I thought she should be bled, but on feeling her pulse, found it so low that I begged them not to venture on it without a better judgment than mine; but they were not willing to consult any *other doctor!*" Under the circumstances, she "boldly prescribed a blister to the afflicted side, with volatile tincture of guaiacum and laudanum, and plentiful cups of flaxseed tea." Despite her family's faith in her abilities, Morris remained uneasy and complained of "a painful, anxious night." She was gratified to find her patient improved the following morning, and to her great relief "this evening they sent me word she was vastly better."[11]

Regardless of her success in this case and others, Morris could not shake her discomfort about directing medical treatment. But she also recognized that her anxiety stemmed in part from the deaths of the physicians in the family. Because of their absence, she and her relatives had been thrust into a position that they found "very hard": "to ask advice, as we never before had occasion to go out of our own little circle for it." In closing the letter she penned a revealing comment on a case where she had been able only to speak to the patient's mother before making her diagnosis. She fretted, "I gave her a little medicine; possibly I may do harm with my quackings, but the intention must screen me from censure." Though family members preferred her judgment to that of "any other doctor," Margaret Morris perceived her ministrations—in person or by proxy—as "quackings," saved from criticism and harm only by her good intentions.

New York merchant John Pintard's letters to his daughter also indicate a great deal about the interpenetration of domestic and professional medicine in early America. Deeply interested in medical matters, Pintard sent a steady stream of remedies and advice for his son-in-law, a New Orleans physician, to test. They were culled from every possible source, professional as well as popular. From the *Evening Post* in mid-1819 he forwarded "a description of the plant skullcap with particulars of its virtues & efficiency in cases of Hydrophobia. The remedy is considered infallible against that most direful disease."[12] Earlier that year he had mailed a "valuable" cure for liver complaint which he had "recd from Mr Furman my president, . . . [who] is very much of a family physician." Two years later he related the success that Mrs. Porter, the sister of the late president Timothy Dwight of Yale and of *Daily Gazette* editor Theodore Dwight, was having: "She is very intelligent, interesting, and has performed wonder[s] in pulmonary cases, by her prescriptions of the Bugle weed."[13]

Though receptive to nonprofessional medicine, Pintard was not hostile to orthodox practice. On the contrary, the merchant had great faith in learned practitioners, especially in the eminent John Francis. In 1819 he praised Francis as "an extraody man, & what is more to me my friend on whose judgment in case of illness, I shd confidently rely." As this assessment intimates, Pintard traced much of Francis's success to his personal warmth, a quality not exhibited by all doctors. A dozen years later, Pintard volunteered a more specific evaluation. Francis, he wrote, "is frank & communicative, & considers it a religious duty to be candid with his patients & families." He was "the very opposite of the late Doctor Post, who was the most cold, heartless man I ever knew. Approached his patient, felt the pulse, prescribed & retired without opening his lips not satisfying the enquiries of an anxious family." Pintard found more than

Post's professional comportment troubling. "His whole stock of books," the merchant marveled, "wd not have filled a wheelbarrow. F[rancis] on the contrary has a very extensive professional Library, also every modern work of dis[tinc]tion & merit." A good physician in Pintard's estimation was kind yet forthright, and he was learned in both ancient and current medical knowledge.[14]

Pintard's wife must have concurred in his estimate. In October 1821, the merchant, plagued by dysentery, confessed to his daughter that he had consulted with Francis partly "[t]o gratify Mama." Eight years later, Pintard expressed the same sentiments as he complained to his daughter about the expense of Francis's house calls. But he concluded that they "will be cheerfully sustained to please poor mother, whose sole confidence rests on Dr F." Pintard also felt, however, "that from intimacy & friendship I think he knows my constitution best. He being young & alert, can in case of emergency move quick and I have the fullest confidence in his judgment." Regardless of Pintard's great faith in Francis, he simultaneously expressed equal confidence in his wife's medical expertise. "I hope," wrote the merchant, "that I shall have little occasion for his advice and less for his physic. Indeed yr mother who understands me well is after all my best physician." Ten years later the refrain was the same, this time as he gave thanks for having survived a threatening case of influenza: "My malady has yielded to the skill of my Physician, Dr Francis, but above all, under Providence, to the tender unceasing care & attention of yr dear mother."[15]

For Pintard domestic and professional medicine meshed harmoniously. His letters demonstrate that he thought that there were benefits attached to each tradition. The well-qualified physician supplemented knowledge drawn from the learned medical canon with experience gained from treating people. The reverse was true for the skillful female healer. Every woman had practical expertise that stemmed naturally from her nurturing functions within circles of family, friends, and community. Pintard assigned equal but different importance to the woman's role, recognizing that nursing patients was as critical as directing treatment.

But not all good nurses were women. Philadelphia merchant Thomas Cope's lengthy diary entry for 20 January 1805 was devoted to his "beloved & excellent" wife, Mary, who five days earlier "had been attacked with rheumatism or gout in the stomach."[16] He traced the illness in minute detail from its inception. "Her pains," he began, "were excruciating, her pulse gone & a death-like cold, clammy sweat had seized her whole frame." Moreover, wrote Cope, "her physician gave me no hopes of her recovery." The prospects did indeed seem dismal, for "that night the disease would not yield to medicine." On the following day the "symptoms were more favourable," and by the seventeenth she was much improved. By the nineteenth she had worsened, "again seized with spasm in the stomach, nausea & vomiting & so great was the irritability of the principal seat of the disease that for several hours the stomach rejected everything thrown into it & it was with great difficulty & constant attention that at last this propensity gave way to medicine & nursing." Cope took hope from her freedom from pain and regular pulse, but he vowed to care for her with diligence. This entailed far more than strict compliance with the physician's orders, requiring flexibility borne of experience and attention. The night before, the merchant had "sat up with her & administered the doses ordered for her relief, persuaded that in a case so critical much depended on a careful & proper attention to passing symptoms, so as to seize every favourable moment for procuring ease." Cope thought it would be impossible to overestimate "the benefits of this kind of attention . . . in her case." In her illness, he explained, "a rigid & literal adherence to the directions of the physician was ineligible. Symptoms would occur in his absence against which no provision had been made & it required great caution to adapt the applications to these unforeseen & varying circumstances." Yet not just anyone should tamper with the physician's instructions. "This," Cope declared, "in the height of the paroxysms, I was not willing to trust to other hands than my own & I have consolation in believing that she has derived great advantage from the caution." Especially in stomach disorders this caution was essential, for "the patient anxious for relief is ready to receive what is offered & nurses are too apt, from a desire to be doing, to do more than is proper & frequently aggravate the symptoms & prolong the disease by premature attempts to restore strength to the patient."

Cope was to have good reason to be wary of the quality of nursing and to be sensitive to the stakes involved. Nearly four decades later he was reminiscing about past calamities, including the death of this wife. "A careless domestic," he recalled, "had given her arsenic instead of magnesia. Speedy medical aid proved unavailing, she closed her mortal career peacefully, but in great suffering."[17]

As Thomas Cope could attest, the value of good nursing was beyond calculation. His diary entries also made clear that an experienced nurse behaved very much like a physician—and indeed stood prepared to modify or countermand the doctor's orders. As the number of formally educated physicians grew in the half-century following the Revolution, they sought increasingly precise definitions of what constituted proper domestic medical activity. In so doing, they challenged woman's traditional healing primacy within the home.

Advice to Mothers

Beginning in the mid-eighteenth century, doctors embarked on a quest to reallocate the health-care responsibilities of physicians and lay people, especially women. Later joined by lay writers, the crusaders relied in part on handbooks addressed specifically to female readers and male physicians. These volumes, devoted to the correct management of women's complaints and childrearing, analyzed and prescribed about matters within the traditional domain of women. The doctors aimed to educate both segments of their audience: women, whom they saw as uninformed and superstitious; and physicians, whom they felt lacked practical experience. The physician-authors had two other overarching goals in publishing these specialized domestic guides. First, they wanted to strengthen their own professional and cultural authority by demonstrating that formal education, not tradition and experience, was the proper source of healing legitimacy. At the same time, they sought to underscore the importance of childrearing and provide the information that they thought was necessary for children to reach adulthood and become model citizens.

Though the precise connection between advice literature and actual behavior is very difficult to establish, it is clear that maternal health guides promoted changes that eventually had enormous consequences for women's roles in the sickroom, the family, and the society.[18] Physicians —most of them men—and eventually other professionals would define appropriate childhood and familial roles and behavior, while mothers would be charged with putting those ideas into action.[19] During the first century of this crusade, however, women played an indispensable part in this role definition, because most physicians had so little experience with infants and young children that they could not stand alone. Women had roles of undeniable importance, both in real life and in advice literature.

Works by British and Scottish authors, heavily influenced by Lockean environmentalism, predominated at first. For Locke the goal of childrearing was to produce rational adults who could deny themselves short-term pleasures in order to pursue long-term aims. As Locke argued in his *Essay Concerning Human Understanding,* human rationality was weak and easily affected by appetite, so it required constant nourishment and protection. It was the parent's task to help the child develop mental and

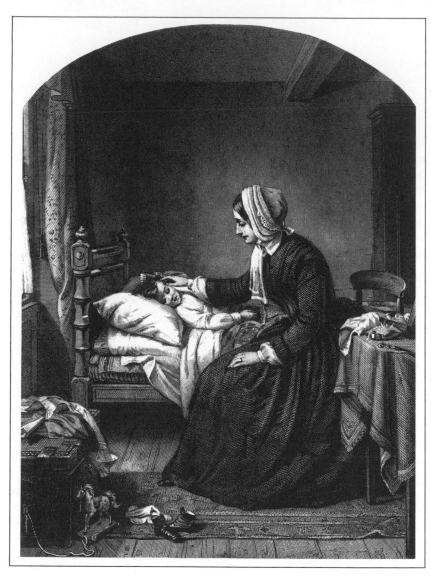

This illustration graced the frontispiece of the March 1858 *Godey's Lady's Book,* but the scene would have been equally familiar to earlier generations. So, too, would the central theme of the accompanying story, which attributed the child's recovery and character not only to his mother's careful nursing but also to her ability to instill in him the moral and physical qualities appropriate to Americans.

physical habits that would strengthen the power of reason. To build a strong body, Locke recommended a light diet, loose clothing, and plenty of fresh air and exercise. To instill good mental habits, he urged early discipline founded on obedience and self-denial.[20]

Household health guides publicized these ideas, and many followed William Buchan's example by including discussion of children's diseases and female complaints. In *Domestic Medicine* Buchan linked appalling childhood mortality directly to parental ignorance or carelessness.[21] Buchan was right about the vulnerability of British children to disease. Half or more of all recorded deaths occurred among youngsters under five, and roughly one-quarter of them never even reached their first birthdays. This was true despite a general late-eighteenth-century fall in mortality rates. No marked reduction in infant mortality occurred until the mid- to late-nineteenth century.[22]

Buchan thought much of the blame rested with parents, and he especially deplored their reliance on wet nurses and other strangers to take care of their children. Though he realized that some mothers were physically unable to nurse their children, he charged that far too many parents were "bring[ing] up their young by proxy." Those who deferred to such outsiders, argued Buchan, were self-indulgent shirkers of their parental duties, "the dupes of ignorance and superstition." Their children experienced irreparable physical and moral damage in their formative years, and a society composed of such maimed citizens faced grave problems.[23]

Both mothers and fathers needed to change their approach to childrearing, wrote Buchan. Women needed to receive a more practical education, since most of them were as ignorant about infancy and childhood "as the infant itself." Men, better educated but traditionally inattentive to such matters, needed to apply their more extensive knowledge to improving their offspring's well-being.

But the fault lay not altogether with parents. Buchan also chided physicians, who had long neglected childhood ailments because they were "generally considered as the sole province of old women." A circular process, this neglect had also encouraged women "to assume an absolute title to prescribe for children in the most dangerous diseases." Doctors thus were "seldom called till the good women have exhausted all their skill," by which time anything they did was certain to be ineffectual. It would be better to reallocate responsibilities and to "have nurses do all in their power to prevent diseases; but, when a child is taken ill, some person of skill should immediately be consulted."

Thus doctors and parents shared responsibility for bringing about change. Doctors had to learn more about children's diseases so that they would be better qualified to give advice about young people in illness and in health. On parents, especially mothers, fell the burden of *preventive living*, of helping their children avoid disease. Buchan discussed bad influences at length: diseased parents; improper clothing, air, food, and exercise; precocious schooling and employment; uncleanliness; and hired nurses. He also suggested that the work involved in prevention was far more important and more difficult than that involved in treatment: "The nurse may, for the most part, do the business of the physician; but the physician can never do that of the nurse."[24]

Other household health guides provided information on the diseases of women and children, but the amount and presentation varied widely. Anthony Benezet and James Ewell, for instance, gave approximately the same space to each.[25] James Parkinson and Josiah Burlingame chose instead to intersperse information about female and childhood ailments throughout their volumes.[26] It was Horatio Gates Jameson who most clearly presented the rationale governing contents. Jameson allocated roughly sixty pages for women's diseases and a third of that for children's complaints, but he reminded his readers that they could find more coverage in handbooks devoted exclusively to midwifery and children's diseases.[27]

In this genre, too, William Buchan was preeminent, sounding familiar themes in his *Advice to Mothers,* first published in America in 1803. Women held the future in their hands, stated Buchan, for "every man is what his mother has made him." Infancy and childhood were such crucial periods that no amount of corrective action in adulthood could neutralize or destroy "the evils occasioned by a mother's negligence; and the skill of the physician is exerted in vain to mend what she, through ignorance or inattention, may have unfortunately marred." The mother's responsibility was formidable, and Buchan's principal objective in *Advice to Mothers* was to teach mothers how to take proper care of themselves and their children.[28]

After a brief chapter providing advice to unmarried women, Buchan covered pregnancy, childbirth, nursing, and childrearing. Throughout he placed a premium on correcting popular misconceptions, which he deemed more damaging than lack of knowledge: "*mere ignorance hath never done any material injury,*" for "*we do not err in things we are professedly ignorant of, but in those which we conceive we know.*" Buchan did not single out mothers as the only ones who had a lot to learn. Nurses and midwives were also major offenders, because they often based their actions on superficial or incorrect knowledge. Doctors likewise suffered from ignorance, though theirs stemmed from lack of experience with child-hood complaints.[29]

To correct misconceptions Buchan gave detailed information about diet, dress, cleanliness, exercise, and other facets of early existence. He omitted treatment information entirely, because he was fully persuaded that proper living was the key. "Medicines," he wrote, "however skill-fully administered, cannot supply the place of proper nursing; and when given without skill, which I fear is too often the case, it must be produc-tive of much mischief."

Physician-philanthropist J. G. Coffin praised Buchan's work in the re-spected *New-England Journal of Medicine*. He believed that mothers should read *Advice to Mothers* to learn how to prevent the harm done every day by "the negligence of physicians, the ignorance of parents, and the rashness of nurses." Not all nurses were bad, he conceded, but Coffin worried about those whose "arrogance and selfishness" led them "to in-vade the province of the physician [rather] than to be useful in their own." Too often custom—and the uninformed nurse—controlled what happened in the nursery. If mothers would only "exercise their own un-derstanding," they would be capable of evaluating and countering the actions of "the despotic leaders of the nursery," who were "too often guided by nothing better than the blind maxims of unthinking tradi-tion." *Advice to Mothers* would be a trustworthy guide.[30]

Despite his success in this field, Buchan was not the pioneer. Instead, he followed a trail blazed decades earlier by physician William Cadogan, a Leyden graduate with considerable experience in Britain's new found-ling hospitals. Anonymously published in London in 1747, Cadogan's short book had gone through at least eleven editions by 1773, and sub-stantial excerpts were reprinted in early nineteenth-century American editions of Buchan's *Advice to Mothers*.[31] As Buchan was to do, Cadogan argued that high infant and child mortality could be reduced by adopting "reasonable and more natural" methods of child care, among them breastfeeding, using cool and loose clothing, and following good habits in diet, ventilation, and exercise. The *Essay Upon Nursing and Management of Children* also suggested that male professionals assume supervision of the nursery. "In my Opinion," declared Cadogan, "this Business has been too long fatally left to the Management of Women, who cannot be supposed to have proper Knowledge to fit them for such a Task, notwith-standing they look upon it to be their own Province." What was needed was "a Philosophic Knowledge of Nature, to be acquir'd only by learned Observation and Experience, and which therefore the Unlearned must be incapable of." "Unlearned" mothers and nurses tended to follow custom, but doctors and fathers, working from informed observation and experience, could comply with the "Design of Nature," understood through reason and common sense. Women were still giving treatment according to "the Examples and transmitted Customs of their Great Grandmothers." People in those "unenlight'd Days" believed in "I know not what strange unaccountable Powers in certain Herbs, Roots, and Drugs; and also in some superstitious Practices and Ceremonies." It was important to begin to take heed of the many things that had made "the Practice of [medicine] more conformable to Reason and good Sense" and had reduced the number of "mysterious and magical" explanations.

Cadogan's book had enormous influence. As Valerie Fildes has explained, Cadogan combined old and new ideas "in [such] a fresh, positive way" that his thinking seemed well in advance of his contemporaries'. But Cadogan's book also publicized and reinforced several significant trends that made British lay and professional audiences more receptive to his work. Most important was the mid-century appearance of two new types of institutions to provide care to the destitute: foundling hospitals for infants and young children, and lying-in wards and hospitals for parturient women. Each setting provided unprecedented opportunities to determine the benefits and perils of various commonplace practices. Publications like the *Gentleman's Magazine* made these conclusions widely available, not only to medical men but to the public at large.[32]

Like Cadogan, other British medical men, most of them active in the emerging fields of pediatrics or professional midwifery, published popular manuals. As had Cadogan, most focused on children's diseases, though some also included advice about pregnancy and lying-in. However individual authors defined the range of their volumes, each argued that it was necessary to reach two distinct but overlapping groups. One was the nonprofessional woman, whose skill in caring for children derived from practical experience and long tradition. The other was the male physician, woefully inexperienced in the actual treatment of children yet a claimant to greater expertise based on theoretical knowledge. Each group had merits as well as shortcomings, and the writers hoped to educate both groups simultaneously. They had two interrelated goals. First, they sought to spread knowledge, both theoretical and practical. By giving women facts derived from learned theory, the physicians hoped to eradicate practices rooted in superstition and tradition. By giving doctors information about infant behavior in sickness and health, the writers hoped to improve diagnostic and treatment skills. Though disseminating knowledge was an important enterprise in its own right, British medical men invested in it another, equally important purpose: reallocating health-care responsibilities. They hoped to promote the ascendancy of the physician in spheres formerly under female rule. Women, newly girded with knowledge, were to assume responsibility for prevention.

Popularizers in Pediatrics and Obstetrics

As other writers joined Cadogan's crusade, they echoed his dissatisfaction with prevailing health care for children, and many voiced similar concerns about the treatment of parturient women. Unlike Cadogan, most did not immediately condemn domestic practice and dismiss lay practitioners from the healing arena. Given the weight of custom, the household setting of treatment, and most doctors' ignorance about children, a strategy predicated on excluding lay healers would have been foolish. Instead, they adopted a more moderate—and more feasible—approach: they sought to use the knowledge acquired through dispensatory work simultaneously to improve domestic practice and to forge a new health-care partnership, one in which professional practitioners would join hands with their domestic counterparts.

The nature of this partnership was not foreordained. In the early manuals, doctors were shadowy figures, occasionally invoked but rarely portrayed as indispensable. Over time, a different conception of professional and nonprofessional roles began to emerge: physicians became the ones who were to direct disease treatment and to educate nonprofessionals about how to stay well, while lay people, having learned correct information, were to apply that knowledge to preventive living and nursing the sick.

Physician George Armstrong, founder of the first children's public dispensatory in Europe in 1769, typified the early architects of the nascent health-care partnership. Armstrong's *An Account of the Diseases Most Incident to Children,* published in London in 1777, was an enlarged, third edition of a work that had originally appeared ten years earlier. In it Armstrong encouraged parents to limit their medical involvement to preventing or arresting disease, and he advised them to consult a doctor for anything more serious. But the thrust of Armstrong's manual ran counter to this division of responsibility, since he focused more on transmitting what he had learned from his hospital work than on defining appropriate treatment roles. In his zeal Armstrong did provide practitioners with more up-to-date information, but he did little to discriminate between professional and nonprofessional responsibilities.[33]

One reason for this blurring of roles was that Armstrong used one text to reach two very different audiences, the professional and the nonprofessional. London surgeon William Moss adopted the same tactic in a 1781 work addressed "to the MEDICAL FACULTY" and "to the PUBLIC AT LARGE; and purposely adapted to a FEMALE comprehension." Moss, whose practice included attendance at the Liverpool Lying-in Charity, also provided information about pregnancy and lying-in in his *Essay on the Management and Nursing of Children in the Earlier Periods of Infancy.*[34]

Moss was more explicit than Armstrong about the existing nature of health care for children and the challenges that physicians confronted. Physicians, wrote Moss, had neglected infants and children for so long that most people assumed that their care fell into "the sphere of domestic control and superintendency." This presented problems, charged Moss, given "the inefficacy and dangerous tendency" of most domestic medical practice, whether drawn "from medical books, and receipts," friends, family, or newspapers. The time had come, Moss argued, for physicians to assert and act upon the superiority of "a knowledge deduced and delivered from facts and experience . . . over that which is founded upon and supported by general usage, custom, or opinion, of whatever authority, date, or origin they may be." But, he continued, superstition and custom could not "be removed . . . by mere *verbal* directions," because by their nature they were "occasionally given, . . . frequently forgot, wilfully neglected, or despised and over-ruled by nurses and various officious advisers." Domestic manuals were, in Moss's opinion, very well-suited for the task.[35]

Of course, he hastened to write, household health guides had to be compiled with great care, because medical knowledge could not be reduced to a few hard-and-fast rules that were always true. Only with years of study and experience could a person learn how to discriminate among disease states, and books for home use should not tempt readers to assume responsibilities for which they were not qualified. Domestic health manuals should therefore "be concise, distinct, and plain," and nothing should be included that might confuse or mislead readers who did not have medical training.

Moss tried to follow his own prescription. He described errors in popular practices and suggested improvements, many of which had nothing to do with administering medicine but instead necessitated changes in diet, clothing, ventilation, and similar matters of lifestyle. Although he did give specific information about treating diseases, he also called attention to areas where he omitted information, a signal that he judged those details inappropriate for lay readers. Moss even carefully earmarked a number of sections as meant exclusively for physicians, but their inclusion obviously made them equally accessible to the interested lay reader. Nonetheless, to a greater extent than had Armstrong, Moss promoted the idea of a clear division of responsibility between doctors and lay people.[36]

Michael Underwood, eminent licentiate of midwifery in the London College of Physicians, also saw the need to correct "vulgar errors" and to distinguish between professional and nonprofessional medical duties. In 1784 he addressed "intelligent Parents . . . as well as the medical world" in his *Treatise on the Diseases of Children,* issued in the first of several American editions in Philadelphia in 1793.[37] Though he took care to explain technical terms when he used them, Underwood did not try to provide answers for every situation. He knew that nonprofessional readers would not understand all of his sections, but, as with Moss, that was his deliberate sign that they should avoid treating cases in those sections. Nor did Underwood expect to please all physicians, for the "prolixity of other parts may be equally disagreeable to professional men." The idea, wrote Underwood, was that parents and doctors had a great deal to teach each other. Given the rudimentary communications skills characteristic of children, doctors had "a very imperfect knowledge" of children's illnesses and needed assistance from women to increase their expertise. Even though women had garnered a great deal of knowledge through experience, Underwood did not think it would be a good idea "to intrust the management of [children's diseases] to old women and nurses." Physicians, who were learned, should direct diagnosis and treatment, while women, who were unlearned, should occupy a necessary but auxiliary role.[38] In Underwood's view, the ideal relationship between parents and doctors would be interdependent and mutually educational, but the physician would have unquestioned diagnostic and treatment authority.

As had been the case with his predecessors' handbooks, Underwood's *Treatise* did not fully support the ideal promulgated by its author. It is true that Underwood repeatedly highlighted the "prejudices repugnant to the ease and health of children" and warned against entrusting treatment to "matrons and old nurses." In addition, Underwood did emphasize the importance of preventive living, an area obviously under lay control. But the doctor also bowed to the exigencies of the times and gave enough medical information so that "the . . . reader may be competent either to superintend and to act, or, at least, to judge of the nature of the case, and its probable termination."[39]

Alexander Hamilton, professor of midwifery in the University of

Edinburgh and a Fellow of the Royal College of Physicians, had just as much trouble designing his handbook to reflect accurately the structure of the relationship he was trying to promote. His *Treatise on the Management of Female Complaints, and of Children in Early Infancy* had been revised for a popular audience from his earlier midwifery guide for doctors, and its 1792 New York publication was the first of many American editions. Hamilton's *Treatise* stressed prevention over treatment, citing the hazards of explaining cures to people who knew nothing about learned medicine. Similarly, he tried to avoid using technical language and references to other books because he thought it would be "improper to refer those for whom this work is intended to medical authors." But Hamilton did give treatment information for those ailments that he felt could safely be handled by lay people, grouping the cures at the end of the volume together with instructions on consulting doctors by letter and choosing nurses. He even provided a section on anatomy and physiology in hopes of improving the lay person's ability to prevent and treat many diseases.[40] Hamilton, then, was not hostile to domestic practice—indeed, the 1793 Worcester, Massachusetts, edition was called *The Family Female Physician*—but he did envision treatment as falling more properly within the physician's realm than the parent's.[41]

London physician Hugh Smith also insisted that doctors should have responsibility for treating disease and that lay people, especially mothers, should assume responsibility for prevention. But "separat[ing] the two provinces" was no easy matter, complained Smith, because of the remarkable extent to which the work of mother and doctor interpenetrated. Nonetheless, Smith's 1792 *Letters to Married Women, on Nursing and Management of Children* reinforced his beliefs, for the book omitted therapeutic details in favor of preventive advice.[42] Even Smith evidently had qualms about the relative paucity of treatment information; he referred readers who needed more guidance to his *Family Physician*.[43]

Like Smith's, James Parkinson's directions to mothers stressed right living and provided few remedies. Yet readers in search of remedies could easily consult Parkinson's more general guidebook, *Medical Admonitions to Families,* since the advice for mothers was appended to it. In Parkinson's view, parents, especially mothers, had the power not only to prevent many illnesses but also to facilitate cure when illness did strike. The key, he argued, was for parents to avoid "the excessive indulgence of children," beginning at birth. The future would be perilous for the child "accustomed to yield to no opposition, and taught that the business of life is not to endure, but only to enjoy." Nervous problems, epilepsy, and insanity were among the legion ailments likely to strike the coddled infant. Moreover, the child who was "intractable" in "temper and disposition" suffered more and longer when ill than one who followed instructions and submitted to necessary confinements and restraints.[44]

Parkinson's format reinforced his message since he did not use the usual organization according to causation, symptoms, and treatment. Instead, each disease entry displayed anew the extent to which undesirable qualities—petulance, forwardness, resistance, and so forth—interfered with treatment and cure. In the malignant sore throat, for instance, parts of the treatment were "disagreeable [and] . . . productive of an increase of suffering, for a time." The point was not to discuss those measures but was to stress that only a dutiful child would submit and thereby promote healing.[45] For Parkinson, parental responsibility in medical matters was obvious. They were to ensure their children's lifelong welfare by establishing in infancy a strong constitution and good temperament. Treatment, however, was beyond the parent's legitimate purview.

The importance of preventive living became a central tenet for many authors, as they struggled to articulate more clearly the boundaries between lay and professional responsibilities in health care. Among them was John Herdman, whose *Discourses on the Management of Infants and the Treatment of their Diseases* was published in London in 1807. A member of London's Royal College of Physicians and Edinburgh's Medical Society, Herdman had also treated children while one of the physicians to the London Dispensary. Herdman took pains to explain the rationale underlying his boundary definitions, and in the process he sketched the structure of the emerging health-care relationship. Herdman's *Discourses* stressed preventive living, because, wrote the doctor, infant mortality was "impious," the result of "the most horrid and culpable mismanagement." Instead of paying "due attention to the laws and institutions of Nature," lay people too often allowed "ignorance, false reasoning, and fancied improvements" to dictate the way they handled children. Since infancy and childhood were the "peculiar province" of mothers, it was with them "that the reformation in . . . treatment must begin and be completed." Herdman upbraided mothers for having "implicit confidence in the judgment and opinions of . . . midwives and nurses." The worst transgression was in allowing them to prescribe, not only for children but for mothers themselves: "You take them out of their own sphere, and you dignify them with the office of the Physician." Midwives and nurses of course encouraged mothers in this behavior, for they considered this "their own peculiar province" and they jealously guarded it.[46]

Women defended themselves by arguing that midwives and nurses had a great deal of experience. This was a weak defense, argued Herdman, because women did not understand what constituted true experience. Even the most practiced midwife or nurse, the physician pointed out, got her knowledge from "her grandmother, her mother, her aunt, or some such motherly woman, and in her common intercourse with society; from those who were educated in a similar manner, and who are equally ignorant with herself." This was *inheritance,* not experience. These were customs and practices, sanctioned perhaps by centuries of use, but simply handed-down nonetheless. What was crucial to the proper definition of experience was "a mind free from prejudice, open to conviction, acute and discerning, greedy of observation, and inured to habits of thinking or reflection." But proper management of infancy depended on more than experience or reason, since it also required adherence to "the fixed and established laws of nature."[47]

Mothers should turn to doctors, who were not swayed by fashion or custom but were guided by facts derived from education and cultivated reason. Herdman did not advocate stripping mothers of all medical authority, and in fact he viewed mothers as central to matters of health and disease in the household. In addition to assuming responsibility for prevention, mothers made or endorsed all of the health-care decisions in their families: they decided when to call in a physician and which one to consult; they administered, monitored, and adjusted treatments; and they acted as liaison between doctor and patient. In order to exercise their duties properly, however, mothers had to educate themselves: "Store your minds with the subject; think for yourselves; and be no longer the dupes of those, who make traffic of your prejudices." As mothers learned more about the human body and the causes and treatments of its diseases, they would also become informed about "what the profession can do, and what it cannot do; of what ought to be done, and of what ought not to be done."[48]

At first glance, Sir Arthur Clarke, another member of London's Royal College of Surgeons, seems to have had a completely different vision of the mother's medical role. "There are few Mothers," he wrote in *The Mother's Medical Assistant,* published in London in 1820, "who are not competent to assume the office of Physician to their own offspring, in a variety of cases; and especially in all those rapid fluctuations of health, so peculiar to Infancy and Childhood." Yet Clarke was no more in favor of having mothers direct treatment than were his medical contemporaries. Like them, he recognized the strength of certain practical considerations. Because delay in treating children was likely "to render every exertion abortive," Clarke thought it was of "paramount importance, to diffuse a

knowledge of the simple, and often efficacious means, which may allevi-
ate the infant's sufferings, and stay the progress of disease, until advice
can be procured." Thus Clarke wanted to educate mothers about what
they should do if disease struck. Using simple, nontechnical language, he
aimed to "[avoid] that unnecessary detail of symptoms" because he
thought too much information "produc[ed] confusion and uncertainty"
instead of "a distinct apprehension of the source and character of the
disease." To make his book easier for lay readers to use, Clarke rejected a
"scientific" order, beginning instead with diseases of the head and working down the length of the body.[49]

Clarke recognized that popularizing medical information might encourage some mothers to enlarge rather than reduce their treatment
efforts, but he urged them to use their newly acquired knowledge in an
auxiliary role. The physical proximity and emotional intimacy of the
mother-child relationship made "Mothers, *if properly directed* in their observations," ideally suited to gather "the preliminary information which
should . . . soften or remove the difficulty." In Clarke's view, however,
prevention, not treatment, was the proper role for mothers. Like his colleagues, Clarke believed that disorders of infancy and childhood—except
for contagious or epidemic diseases—generally could "be inferred to the
mismanagement of those who have the care of them." Medical aid would
sometimes be advisable, but primarily people should "regard the best
efforts of medical skill, but as auxilliary to the operations of Nature—in
all cases the safest and most powerful physician." Improvement depended largely upon the mother, who was always at hand, rather than the
doctor, who was often too late to influence the outcome.[50]

British authors continued to publicize and refine the idea that there
were distinct lay and professional responsibilities in health care. In 1840
Thomas Bull, physician-accoucheur at the Finsbury Midwifery Institution, had no trouble describing the ideal division of responsibilities in
The Maternal Management of Children, in Health and Disease.[51] Mothers, he
wrote, had two roles. Their first responsibility and "especial province"
was to prevent disease, work that the dissemination of correct information made them better equipped to handle. Of equal importance were
"those duties which constitute the maternal part of the management of
disease." By this, clarified Bull, he did not mean to suggest that mothers
had responsibility for treating disease, for treatment fell entirely within
the doctor's realm of responsibility. But physicians should be able to
count on mothers to exercise "vigilant maternal superintendence."
Mothers should give "a firm and strict compliance with medical directions in the administration of remedies, of regimen, and general mea-

sures, . . . [and] an unbiased, faithful, and full report of symptoms to the physician." Bull envisioned a transformed health-care partnership: not only were male doctors newly involved in caring for women and children, but they were directing all aspects of that care.

Long before Bull's book appeared, other voices had begun spreading the same message. British medical men were no longer alone in seeking to educate the population about the management of children, and the emphasis on domestic responsibility for prevention was growing stronger.

Health Care for the Republican Family

In the first decade of the nineteenth century, American physicians also began to use domestic health guides specifically to educate wives and mothers. But only one of the American authors, transplanted Briton Joseph Brevitt, boasted credentials in midwifery or pediatrics. Furthermore, the appearance of these books in America antedated the appearance of children's and lying-in hospitals in the United States.[52] The character of the manuals and the qualifications of their writers reflected the American social and medical milieu. Yet for them, as with the British, the goal of raising healthier children was inseparable from the task of reallocating the child-care responsibilities of parents and physicians.

Many people in the decades following independence invested childhood and motherhood with greater cultural significance than ever before. When Benjamin Rush linked the "perfection" of the new American republic to the inculcation of civic "principles, morals, and manners," Americans envisioned an educational effort that literally began at birth. At the same time, they assigned growing importance to the mother's role in childrearing.[53] Clergymen, reform-minded individuals, and physicians on both sides of the Atlantic produced a flood of books and magazines to advise women about moral upbringing, discipline, and both practical and intellectual education. The appearance and popularity of this literature mirrored social changes, especially the removal of the father's workplace from the home, that were slowly realigning the familial division of labor, particularly among the literate, middle-class groups that also provided the largest literary market. As more and more people defined women as the primary childrearers, mothers came to be viewed as powerful agents for social betterment.[54] This in turn had important consequences for women's education, since it seemed illogical to believe that the "Republican Child" could be raised by a woman who did not embody all the characteristics of the ideal republican citizen, including independence, rationality, benevolence, and self-reliance.[55] Religion—

benevolence, piety, and morality—melded with science to shape the conceptual framework and motivate social activism.[56]

Like the British writers, American authors gave practical advice on day-to-day living, child care, and disease management. But they went beyond these areas to spell out in greater detail the nature and scope of the mother's and doctor's respective responsibilities. Since their works provided so much information about disease *treatment,* this attempt to clarify boundaries was particularly important. These publications should also be differentiated from those of a slightly later group of physician-authors. The later writers, to be discussed in chapter 4, focused on disease *prevention* and infused their advice with moral lessons, which they found impossible to disentangle from matters of healthy living. The moral underpinnings are certainly not absent from the early literature, but the morality is embedded in a larger concern: dispelling ignorance and replacing it with correct information. This group of writers felt that once people had acquired knowledge through education, they would have the tools to live properly. The writers discussed in chapter 4 started from a different vantage point: what was most critical to them was to define the right way to live, which would then determine what information had to be provided to citizens so that they could perform their duty.

Samuel K. Jennings was probably the earliest American contributor, publishing *The Married Lady's Companion, or Poor Man's Friend* in Richmond in 1808. Jennings, a native of New Jersey and a medical graduate of Rutgers, spent the first quarter-century of his professional life in Virginia practicing medicine and promoting his patented vapor bath. Moving to Baltimore in 1817, he soon became a prominent member of the state's medical profession, and in 1827 was one of the founders of the Washington Medical College in Baltimore.[57]

As the title of his book suggests, Jennings wrote for a broad audience, and he even addressed one section to midwives. The volume gave advice on marital duties, pregnancy, childbirth, and midwifery as well as the management of children in health and disease. Jennings rhapsodized that "the greatest revolution in the morals and health of the world" would be achieved if "every woman" were "properly qualified, and would faithfully perform her duty in bringing up her children." Jennings tried to educate matrons about the scope of their responsibilities in medical matters, using two familiar reference points—midwives and physicians—to do so. Most midwives, he maintained, were "exceedingly ignorant and self-conceited." He did not advocate trying to eradicate them, however, because he felt that their "expediency and . . . popularity" would doom such an effort. The solution, argued Jennings, was for them

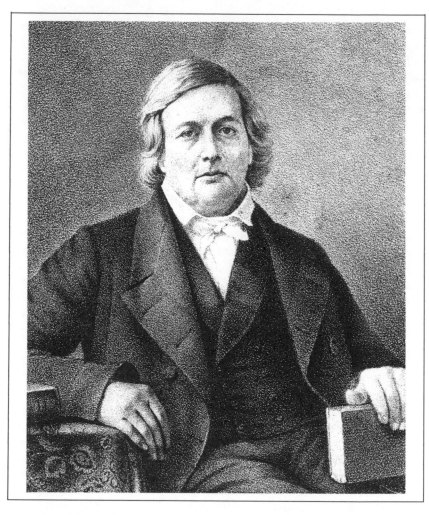

Portrait of Samuel K. Jennings, author of *The Married Lady's Companion, or Poor Man's Friend* (Richmond, 1808), from the frontispiece of his *A Compendium of Medical Science* (Tuscaloosa, 1847).

to "[submit] to their own proper station . . . ," since "within the limits of a certain sphere, they might be useful and respectable."[58]

   At the other end of the spectrum was the physician. Unlike most of his British and American counterparts, Jennings believed that parents usually depended completely on a doctor whenever their children fell sick. He approved of this practice when the case was "difficult and dangerous" because the family would then be assured "the most judicious advice." Not all maladies, however, were life-threatening or complicated. Moreover, there were some diseases, like croup, that "requir[ed] immediate assistance," because they "frequently carri[ed] off the patient so speedily, as not even to admit of calling in a physician from a distance of one mile." Regardless of how rapidly or slowly they progressed, all diseases were more easily recognized and treated in their formative stages; obviously, wrote Jennings, children would benefit from having parents who were able to spot early signs of trouble. In addition, since the people who had the greatest emotional investment "in the health and happiness of . . . children" were parents, not doctors, Jennings thought that informed mothers and fathers would be the most appropriate people to treat their children.[59]

How were parents to equip themselves to care for their children properly? They should, wrote Jennings, be unceasingly and minutely observant of their children's behavior and habits. Every bodily function should be monitored, including appetite, elimination, exercise, energy, respiration, complexion, and pulse. If parents understood the signs of health in their children, they would be able to evaluate the seriousness of any deviation. Jennings also reminded parents to be on the lookout for the sorts of minor aches and pains that often preceded disease, and he added suggestions for preventive living.

Some authors focused more on the care of women than on the management of children. One was Joseph Brevitt, an Edinburgh-trained Englishman practicing in Baltimore, who published *The Female Medical Repository* in his adopted city in 1810. Writing for "female practitioners and intelligent mothers," Brevitt devoted most of his volume to "practical midwifery," to which he appended some discussion of infancy. In addition to providing instructions about the proper management of pregnancy and childbirth, the handbook presented some guidelines about the roles and qualities of the participants in health care: lay and professional practitioners; family and friends; and patients.[60]

Brevitt, formerly a London licentiate in midwifery, took for granted the existence of midwives and other female practitioners, but he argued that they needed different kinds of knowledge than did mothers or nurses. The most critical difference, Brevitt thought, was that mothers and nurses could skip the anatomical section of his book but female practitioners could not, without being branded "reproachfully ignorant, and consequently dreadfully to be feared and avoided." Without this knowledge, female practitioners would be assuming a prerogative that was not theirs to assume; fortunately, he thought, the dissemination of learned works for popular audiences was helping to change things, even if the changes were slow and incremental.

Brevitt also had instructions for practitioners about their approach to childbirth and its aftermath. One area of special concern was "the frequent and imprudent practice of the generality of female acquaintance imprudently crouding into the patient's apartment immediately they learn she is in bed." However good the intentions, Brevitt said, "It is the cause of a continual succession of disturbance to her when she should rest." The doctor had to exercise good judgment and then stand firm in seeing that his directions were executed. The physician could not let his own emotions interfere with his judgment, even when his "own sympathy and anxiety for the sufferer" were "spurred up by the importunities of her friends." Even if accused "of being cold and unfeeling, and not enough alive to [the] patient's welfare," he should stand firm, advised Brevitt. Yet physicians had to be careful not to be aloof or haughty, and sometimes they would be advised to "condescend to lower [their] own self propriety, or the vain imaginations of [their] own superior knowledge, to a level with the interested sympathysing friends." Such "condescension . . . ," he continued, "is the mark of a great and cultivated mind, and never fails to secure . . . tranquillity and resignation, in a full and endearing confidence of [the physician's] correct and better judgment." Once the friends understood "the *why* and *wherefore*," their resistance to the doctor's course of action would be sure to vanish.

Though Brevitt thought that it was important to establish qualifications and to define roles in caring for women, he believed that success in these areas was largely dependent on fostering changes in another area: the responses of individual women to the prevailing canons of modesty. He warned women that modesty was excessive if it kept them from seeking medical attention early in an ailment. Brevitt recommended that an "aged and experienced matron" be asked to "make a strict examination, in an early stage of the complaint," and if she recommended consulting "an experienced physician," then one should be called in immediately. Of course, once consulted, the physician should be thoroughly informed and consistently obeyed.

The issues of modesty and propriety pervaded women's health care, as naval surgeon Thomas Ewell revealed in a series of manuals written during the first third of the nineteenth century.[61] Indeed, Ewell expected criticism for daring to discuss women's complaints in volumes that also included men's diseases.[62] The University of Pennsylvania graduate thought such a dichotomy so artificial as to be ridiculous. Women, he wrote, "are almost always the first to prescribe in their families; they generally act as attendants on the sick;" and as such they could "collect much useful information for the faculty." Yet both sexes, counseled Ewell, should avoid the habit "of seizing at extraordinary means in emergencies," and instead should "deliberately, previously acquire qualifications for acting." To encourage being prepared, he recommended materials to stock the family medicine chest.[63]

Education, especially for women, was the answer, argued Ewell. Citizens had to understand learned medical practices so that they could follow them when necessary and proper. As Ewell explained in his 1824 *American Family Physician,* revised and expanded two years later, this meant that people needed access to reputable domestic guides, which "to be most serviceable, should be plain, intelligible, and systematic." These guides would also help the doctor: families that had "rational" and "correct" medical information would be more likely to follow his instructions, while "unenlightened" families, "with [their] usual attendant, presumption, will be perpetually intruding doubts and countervailing doses." The enlightened family would also exhibit "diffidence, and consequently an early appeal to physicians of skill."[64]

Ewell, still smarting from an earlier review that had criticized his work for its derivative nature, thus provided the perfect rationale for the character of his manuals. As he explained about his 1818 *Ladies Medical Companion*, its value came from the very fact that it did not have "something new to communicate." His enterprise was legitimate because his primary objective was to educate "the uninformed" about learned medical knowledge.[65] More specifically, Ewell argued, "an essential part of the education of every male and female . . . should be a general knowledge of the outlines of the nature of their bodies, and the principles of the cure of their disorders." The goal was not to prepare nonprofessionals to practice medicine. The aim was rather "to enlarge the mind; to habituate it to think rationally on the subject, and to guard against the innumerable impositions of the quacks, . . . as well as those of vast boasting experience."[66] Furthermore, as he said elsewhere, anatomical knowledge, especially of the female generative organs, would encourage women in "the rational treatment" of their own "peculiar disorders, often so injudiciously conducted[,]" and "the prevention and cure of children's complaints."[67]

Ewell thought that properly educated mothers would be well equipped to dispense "occasional relief [to their children], when a physician cannot be had." They would also be knowledgeable enough "to prevent injudicious meddling" and promote "the application of the principles of medicine to their particular case." By educating women, Ewell thought he could convince them that "the great variety of prescriptions for the diseases of children, in almost every old woman's head, should be abandoned; but few medicines, and those of the most simple kind, are wanted for them."[68] Likewise, women's diseases were "to be cured according to principles," and they should be treated only by "the man of sound mind, who reads the books of his profession."[69]

Ewell also spelled out proper conduct for sickroom attendants. Remember, he said, that "refraining from officious interference" was as critical "as giving timely attention." The nurse's responsibilities included ensuring the patient's comfort with fresh and pure air, cleanliness, and an appropriate diet. Most fundamentally, however, the nurse was to obey and assist the physician.[70]

In prefatory remarks to an 1827 reprint of *Letters to Married Ladies*, Hugh Smith's American editor thought it necessary to delineate further the respective duties of mothers and doctors. The most common objection to guides for mothers, he explained, was that "they contain directions and instructions better calculated for physicians than for mothers; and thereby bewilder and alarm."[71] The editor agreed with Smith that it was difficult "to determine the precise line of distinction, and completely separate the duties of the one from those of the other." One rule, however, was clear and unquestionable: *"No direction should ever be given to the mother, calculated to make her the physician of her child."* Here most authors had erred, even notable ones such as Herdman, Buchan, and Burns. Their books he thought better suited for doctors' libraries, despite the valuable information they provided. For nonprofessionals "to acquire the knowledge necessary" to use these resources appropriately, argued the editor, would require them to have had "as many years of laborious study, and hard earned experience" as physicians had had. Without these credentials, Smith's editor feared that readers were not likely to exercise sufficient caution in taking medical action. For this reason he advised parents and nurses "NEVER TO ASSUME THE RESPONSIBILITY OF THE PHYSICIAN."[72]

Smith's anonymous American editor chastised his readers about specific offenses. One of the most worrisome was concealing the truth from the doctor. It was essential, he said, that the physician be completely informed. As he wrote, "It is not for you to judge what symptoms are essential, and what are not, to influence his prescription; and no one can tell the amount of evil this folly may bring upon the patient." This did not mean that his readers had to ignore canons of modesty, but they might at times have to adjust them since "true modesty never interferes . . . with health." Another common mistake was failing to obey the doctor scrupulously. Avoid "deviating from the prescriptions of your physician," advised the editor, "or in any way interposing your own judgment, which may serve to counteract his." In addition to harming the patient, such action would damage the trusting relationship that should exist between patient and physician: "Let me ask you; if you have no confidence in your physician, why employ him? And if you have,—why act as if you had not? Why trammel him, and fetter him in this manner?"[73]

Dr. G. Ackerley's *On the Management of Children in Sickness and Health,* an 1836 New York publication, reinforced and extended the instructions given by Smith's American editor. Three times the size of the first edition, the book was still slender at seventy-eight pages. Because his book was for the general reader, Ackerley promised to omit technical and theoretical discussions and to include information on preventive measures, "which clearly fall within the province of the parent to carry into effect."[74] Like his medical colleagues, Ackerley thought prevailing rates of childhood mortality were lamentable and avoidable. People had been endowed by the Creator "with moral sentiments and reflecting faculties," but they had to cultivate and exercise those faculties. Thus fathers as well as mothers should be knowledgeable so as "to avoid gross error." It was not necessary for the father to "take upon himself the duties of the physician, nor the office of the nurse, but . . . a knowledge of the *common* errors that prevail."[75]

Ackerley had more specific and detailed guidelines for the mother. To begin with, she should refrain from "trying one experiment after another" because early professional attention to sickness was crucial. In line with this advice, Ackerley's volume did not encourage self-treatment. He argued that it was difficult to use curative details "with advantage, without a correct knowledge of disease, and unless applied with judgment, and adapted to the varying states of each individual case." Moreover, no two cases were exactly alike. This challenged even the doctor, who had the benefit of "the accumulated knowledge of ages" and of judgment acquired through experience. This point was critical, because "it is in this nice perception of the *really* different, although apparently *similar,* states of disease, and the adapting of his remedies to the peculiarities of each, that the physician evinces his superior skill."[76]

As his comments intimate, Ackerley had definite ideas about how mothers should choose their physicians: "One should be selected, if time and opportunity permit, in whose *skill* and *integrity* we have entire confidence. It is certainly desirable to have gentleness and mildness of manner combined with skill if it can be obtained, particularly in the treatment of children; but, although we should never countenance coarseness and vulgarity, by allowing it to pass for eccentricity, we should never reject a man because his personal appearance, his manner or his dress, does not exactly accord with any preconceived notions we may have as to perfection in these matters, for they are small matters."

Selecting a suitable physician was only half the formula for good medical care. Once located, the doctor had to be given full cooperation, beginning with absolute honesty. There should be no secrets and no exaggerations; there should be only "the whole truth, and nothing but the truth." Full cooperation entailed much more from the patient and his caregivers. "Whatever remedial means are advised, . . . however trivial or unimportant they may appear, ought to be fulfilled with the most scrupulous care and exactness." There were good reasons for this. Most fundamentally, "the most judicious measures, prompted by the wisdom of the best experience, and approved by the soundest judgment, are often rendered entirely nugatory by imperfect fulfilment, arising through negligence in those who have the care of the child, or the kind but injurious interference of friends." To reduce or eliminate meddling, a competent doctor seldom welcomed friends in the sickroom. "All persons not really necessary ought to be excluded," stated Ackerley. He was precise in his advice: in addition to the parents, the sickroom should contain no more than one "quiet" nurse. Far from being an unkind practice, barring visitors had two equally important purposes: to enable treatment to proceed as directed and to shield parents from the distress that would arise from exposure to conflicting opinions.[77]

Orthodox medical men tried to instruct women in other ways. One was through periodicals like the *Journal of Health,* first issued in Philadelphia in late 1829 by "An Association of Physicians." There they proposed to "[lay] down plain precepts, in easy style and familiar language, for the regulation of all the physical agents necessary to health, and to point out under what circumstances of excess and misapplication they become injurious and fatal." Nonprofessionals should confine themselves to the realm of prevention, they argued, for the physician alone was competent to diagnose and treat disease.[78] Particularly when a child was stricken, the doctor should be summoned immediately, since most childhood diseases progressed so rapidly.[79] In justifying this separation of duties, they also voiced doubt about the widom of publishing domestic health guides, because "without exquisite knowledge, to work out of books is most dangerous." The hazard was "incurred by mothers and nurses, who, assuming a symptom as indicative of the entire disease, administer to children medicines recommended in books of Domestic Practice, which a skilful physician would be fearful of prescribing after a careful examination of all the symptoms, or if he did recommend them, it would be with a great many restrictions and cautions to guard against unpleasant consequences." Parents and nurses, for instance, might give an opium-based remedy to a fretful child, unaware that the symptoms could have been caused by a number of different conditions, "and consequently require a diversity of remedies, or that they [should] be administered at different periods, according to the nature of the malady." Even worse, family members often deluded themselves about a child's condition; when it became clear that the child was not improving, "they send messenger after messenger for the doctor, each one more urgent than the former." Upon the doctor's arrival, it would be his "melancholy discovery that the time for efficient medicine [was] past." This contributor bemoaned not only the family's use of "the 'Family Oracle' or 'Domestic Medicine' or the like," but also seeking and heeding advice from the neighbors.[80]

The editors' skepticism of domestic guides as the basis for treating children's complaints also reflected, as we shall see in chapter 4, mounting criticism of the genre. Increasingly during the middle third of the nineteenth century, American physicians began to reevaluate the kind of information that they were giving to the public. Orthodox doctors worried that these early nineteenth-century handbooks undermined the reform effort that they were published to promote. To be sure, they did delineate a healing relationship in which lay people granted treatment responsibility to doctors and assumed or retained for themselves responsibility for prevention and nursing. But most of the manuals also included treatment details, since they were written not only for the uninformed lay person but also for those living in remote areas or faced with emergencies. Though authors continued to think that it was laudable to provide correct information to replace what was erroneous, they began to recognize the extent to which that information also eroded the ideal image that they were trying to support.

Anthony Todd Thomson probably came closest to reflecting the reality of the healing relationship in his 1845 *Domestic Management of the Sick-Room*.[81] Thomson did begin with the standard disclaimer that he did not intend "to enable any one to undertake the treatment of disease," and he did depict lay people as responsible for preventing disease and assisting the doctor. But Thomson also gave treatment details, using as his rule of thumb a criterion that seemed to contradict or at least blur this image: whether the illness should be "regularly or domestically treated." Especially in tandem with providing information about therapies, choosing this kind of language perpetuated confusion about where authors equally well for insane persons, when they refuse to take food or medicines. It consists of a spoon (*a*), with

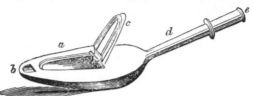

a hollow handle (*d*), opening at the top (*e*), and also into the bowl of the spoon, which is covered with a hinged lid (*c*), but is open at the apex (*b*). The spoon is made in the form of a wedge, in order to force the teeth apart when resistance is made to its introduction into the mouth ; and it is rounded at the corners to avoid injuring the tongue and gums. When any fluid is poured into the spoon, and the lid shut down, the pressure of the atmosphere, at the opening (*d*) near the apex, prevents the fluid from running out of the spoon, as long as the orifice at the upper end of the handle is firmly compressed by the thumb of any person ; but as soon as the thumb is removed, the fluid is projected with considerable force from the spoon. When the spoon is to be used, the head of the child must be steadied by an attendant, who should also gently compress the nostrils, which obliges the mouth to be opened for the facility of breathing.

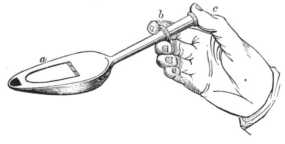

Proposed design for a spoon to facilitate domestic administration of medicines, from Anthony Todd Thomson's *Domestic Management of the Sick-Room* (Philadelphia, 1845), p. 174.

thought the lines of responsibility should be drawn. As the century advanced, more and more American physicians were to advocate that popular instruction in medicine take the form of treatises on prevention rather than on treatment. Early writers laid the groundwork for this shift.

Mothers as Advisers

Physicians were not the only ones who disseminated handbooks for women's and children's diseases. Lay writers, particularly women, joined the crusade, most noticeably in the 1830s. They blended folk customs with high culture, experience with learning. Though they seemed traditional in the stress they put on the healing authority derived from the mothering experience, they echoed the new note being sounded by physicians. That is, lay writers agreed that the woman's medical sphere was indeed circumscribed in the face of the physician's more extensive and scientific knowledge. Yet along with orthodox practitioners, they staked new claims for women: not only were women to be acknowledged as invaluable helpmates to doctors when illness struck, but, more importantly, their duties in many ways superseded those of the physician, charged as they were with ensuring a healthy population.

Typical of the lay writers was "An American Matron," who encapsulated her vision of the mother's medical role in the title of her 1811 *Maternal Physician*. Although she believed her qualifications unassailable as "the result of sixteen years' experience in the nursery," she thought it wise to emphasize that the book included "extracts from the most approved medical authors" in case some readers doubted her legitimacy. She did in fact rely heavily on excerpts from learned works—particularly those by Buchan, Underwood, and Wallis—but she made no pretense of "[being] scientific enough to describe technically," nor did she "profess to write systematically." Instead, she used quotations liberally and sprinkled her own observations "when and where they strike me most forcibly." Pragmatically deferential, she nonetheless filtered medical advice through her own experience. Not only did she report practitioners' differences of opinion, but she adjudicated their claims.[82]

The introductory heading set the tone for the book, proclaiming "every mother her child's best physician." This seemed a natural conclusion to her, a role inherent in the special relationship between mother and child. "Who," she asked, "but a mother can possibly feel interest enough in a helpless new born babe to pay it that unwearied, uninterrupted attention necessary to detect in season any latent symptoms of

disease lurking in its tender frame, and which, if neglected, or injudiciously treated at first, might in a few hours baffle the physician's
skill, and consign it to the grave[?]" To maximize maternal effectiveness,
it was crucial that "every intelligent mother" read "the most approved
medical books on the treatment of children and [pay close] attention to
their [children's] constitutions and complaints." With this preparation,
mothers would be qualified "to judge when nature really requires assistance, and how to administer it with propriety, in all *common complaints.*"[83]

But the American matron was careful to explain that she envisioned a
very restricted treatment role for mothers. "For this reason," she wrote,
"a mother is a child's best physician, as *it is better by care to prevent disease
than to be ever so well skilled in curing it.*" Mothers usually could and
should cope with minor ailments, but diseases such as quinsy and croup
required immediate professional attention. In the case of such "complicated disorders," she thought it would be as foolhardy for her to give
remedies as it would be for her readers to use them. She accordingly
confined her directions "to very narrow limits," which she defined as
"only . . . such complaints as I frequently manage successfully in my
own family, and which every lady ought to understand enough to administer the first remedies, by which she may often save herself many
groundless alarms, and her children much suffering." She clarified her
meaning in speaking of the management of whooping cough: "What is
said here is enough to enable us to know when more assistance is *requisite,*
and this is absolutely necessary for every mother to know."[84]

In order to exercise their responsibilities properly, mothers obviously
needed the good judgment acquired not only from experience but also
from education. Thus the American matron disagreed—and cited
Buchan in support of her view—with those physicians who "assert that
women never ought to open a medical book, or presume to meddle with
medical knowledge in the least, lest they become fanciful, and conceit
themselves and families ill with every disease they read of." In fact, she
hoped her book would become "a pocket companion, always at hand,
and always faithful." Her aim was "to render it so far scientific by quotations from respectable medical authors, as will enable every intelligent
reader to proceed with confidence when called upon to administer the
cordial or the drug, for the relief of any complaint here specified, and
with the aid of the rules given." She included plant remedies as well,
similarly basing that section on approved medical works.[85]

Echoing the Ewells, she recommended that every woman keep a well-
stocked medicine chest and a good set of weights and scales. But she

cautioned her readers to remember that "medicine does not work by magic, and therefore cannot be expected to cure any complaint instantaneously." The American matron warned people not to cut short a course of medicines just because they seemed to have produced a rapid improvement. If they did so, instead of the expected cure, "the disease [would return] with renewed energy, like a baffled enemy, who, perceiving his opponent off guard, or wholly withdrawn, returns to the attack with renovated courage, confident of victory." Mothers should have enough confidence in the nature and course of the doctor's treatment plan to execute the doctor's directions fully and faithfully.[86]

The importance of motherhood as a credential for authorship was evident in other works. In 1833 the first American edition of *Advice to Young Mothers on the Physical Education of Children* appeared. "By a grandmother," its writer, Margaret Jane King Moore, Countess of Mount Cashell, described her qualifications as impeccable. "Having suckled many children," she boasted first-hand knowledge that no male physician could equal. To this expertise she had added familiarity with "the best books . . . on the management of children." Though she considered herself well educated in this sphere, she nonetheless agreed with medical writers that mothers should relinquish control of treatment to doctors and take responsibility for prevention. This would be an important role, she stressed, because so many illnesses resulted from "imprudence and neglect" of physical and moral education in early life.[87]

Advice to Young Mothers did give suggestions for early treatment of infant disease, but it also advised calling a doctor immediately if the therapy seemed ineffective. A doctor was the appropriate person to direct treatment in "dangerous" situations because he had the advantage of years of study. Picking a good physician was not a simple task, though:

> To choose a physician well, one should be half a physician one's self: but as this is not the case with many, the best plan which the mother of a family can adopt is to select a man whose education has been suitable to his profession; whose habits of life are such as prove that he continues to acquire both practical and theoretical knowledge; who is neither a bigot in old opinions, nor an enthusiast in new. A little attention in making the necessary inquiries, will suffice to ascertain the requisites here specified; to which should be added (what is usually found in medical men of real merit,) those qualities which may serve to render him an agreeable companion: for the family physician should always be the family friend.

Once the doctor had been selected, mothers and attendants should rely fully on his skill and treat him with complete candor and unquestioned obedience. If the physician prescribed something "that the child particularly dislikes, or which has before disagreed with it," the mother would be responsible for explaining the relevant medical history to the practitioner; a sensible physician would substitute another medication or justify the need for the original one. If "unexpected resistance" from a sick child prevented the full execution of the doctor's orders, it was the mother's duty to notify the practitioner. Nor was the mother to give medicines of "old nurses, or of quacks" unless she had obtained prior permission from the physician. Breaking these rules might lead to "the greatest injury by deceiving the medical attendant" and negating the value of having consulted qualified personnel.[88]

Lydia Maria Child elaborated on the lessons presented by these lay women. Abolitionist, reformer, and prolific writer of women's books, Child was one of the best known of the authors of manuals treating the diseases of women and children. When *The Family Nurse* appeared in 1837, the subtitle identified it as a "companion" to her enormously successful *Frugal Housewife*. The commercial association alone was evidently not endorsement enough, since the title page also boasted that the volume had been "revised by a member of the Massachusetts Medical Society."[89] This revision, she explained in her preface, was intended "to make the book *safe*" and to make certain that "it contains no prescription that can endanger life or health, if a common degree of judgment be exercised."[90] Moreover, the book was about elements of nursing and was not meant to supersede the physician. "It is simply a household friend, which the inexperienced may consult on common occasions, or sudden emergencies, when medical advice is either unnecessary, or cannot be obtained."

Child saw herself primarily as a conduit for learned opinion, which she stressed by listing the medical authorities upon whom she had depended. When speaking of children's diseases, for instance, she confessed to "have almost uniformly followed Dr. [William P.] Dewees, who is very celebrated in that branch of his profession." She broke her allegiance to Dewees in her discussion of croup, where she adopted the advice of learned physicians who thought his remedies were not rigorous enough for the New England climate. Nor did she prescribe calomel. This was not because of a prejudice against its use, she assured her audience, but because it could not be safely "administered by inexperienced hands." Tinctures she advocated "sparingly and reluctantly," and she cautioned the untutored against "meddl[ing] with medicines." Even when Child used medical terms "for the sake of brevity and convenience," she referred her readers to the "clear and simple" explanations for them at the end of the book.

In keeping with her title, Child gave considerable attention to nurses' duties. "The first and most important duty," she declared, "is to follow scrupulously and exactly the directions of the physician." On avoiding misunderstanding, she was more precise: "Let no facts be concealed from him, or half told. Let no entreaties of the patient, or faith in your own experience, induce you to counteract his orders." Nurses did have some discretionary responsibility, but it was limited. Only in "common cases," she wrote, could "a good nurse . . . judge when a gentle emetic, or cathartic, or cooling beverage, is necessary; how much exercise is salutary; and when a cheerful guest may be admitted." She warned against different persons "trying experiments unknown to each other. If you think of anything which seems an improvement upon [the doctor's] practice, suggest it to him, and mention your reasons." Her detailed instructions about managing sick people also included some specific advice about how to administer medicines: "Be very careful to get exact directions of the food and medicine to be taken during the night: it is prudent to make a memorandum of them. Be scrupulous in measuring medicines: it is best the physician should see the size of the spoon you intend to use. In extreme illness important results often depend upon not varying five minutes in the prescribed time of giving medicines. It is well to keep a record of what occurs between the physician's visits, that he may accurately know the progress of the disease."[91]

Despite the practicality of *The Family Nurse,* Child's previously loyal readership balked at buying her book. Half a dozen years of radical abolitionist campaigning had injured her reputation, and sales of her subsequent works suffered.[92]

Louisa Mary Bacon Barwell, British musician and popular education writer, met only marginally greater success when her *Infant Treatment* appeared in its first American edition in 1844, eight years after its original London publication. "Addressed to mothers and nurses," the book had been endorsed by prominent American doctors, including Valentine Mott and Charles A. Lee. Lee, himself the author of a popular physiology textbook, especially praised the fact that the volume had been written "in accordance with the established principles of physiological science."[93]

In line with this emphasis on physiology, Barwell provided guidelines for proper living instead of printing specific remedies. Experience and common sense, she wrote, should be supplemented by "study[ing] the organization and functions of the human frame, as without that knowledge, there can be no certain or consistent attention to the rules of health, while, with it, attention to those rules becomes comparatively simple." It was especially important that women acquire this knowledge, because it was women's responsibility "to guard and nurture the physical, as well as the moral well-being of our race, during the most helpless period of existence." Such knowledge would also improve the management of pregnancy, essential to the child's good health.[94]

Moral and physical well-being were closely intertwined, and both should be inculcated from birth. This was the responsibility of the mother, not of a wet nurse. "A hired person," Barwell remonstrated, "cannot be expected to feel like a parent; she has not the motives for subduing her passions, restraining her appetites, sacrificing her pleasures and her rest—in short, for practising the self-devotion and self-control which the office of a nurse demands." When a child did get sick, Barwell advised that "the family physician should be immediately summoned, and the whole medical treatment committed to his hands. The mother and the nurse, have now no other duties, than faithfully to conform to his instructions and carry out his advice. No remedy should be given, without his knowledge, no medicine given, except by his prescription." Both the patient and the parent should have faith in the practitioner and his remedies. This meant that the parents should avoid "the practice of rendering the physician a *bug-bear,* or object of terror to the child, to frighten it into obedience, when other measures have failed." This would make the situation difficult for the doctor, "whose presence should rather soothe and tranquillize, than irritate and frighten."[95]

Infant Treatment closed with a supplementary chapter by the American editor on infant mortality, diseases, and other matters. "Americans," he said, "have been accused of undervaluing human life, and of manifesting great indifference to its preservation." It was a just charge, the proof lying "not in the frequency of duels, of savage personal combats, Lynch law, the bursting of steamboat boilers, or the destruction of rail-road cars, but rather in the general, and we fear, wilful ignorance of the laws of life." This should be corrected, the editor explained, for it was not part of "the established order of nature, or the systematic arrangements of Divine Providence."[96]

Yet there were discernible reform efforts underway. Changes would not be sweeping or rapid, but the early outlines could be seen in domestic health manuals, particularly in those devoted to the diseases of women and children. Initially written by British physicians involved in pediatric or obstetrical work, by the first decade of the new century the books bore the names of American doctors as well as nonprofessional women from both sides of the Atlantic. Like disseminators of the general household health manuals discussed in chapter 1, these writers were striving toward a more precise articulation of the scope and nature of professional and nonprofessional health-care responsibilities. Physicians, to be sure, were trying to win treatment control in a sphere traditionally governed by women. But they did not intend to rob women of all responsibility for health care. Instead, doctors delegated to women a set of responsibilities that they deemed more crucial to the nation's survival: the moral and physical well-being of children, to be nurtured from birth through an all-encompassing program of preventive living. As the century progressed, the campaign gained adherents and became more influential.

Starting in the late 1820s, popular magazines, particularly those such as *Godey's* and later *Petersons'* that were intended for a female audience, also published articles about health care for women and children. Treatment information, however, was usually omitted from the pages of these periodicals, the stress instead placed on attaining and maintaining health. The extent to which household manuals continued to focus on treatment owed much to persisting ambiguities and tensions in defining the parameters of domestic and professional health-care duties. The magnitude of the problem was highlighted, politicized, and recast by the early nineteenth-century popularity of the unlearned Samuel Thomson's "every-man-his-own-doctor" system of medicine, to which we next turn.

3 'Every Man His Own Doctor'

Post-Revolutionary health guides, whether meant for all family members or women and children only, sought to enlighten nonprofessionals about disease causation and treatment. Information about prevention increased over time and was an especially pervasive theme in works addressed to mothers. Though the authors stressed that lay people should defer to physicians because of their learning and skill, the writers recognized as well the expertise conferred on every human being by individual experience. Thus they portrayed the optimum healing situation as one characterized by a spirit of cooperation among all parties involved. In this scenario, however, the doctor retained supervisory authority, entitled to full obedience from the patient and other participants in the healing process. No hard-and-fast delineation of lay and professional responsibilities was possible, and these books tried to mediate between potentially incompatible expectations and perspectives. On the one hand, writers admonished nonprofessionals to summon and obey the doctor when illness struck; on the other, writers firmly believed citizens needed to know enough about treatment so that they could cope in emergencies. As a result, the disease information they provided in domestic handbooks—while path-breaking in its attempt to educate according to the learned medical tradition—simultaneously gave nonprofessionals new means to preempt the doctor's role.

Nonetheless, physicians expressed a naive faith that enlightened lay people would adopt appropriately subordinate and supportive roles. This faith began to crumble after 1800, when Samuel Thomson's root-and-herb medical system emerged as the first of a succession of popular medical sects. Like the homeopaths and hydropaths to be discussed in chapter

6, Thomsonians challenged regular medicine. They rejected orthodox therapeutics with its reliance on "heroic" bleeding, blistering, and purging. The sects loomed even more formidably because each also boasted its own organizations and doctrines, thus further calling into question the extent to which there were meaningful differences among educated physicians, quacks, and empirics.

Many orthodox physicians scoffed at Thomsonianism and, especially after the 1830s, tried to dismiss it as the embodiment of crude popular delusions. For them it was a manifestation in the medical arena akin to the religious enthusiasms of the day, such as the Millerite movement and Mormonism, the perfectionist impulse gone awry. Yet Thomsonianism's very popularity made it great cause for concern. Medical historians, chief among them Joseph Kett and William Rothstein, have attributed Thomsonian success to contemporary medical inefficacy and the democratic temper of the times. Thus the movement was doubly threatening. It was an organized alternative to regular medicine, and it fueled societal tendencies to democratic excess.[1] But historians have only tangentially addressed another, equally serious threat Thomsonianism posed: the restructuring of health care.

Learned doctors charged that Thomson, an uneducated man, perverted republican ideology by insisting that every person could be his or her own practitioner, thereby removing domestic practice from the overarching learned tradition that gave it meaning for orthodox physicians. In defending orthodox medicine against Thomsonians and other unorthodox healers, the regulars tried to use legislation to exclude or penalize sectarian practitioners. Yet historians have failed to look beyond legal tactics to chronicle a more successful strategy that was increasingly deployed. Gradually orthodox physicians recognized and articulated an antidote for sectarianism: to educate the population about medical matters. In so doing, learned doctors became increasingly aware of the risks of focusing their educational efforts primarily on disease *management*. Thomson and his followers helped reinforce the orthodox belief in the importance of spreading knowledge about disease *prevention*. At the same time Thomson's lieutenants, becoming more and more disenchanted with their zealous leader, worked toward many of the same goals espoused by their orthodox opponents.

The Botanic Tradition Endures

Nineteenth-century American botanic medicine was a reputable subject, having emerged from colonial popular and learned traditions.[2] Household use of English folk remedies, which had flourished for centuries, continued unabated in the New World. British emigrants also embraced Indian materia medica, as John Josselyn first chronicled in his 1672 *New-England Rarities Discovered*. Herbal medicines constituted major portions or entire texts of self-treatment manuals, as in the prolific Gervase Markham's *The English Housewife,* which was reprinted frequently in the mother country after its 1613 appearance. Equally popular was Nicholas Culpeper's 1652 *The English Physitian,* which remained in use for more than a century after its colonial debut in Boston in 1708.[3] John Wesley's 1747 *Primitive Physick,* reprinted at least eleven times in the colonies between 1764 and 1795, was another repository of herbal information for the lay person. Wesley's volume was frequently bound with other works, such as the 1770 colonial edition of John Theobald's *Every Man His Own Physician.*[4]

There were also indigenous proponents of herbal medicines. In Virginia the controversial John Tennent, physician-author of the 1734 *Every Man His Own Doctor,* mounted a transatlantic crusade in the 1730s on behalf of the seneca snake-root.[5] Equally notorious was the peripatetic doctor and loyalist, Samuel Stearns, who introduced his *American Herbal* in 1801.[6] Colonial ministers, who often studied and practiced medicine, relied on plant remedies as well. Included among this distinguished group were Cotton Mather, Thomas Harwood, and, most notably, Manasseh Cutler. Educated at Yale and a student of law and theology, Cutler published in 1785 *An Account of Some of the Vegetable Productions Naturally Growing in This Part of America.* Though technically an amateur investigator, Cutler corresponded with many respected students of botany, including Benjamin Smith Barton and C. S. Rafinesque, both of whom were physician-professors beginning to examine indigenous materia medica.[7]

Regular practitioners also compiled or reprinted botanical pharmacopoeias, among them Thomas Short's *Medicina Britannica* in 1751 and Johann Schoepf's *Materia Medica Americana* in 1787.[8] In addition, they offered botanical instruction at the country's first medical schools, beginning with John Morgan's lectures at the University of Pennsylvania. Adam Kuhn, a former student of Linnaeus, succeeded Morgan for a brief tenure, after which came a long incumbency by the highly regarded Benjamin Smith Barton. Similarly qualified individuals taught at Harvard Medical School, starting with Benjamin Waterhouse. Waterhouse's successor, Jacob Bigelow, was the author of the three-volume classic, *American Medical Botany,* which appeared between 1817 and 1820. In 1820 he also chaired the committee that produced the first *United States Pharmacopoeia.*[9]

The popular botanic tradition endured beyond the turn of the nineteenth century, finding expression in several different veins. Indian medicine and its reliance on plants enjoyed great vogue. In the latter half of the century patent medicine advertisements exploited Indian themes, while during the antebellum period a number of handbooks of Indian medicine appeared, particularly in the Midwest.[10] One of the most popular manuals was Peter Smith's *The Indian Doctor's Dispensary,* published in Cincinnati in 1813.[11] Among Smith's competitors were Jonas Rishel's 1828 *The Indian Physician* and Samuel North's 1830 *Family Physician and Guide to Health,* which closely imitated Rishel's volume.[12] Botanic remedies were also featured in "pow-wow" books, which drew upon superstition, as did John George Hohman's 1820 *Long Lost Friend or Book of Pow-Wows.*[13]

Botanic cures also reached a wide audience through popular health guides. Orthodox physicians played a part in this popularization by including plant remedies in the household manuals they published, though mineral prescriptions remained more central to their materia medica. Health writers outside orthodox ranks depended more on plant remedies and featured them in their guides. Little is known about the writers of most of these herbal manuals, though Madge Pickard and Carlyle Buley are probably correct in concluding that the majority had limited formal training and education. Lending credence to this view is the fact that few popular herbalists followed the standard practice of displaying their qualifications on the title pages of their books.

Authors of these botanical guides seldom directly opposed the regular medical profession. Some, like Samuel Curtis's 1819 *Valuable Collection of Recipes* or Samuel Henry's 1814 *New and Complete American Family Herbal,* ignored the issue altogether, presenting works unencumbered by defense or explanation.[14] Such volumes also typically omitted discussion of disease causation or treatment rationale; as handbooks of curatives, their utility was assumed to be self-evident.[15]

Even herbalists who carefully justified their pursuits did so without attacking the regulars. Josiah Burlingame made "no pretentions to erudition or eloquence, but in a plain and simple manner . . . compiled [*The Poor Man's Physician*], that every person may read and understand." The intention of his 1826 work was to serve the public by collecting as many useful remedies in one place as possible.[16] A. G. Goodlett stressed his credentials as a former Army surgeon and serious student of learned medicine. "I am writing," he said of his 1838 domestic manual, "a book not for the learned but for the unlearned, . . . to explain, in plain language, the diseases to which we are subjected, and the method to obtain relief from pain and sickness."[17]

Many early nineteenth-century American herbalists interpreted disease

STRENGTHENING CAKE.

Take life everlasting, chop it fine, boil it and make a strong tea thereof, thicken all together, with chopped rye, to the consistency of dough; apply it in a cake to the stomach in case of dissentery or any relaxation of the bowels, or weakness of the lower extremities.—*Proved.*

DROPSY.

Treatment.—Fill a quart bottle half full of the inside bark of white elder; then fill the bottle with wine, add two teaspoons full of hot powder; let the patient take plentifully of it daily; steam twice a week.

BILLIOUS PILLS.

Take two bushels of white walnut bark of the tops or roots, and half a bushel of thoroughwort, (or boneset;) put it in a copper kettle, fill the kettle with water, and boil it till the strength is out of the bark, then strain, and boil it down to a less quantity; then put it into a new earthen vessel and simmer it over a slow fire to the consistency of molasses, thickened with cayenne & wheat flour, equal quantities; make it into pills the size of a pea, give eight or ten for a purge.

TO MAKE HAIR GROW.

Take peach meats, pound them fine; (one gill,) and a pint of vinegar, put the peach meats and vinegar, together into a bottle; wash the place where the hair has fallen off, three times a day, and it will soon grow.—*Proved.*

CANCER WART.

Treatment.—Take a lobster, (or fresh-water

crab;) pull off the pincers and tie it on the cancer, with the back downwards; so repeat for three days, leaving it on all day. A toad, or the spawn of a toad, will do the same.—*Proved.*

SMALL STOMACH WORMS.

Let any person who is troubled with this complaint, eat plentifully of whortleberries and they will carry them off, if continued four days.—*Proved.*

TAPE WORM.

Treatment.—To know for certain if a person has one, take a hickory nut shell, fill it with paste made of wheat flour and milk, close the shell tie it on the navel, over night; if the person has one, the paste will be out when taken off in the morning; then take white glass, pulverize it very fine, mix it with the paste and tie it on as before, this will weaken the worm, then give plentifully, a tea of the bark of white oak, rock oak and shumake, roots: equal quantities. Then at the same time, to kill and carry off the worm, give a tea spoonful of spirits of turpentine, twice a day.

HOEMORRHAGE,

Or involuntary bleeding from the lungs, or otherwise.

Treatment.—Take a new earthen pot, put a quantity of burning coals in it, and throw in a spoonful of yellow rosin, made fine, let the patient inhale the smoke through a funnel, and swallow part of the fume, this will stop any bleeding.—*Proved.*

HOEMORRHOIDS, or PILES.

Treatment.—In the first place a regular

Recipes from Jonas Rishel's *The Indian Physician* (New Berlin, Pa., 1828), pp. 54–55.

within a religious framework and saw their enterprise as part of a much larger mission. Still their message was not inherently antithetical to orthodox teaching. Burlingame explained disease in terms of man's fall from God's grace. When created, Burlingame wrote, people were "pure in . . . nature, not subject to death, sorrow or pain." The fall changed everything. Said Burlingame, "We are now infested with pestilential damps, poisonous effluvia, noxious vapours, harbingers of death, pointing us to dissolution." Burlingame's remedy was temporal as well as eternal. As he assured his readers, "That same Jesus who could heal the sick with a word hath given healing virtue to each herb and flower, suitable to our various complaints, an antidote to all our pain."[18]

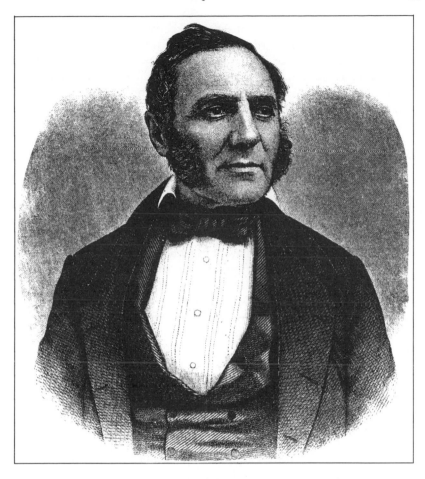

Portrait of John Gunn, author of the enormously popular *Domestic Medicine* (Knoxville, 1830), from the frontispiece of the "207th revised, centennial jubilee edition," *Gunn's Newest Family Physician* (Chicago, etc., 1883).

John Gunn agreed. His variously titled *Domestic Medicine,* first published in Knoxville in 1830, reached its so-called hundredth edition in 1870, enjoying enormous popularity reminiscent of Buchan's book of the same name.[19] The typical small library on the southern Indiana frontier, for instance, boasted a Bible and a hymnbook; if there were a third title, it was often Gunn's health manual.[20]

Man, wrote Gunn in the 1839 version of his book, had been healthy in body and mind until he had transgressed the laws of God: *"His days are now shortened, and encumbered with disease."* Gunn's lament would have had widespread resonance among his contemporaries, as would his firm belief that civilization had compounded the problem. While civilization had polished humans, explained Gunn, it had simultaneously enervated them and had generated artificial needs and desires, "a frightful and inexhaustible source of calamities." In this situation, Gunn preached, most people could blame only themselves when they fell sick; fortunately, however, "the great Father of the Universe, has clothed our soil with means, and those means powerful ones, of curing our diseases."[21] To a markedly greater extent than early orthodox writers, Gunn and other popular herbalists—and, it should be noted, the Thomsonians—linked together themes of nature, providence, and nationalism to legitimize their efforts. In so doing, they tapped and contributed to a widespread tendency of the time to view nature in romantic terms.[22]

Richard Carter shared Gunn's and Burlingame's belief that disease was a product of man's original sin, and he agreed that God healed physical as well as spiritual ills.[23] Born in Virginia in 1786 to an English father and a half-Indian mother, Carter spent his adult life seeking health and practicing medicine, presumably without regular medical training, in different parts of the country.[24] God, Carter maintained in 1815, had given the herb angelica "and all other blessings, for health here, and for salvation of the soul hereafter; for God has fixed a way to heal both body and soul." Carter had no doubt that he was one of God's emissaries, and this certainty gave him strength as he treated people. As he explained, Christ was the greatest physician of all time, and "as long as he stands by me, and blesses my means, I shall feel it my duty to continue my practice let man say what he will; for if God is for me, who can be against me, for I presume it is better to obey God than man."[25]

Carter traced his defensive tone to the ridicule and defamation he had received from gentry in the area. This reception arose, he thought, because his station in life and the way he practiced were "so simple and unrefined."[26] Yet these postures were not incompatible with regular medical tenets. In fact, Burlingame, Goodlett, Gunn, and Carter, like most other herbalists of this period, were careful to ally themselves with learned medicine. Their goals were pragmatic rather than adversarial; in an age of therapeutic uncertainty, their yardstick for recommendation was potential benefit rather than medical classification. Accordingly, they drew not only from the botanic tradition but from learned and folk traditions as well. As Gunn's apt subtitle proclaimed, he offered a book "describing, in plain language, . . . diseases . . . and the latest and most

INDEX.

—※※※—

Regardless of therapeutic affiliation, most authors firmly believed that there was an inextricable link between spiritual and physical well-being. The index from Richard Carter's *A Short Sketch of the Author's Life* (Versailles, Ky., 1825) succinctly but eloquently conveys this relationship.

approved means used in their cure; . . . [and] descriptions of the medical roots and herbs of the United States, and how they are to be used in the cure of diseases." A. G. Goodlett also delineated his therapeutic position in his 1838 title claiming to be "a compilation from the most approved medical authors . . . to which [he] added an account of herbs, roots, and plants, used for medical purposes."[27]

This sympathy for the regular medical tradition extended beyond the book covers of botanic health manuals. It was evident not only in the authorities cited, but also in the depiction of the doctor-patient relationship and of the nonprofessional's role in medical and health care. Richard Carter's unusual work provides a fitting example. In 1825 he published *A Short Sketch of the Author's Life,* appending to it a revised version of his 1815 *Valuable Vegetable Medical Prescriptions.* It has rightfully been labelled "a classic, unequalled for variety, originality, and completeness . . . a composite of Indian medicine, regular practice, poetry, mysticism, advice to the lovelorn, and Carter."[28]

Like the regulars who were writing health guides, Carter expressed a dual motivation: to provide medical advice for the poor and isolated, and to spread medical knowledge. His intention, indistinguishable from theirs, was to facilitate domestic treatment in minor illness, emergency situations, or the absence of professional aid. Despite his preference for plant remedies, he did in fact print remedies from the regulars' pharmacopoeia when he judged appropriate. Carter grounded his advice in a reference library of "the most approved Medical Authors," and he zealously recommended additional reading of the eminent medical authorities of the day.[29] Carter also recognized that there were limitations to the lay person's expertise in medical care. "With care any common man may manage in his family," stated Carter, but "in time of need, and a complaint you do not understand, apply to a physician that is always in full practice of these things." For the physician to be successful, it was essential that he "understand the cause and nature of a disease." In addition, he had "to get the confidence of the patient," which Carter said could be done "by letting the patient know what you are agoing to give him, and how it is to operate[;] and if you are agoing to give him anything dangerous you should let him know it, and carefully caution him against violating your directions, informing him of the dangerous consequences which are liable to ensue thereby." Carter's advice sounds very similar to that being giving by orthodox physicians: though it was the doctor's responsibility to inform the patient about his treatment, it was also the patient's duty to follow the doctor's instructions.[30]

This does not mean that Carter withheld criticism of the regulars; his certificates of cure alone, even if exaggerated, testify to the therapeutic failures of nineteenth-century learned medicine. He also had some very pointed remarks about the shortcomings of regular medicine. Though he criticized orthodox remedies, he recommended whatever he thought would work: vegetable remedies, Indian cures, folk prescriptions, and even orthodox therapies. Most important for the patient in Carter's eyes, no matter what the remedy of choice, was that both the patient and the doctor have faith in God.[31]

John Gunn likewise offered an amalgam of botanic, learned, and folk prescriptions. His descriptions of disease symptoms, causation, and treatment were culled from the respected medical writings of the time. Gunn cast a wide net for remedies, and his citations reveal acquaintance with standard American and European authorities as well as perusal of medical journals and newspapers. Despite some reservations about the use of heroic remedies, he realized that "the life of man [stood] greatly indebted [to the medical profession] through all its ages, from the cradle to the grave."[32]

But Gunn also criticized physicians for trying to monopolize the art of healing. God, he argued, had stocked nature with countless remedies for illness. They were accessible to everyone and should be used by everyone. Moreover, he charged, there was not much difference between the common person's ability to heal and that of the learned physician. Learned practitioners used technical language and obscure words "to conceal the naked poverty and barrenness of the sciences." The hypocrisy of learned physicians made Gunn angry, and his anger was fed by the parallels he saw in other areas, especially religion and law. Like other crusaders in the battle against privilege and elitism, Gunn aimed to reduce learned tyranny and popular submission by spreading knowledge. Medical science, Gunn repeatedly insisted, was common sense stripped of its *"mysticisms"* and rendered *"intelligible."*[33]

Yet Gunn's faith in the average citizen's treatment ability did not lead him to repudiate the orthodox practitioner or his remedies. He encouraged people to learn enough about simple treatments and surgical techniques so that they could take appropriate action in minor illnesses and emergencies. This meant that they had to understand how to diagnose, prescribe, bleed, use catheters, give enemas, administer medicines, and perform some surgery.[34] But Gunn recommended physicians' services in dangerous or difficult cases, such as lockjaw and convulsions in children.[35] Plant remedies he presented as valuable supplements to—not replacements for—the regulars' lexicon. He had no doubt that God intended humans to use botanical substances. "Behold," he wrote, "the spontaneous gifts of nature, yielding in almost every fragrant herb and flower, medicine to heal and relieve our maladies, recalling to our minds the splendid proofs of the Divine Majesty, showing the incomparable superiority of nature over the most elegant works of human contrivance." Regardless of nature's bounty, Gunn recognized that medical practitioners were necessary and that they had to be educated. He reported with regret his consultation with a Virginia doctor, "a man of the highest native genius, a man who must have stood at the head of his profession, had his great intellectual powers been aided by adequate opportunities of education."[36]

A. G. Goodlett's work also straddled the botanic and orthodox traditions. His 1838 *Family Physician* imitated Gunn's work to the extent that it repeated verbatim and without attribution many of Gunn's words. Even more striking is Goodlett's appropriation of texts published by orthodox physicians William Buchan and James Ewell. After an introduction modeled very closely on Buchan's 1811 *Domestic Medicine,* Goodlett followed the text of Ewell's 1816 *Medical Companion* almost exactly, so much so that he reproduced the same lines of verse and the same anecdotes. Goodlett did conclude with several sections that had not appeared in the work of Gunn, Buchan, or Ewell, and they are presumably his own.[37]

Not surprisingly, Goodlett did not see himself as an opponent of orthodox medicine. On the contrary, he thought he and the regulars were working toward the same goal: to "[check] the career of empiricism" by spreading medical knowledge. Household health guides would equip people "to detect ignorant pretenders in the healing art." Goodlett did feel that the regulars had neglected indigenous substances, and he was as nationalistic as Gunn about their medical use. Enthused Goodlett, "in no department of [God's] works do mingled *wisdom* and *goodness* shine with greater lustre than in the vegetable kingdom." America had been greatly blessed, since, "embracing almost every climate and soil of the globe, it richly abounds with drugs of every healing quality." Like Gunn, though, Goodlett simply incorporated plant remedies into the existing orthodox materia medica.[38]

Orthodox physicians showed little concern about these herbalists, either in professional journals or in medical society transactions. Combining botanic, learned, and folk therapeutics was not uncommon even among the regulars, and these herbal guidebooks were evidently not perceived as undermining the profession. The response was dramatically different to another disciple of botanic remedies. This was because Samuel Thomson did not envision his treatments as an adjunct to orthodox medicine but as a replacement. Though eventually rejected even by his own followers for being too fanatical, Thomson experienced great success until the late 1840s, before then both harnessing and sparking the prevailing meliorist and perfectionist temper of the times.[39]

The Birth of Thomsonian Medicine

Samuel Thomson was born in 1769 in Alstead, New Hampshire, the son of a pious Baptist farmer.[40] Curious about herbs from an early age, Thomson explored indigenous plant life as he reluctantly helped his fa-

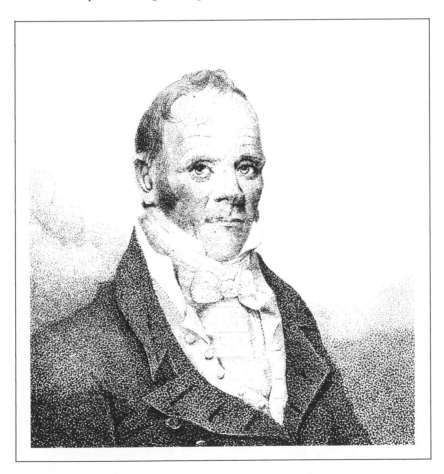

Portrait of Samuel Thomson, founder of the popular root-and-herb system that bore his name, from the frontispiece of *A Narrative of the Life and Medical Discoveries of Samuel Thomson* (Boston, 1822).

ther in the fields. It was at the age of four, Thomson recounts in his *Narrative,* that he stumbled on his major discovery by tasting *lobelia in-flata,* a common emetic. He delighted in persuading other boys to sample it, "merely by way of sport, to see them vomit."

Years passed, and he did not realize the medical potential of lobelia until he gave a fellow laborer a sprig to eat. Then Thomson reported, "[the man] believed what I had given him would kill him, for he never felt so in his life. I looked at him and saw that he was in a most profuse perspiration, being as wet all over as he could be; he trembled very much, and there was no more colour in him than a corpse." Soon, continued Thomson, the man vomited several times and about two hours later ate "a very hearty dinner, and in the afternoon was able to do a good half day's labour. He afterwards told me that he never had any thing to do him so much good in his life; his appetite was remarkably good, and he felt better than he had for a long time."[41]

Thomson's skill with botanical remedies increased, aided by informal lessons from a local female herbal practitioner. At the same time his dissatisfaction with orthodox medicine deepened. Too frequently, he thought, regular doctors bungled in treating disease, and Thomson renounced orthodox medicine in favor of botanical treatments and steam baths for himself and his family. His neighbors also began to rely more and more on him when they fell sick. "All this time," he maintained, "I had not formed an idea that I possessed any knowledge of disorder or of medicine, more than what I had learned by accident." But as word of his successes spread and the number of his patients grew, he began to think about giving up farming to practice medicine. He hesitated because of "my want of learning and my ignorance of mankind," but finally he decided "to make use of that gift which I thought nature, or the God of nature had implanted in me; and if I possessed such a gift, I had no need of learning, for no one can learn that gift." He did not mean to suggest, he added, "that learning is not necessary and essential in obtaining a proper knowledge of any profession or art; but that going to college will make a wise man of a fool, is what I am ready to deny."

Working as an itinerant herb doctor during the first decade of the nineteenth century, Thomson enjoyed considerable success in the area around southern New Hampshire, southern and eastern Maine, and northeastern Massachusetts. Now that he had decided "to make a business of the medical practice," he thought he should adopt "some system or plan," since what he had done previously "had been as it were from accident, and . . . necessity." In so doing, Thomson prided himself on having had "no other assistance than my own observations, and the natural reflections of my own mind, unaided by learning or the opinions of others." Boasted Thomson, "I took nature for my guide, and experience as my instructor."[42]

Despite his claims to originality, Thomson's theory was based on traditional medical doctrines, some of which dated from antiquity. His system was predicated on the idea that all animals are formed of earth, fire, air, and water. "Earth and water constitute the solids," he explained, "and air and fire, or heat, are the cause of life and motion." When the elements were in balance, the body was healthy; if the balance were destroyed, sickness resulted. From these beliefs Thomson extrapolated the key to maintaining equilibrium and therefore health. All illnesses, he said, came "directly from obstructed perspiration, which is always caused by cold, or want of heat." By logical extension, "to restore heat to its natural state [is] the only way by which health [can] be produced." The foundation on which the system was built was, in short, that "Heat . . . was life; and Cold, death."[43]

Formulating an explanation for disease and health was only the first step. Thomson's next task was to develop and systematize therapies that would "increase the internal heat, remove all obstructions of the system, restore the digestive powers of the stomach, and produce a natural perspiration." The Thomsonian course of medicine began with lobelia, or Number 1, designed to "cleanse the stomach, overpower the cold, and promote a free perspiration." Steam baths often were used in conjunction with lobelia, particularly in serious or longstanding cases.[44] But lobelia's action, though intense, was usually too brief to prevent the cold from "return[ing] again and assum[ing] its power." To restore the proper internal heat, the patient then moved on to Number 2, cayenne pepper. Number 3 was necessary to "clear the stomach and bowels from canker . . . and putrefaction," which, untreated, often terminated in death. Number 4, used to "correct the Bile and restore Digestion," was, like Number 3, some variety of tea or tonic concocted from roots, leaves, barks, or other botanic substances.[45] Thomson cataloged other, mostly unnumbered plant remedies, always giving detailed advice and instructions on identification, selection, and preparation. This system was foolproof, Thomson promised, for lobelia would not work "when the patient is dying, and when there is no death." His reasoning was simple and evidently appealing. Lobelia would be "silent and harmless" in the healthy system, because "there can be no war where there is no enemy."[46]

As his success continued, the herbalist was accused by regular doctors of being a quack, but Thomson countered by asking his readers to decide

"Which is the greatest quack, the one who relieves . . . sickness by the most simple and safe means, without any pretentions to infallibility or skill, more than what nature and experience has taught him? or the one who, instead of curing the disease, increases it by administering poisonous medicines, which only tend to prolong the distress of the patient, till either the strength of his natural constitution, or death relieves him?"[47] Given prevailing uncertainties in medicine, this seemed an irreconcilable issue. The debate, however, soon extended beyond rhetorical wrangling and personal choice. Rumors circulated that lobelia had killed some of Thomson's patients, and in 1809 the herbalist was arrested in Salisbury, Massachusetts, for murder. Brought to trial after a month in jail, Thomson at a key point called in botanist Manasseh Cutler, who testified that the plant alleged to be lobelia was in fact only marsh rosemary, a harmless if ineffective remedy. He was acquitted.

The trial was a turning point in Thomson's life. Exasperated by the incessant persecution, he sought and in 1813 received a patent for his therapeutic system. Armed with this document, which he renewed twice before his death, he recruited lay members for "friendly botanic societies." Twenty dollars bought "family rights," which included a copy of Thomson's *New Guide to Health* and access to groups to learn about Thomsonian cures. As his system gained converts, Thomson hired agents and managers, and they all sold family rights, crude ingredients, prepared remedies, and Thomsonian literature.

To try to reach as large an audience as possible, Thomson and his lieutenants used aggressive promotional techniques similar to those being employed by the enormously successful American Tract Society. Early nineteenth-century American book buyers normally procured their volumes from booksellers, general merchants, or peddlers. Often they were sold by subscription to reduce the financial risks, but this practice became less frequent as the nineteenth century advanced and the activities of bookseller, publisher, and printer grew increasingly separate. Thomson, however, eschewed established publishing channels and instead marketed his literature through a cadre of hand-picked agents. The local agent canvassed his area to promote the Thomsonian system, sell family rights, solicit journal subscriptions, and market Thomsonian handbooks and medicines. General agents, on the other hand, rarely traveled. They usually took responsibility for advertising and retail selling of Thomsonian books and medicines, enrolling family practitioners, providing instruction in the Thomsonian system, and running infirmaries. Even early publishers and printers of Thomsonian manuals often had affiliations with the sect, among them authors Elias Smith and Horton Howard. It is, however, unclear how long Thomson was able to sustain an independent distribution system, especially once his authority began to dwindle in the 1840s. Certainly by the 1870s, as Michael Hackenberg has shown in his study of the subscription marketing of Horton Howard's 1868 *Domestic Medicine,* salesmen no longer limited their merchandise to Thomsonian literature but also hawked a wide range of popular works.[48]

The Thomsonian movement spread rapidly in the East, Midwest, and South. In the late 1820s a Boston physician lamented that one-sixth of that city's sixty thousand inhabitants were using Thomson's system. Thomsonians claimed that one of every two Ohio residents supported Thomson, while regular doctors conceded one-third of that state's population to the movement. In the South, Mississippi's governor claimed in 1835 that one-half his constituents were Thomsonians.[49] Thomsonians also canvassed German immigrants, assisted by a German translation of Thomson's *Narrative,* which appeared in 1828.[50] In addition to the friendly botanic societies, Thomsonians offered journals, lectures, and conventions. Despite these visible signs of success, all was not smooth sailing. The first convention was held in 1832, and each succeeding one exacerbated tension over Thomson's personality and behavior. The founder was litigious, distrustful of education and the educated, protective, vindictive, and temperamental. At the last Thomsonian convention, in 1836, Alva Curtis, editor of the *Thomsonian Recorder,* split with Thomson and formed the "Independent Botanic Society," while those loyal to Thomson renamed themselves as the "United States Thomsonian Society."

The Orthodox Response

Despite the sect's internal problems, Thomsonian success made the regulars uneasy. As Daniel Drake observed, the devotees of Thomsonianism were not "limited to the vulgar. Respectable and intelligent mechaniks, legislative and judicial officers, both state and federal barristers, ladies, ministers of the gospel, and even some of the medical profession 'who hold the eel of science by the tail' have become its converts and puffers."[51] How was it possible, orthodox physicians worried, that these people had been duped? Thomson's therapies, charged the regulars, were no more effective and were often more dangerous than their much-maligned ones. Thomson did grant that his course of treatment was powerful, depicting the spasms in one early case as "so violent that [they] jarred the whole house."[52] Others attested to the strength of the Thomsonian treatment in less exaggerated terms. In his 1842 *Guide to Health,* Thomsonian J. H. Smith related the experience of Henry M. Chase. Deaf to the remonstrances of friends, Chase consulted a Thomsonian practitioner and then vividly described the treatment directed by this "very courteous and civil gentleman."

While under the operation of the Lobelia, I must confess that of all the queer sensations I ever felt, this was the queerest; for it was right down the middle of me—up again[,] cut off hands right and left—a pigeon wing in the feet—up again; down again, and so on. . . . The truth is, I was most terribly frightened; for I had heard that, if it refused to come up again, then it was all over with me. . . . Thousands of ideas . . . rushed through my brain in about thirty minutes, when the Lobelia, having done its office, came up in one of the most delightful vomits I ever experienced. I felt like another man; the sun seemed to shine brighter than it had done for a long time before; and, in about six hours, I had gone through what was termed a Thomsonian course of medicine.[53]

Another patient recalled being steamed until "the sweat rolls off as thick as your finger," after which a "powerful vomitive" and warm water were administered, "until there has ensued the most extraordinary vomiting." The patient, insistent that "this horse-cure" had given him "strength and color," admitted that the eleventh treatment "was worse than the others."

I was given an injection of lobelia when I had the vomitive on my stomach. This made me so sick that for 3 hours I gave no sign of life. My children and the neighbors thought me dead. At the end of that time I vomited forth more than 3 gallons of bile, mingled with a sort of thick, heavy skin. . . . But here is the last straw. . . . Sick as I was, they made me take my steam bath. . . . [I]n the night an abscess burst internally and I gave up at least a pint of matter. . . . Today . . . I [am] still spitting up matter and blood, but the pains are over and I feel a great deal improved.[54]

Though contemptuous of Thomsonian therapeutics, the regulars were more troubled to see that Thomson was taking the republican ideology to its most extreme form, and in the process perverting a heritage that accepted natural differences in talent and therefore position. They agreed that the desire to educate the population more thoroughly about medicine and disease was laudable, but they balked at Thomson's aim to make "every man his own physician," which they found subversive.

Regulars had no quarrel with the domestic management of disease, provided it was informed by the learned medical tradition. Thomson, however, sought to wrest control of medicine from orthodox doctors and to bestow it on the people. "In ages past," Thomson explained, "[Religion, Government, and Medicine] were thought by millions to belong to three classes of men, Priests, Lawyers and Physicians. The Priests," he continued, "held the things of religion in their own hands . . . and kept the Scriptures in the dead languages, so that the common people could not read them." There was reason to rejoice, though. "Those days of darkness" had now gone; the Scriptures had been translated into English and ordinary citizens knew how to read. A similar process had occurred in political life, where the common man now chose the country's public servants. But progress on the medical front had lagged. "The knowledge and use of medicine," he complained, remained largely "concealed in a dead language, and a sick man is often obliged to risk his life" because of his ignorance. Here Thomson, in one of his rare direct and positive allusions to orthodox medical opinion, invoked Buchan to endorse his views on the necessity of "laying medicine more open to mankind."[55]

People had to learn more about medicine, Thomson argued, *and* be prepared to take charge of their own medical care. This did not necessarily mean that people would need more formal training, because he believed that formal education was often more of an impediment than an advantage. While the study of anatomy and physiology might be "pleasing and useful," it was "no more necessary to mankind at large, to qualify them to administer relief from pain in sickness, than to a cook in preparing food to satisfy hunger and nourishing the body." Book learning, he maintained, just as easily could be used to obfuscate and deceive as to enlighten and promote truth. All that was really necessary, said a New York state senator in defense of Thomson in 1844, was "reading the great book of nature, which a wise and bountiful providence has spread before [humans]." From this study would come "as great a knowledge of the healing qualities of the roots of plants, flowers and leaves, which God has designed for . . . healing . . . , as can be obtained from the study of musty books in the halls of institutions of materia medica."[56]

It was the inherent talent that was crucial. The telling analogy, Thomson suggested, was to be found in the animal world. If God had given animals such good instincts about caring for themselves in health and in sickness, then surely human beings had comparable innate knowledge.[57] But learning could pervert those natural instincts, bestowed by God to guide and protect each person. In the 1832 edition of his *Narrative,* Thomson added several sections to decry more loudly the extent to which "mankind [had been] reduced below the grade of the beast by the force of education." For Thomson, the proof that human instincts had been corrupted or dulled lay in the widespread failure to recognize that heroic therapies rarely cured patients and often killed them. As the botanic practitioner wrote, "If *arsenic, mercury,* and *nitre,* are in their nature poison, can they in the hands of a physician, be medicine? If, when taken by accident, these things kill, will they cure when given designedly?"[58]

Enormous benefits would accrue, he argued, if only people were "to be brought back to [their] proper grade, that of other animals, and at the same time to exercise all their natural faculties." He was confident that "the people . . . would improve in stature and vigor, and become 'mighty men of renown;' such as we read of in olden times." But, Thomson warned, disaster loomed, for he feared "the hood-winking system" was going to endure. If that were to be the case, he predicted degeneration would continue, and people would "become more like a race of monkeys than like human beings."[59] For Thomson more was at stake than disputed therapeutic systems; the very future of the race depended on his crusade. Many people shared Thomson's concern about the inefficacy of orthodox medicine, but even those sympathetic to his blueprint for change grew disaffected as his views became more extreme and inflammatory.

The Struggle for Professional Standards

In 1837 orthodox physician Sumner Stebbins published an attack on Thomsonianism. In it, he, like most other established physicians of the day, admitted that learned medicine was "somewhat uncertain." Despite the inadequacies of orthodox medicine, Stebbins could not believe Thomsonianism was the solution. Asked Stebbins, "Will the casting away the recorded experience—the well-attested facts—the collected wisdom of the ages—and launching, without compass or rudder, upon the ocean of empiricism, with no guide but blind and ignorant conjecture—have a tendency to improve the healing art?"[60]

The situation was both more volatile and less clear-cut, for Stebbins neglected to mention the extraordinary amount of debate that characterized the medical profession in the decades between the American Revolution and the Civil War. Intrafaculty acrimoniousness splintered the profession and highlighted medical uncertainty. Feuds were notorious. One, between John Morgan and William Shippen, Jr., the most eminent professors in the country's first medical school, eventually divided both the school and the medical department of the Continental Army. Another erupted most virulently during the 1793 yellow fever epidemic in Philadelphia, when Benjamin Rush and his opponents exploited the press in a vitriolic battle over therapy. "A Mahometan and a Jew," Rush wrote, "might as well attempt to worship the Supreme Being in the same temple, and through the medium of the same ceremonies, as two physicians of opposite principles and practice, attempt to confer about the life of the same patient."[61] Rivalries were no less common in the nineteenth century, and medical schools were plagued by schisms, conspiracies, and coups, which often destroyed careers and institutions in the process.[62]

Feeding this internecine warfare was the uncertainty of medical practice itself. Southerner J. Marion Sims became a world authority in gynecological surgery, but his entry into practice was chastening.[63] Upon graduating from the Jefferson Medical College in Philadelphia in March 1835, he worried, "I felt absolutely incompetent to assume the duties of a practitioner." When he set up his office in his South Carolina hometown two months later, his anxiety deepened, for he was acutely conscious that he "had had no clinical advantages, no hospital experience, and had seen nothing at all of sickness."

His first case was an emaciated child of about eighteen months who was suffering from chronic diarrhea. After an exhaustive examination, Sims lanced the baby's swollen gums in an effort to ease teething pains. Then, however, he was stymied. As he explained, "When it came to making up a prescription, I had no more idea of what ailed the child, or what to do for it, than if I had never studied medicine. I was at a perfect loss what to do, but I did not betray my ignorance to the mother." Instead, he promised her that the medicine and directions for its use would be ready in an hour. Sims hastened to his office, "and took out one of my seven volumes of Eberle, which comprised my library, and found his Treatise on the 'Diseases of Children.'" Though he pored over the eminent doctor's article on "Cholera Infantum," he still did not know what to prescribe. "But," Sims recalled, "it was my only resource. I had nobody else to consult." He was able to take action, though, for Eberle "had a peculiar way of filling his books with prescriptions, which was a very good thing for a young doctor." Though he finally compounded one of Eberle's remedies, the child's condition did not change. In desperation Sims prescribed a new medicine from the following chapter. "Suffice it to say," he lamented, "that I changed leaves and prescriptions as often as once or twice a day."

The baby failed to improve. As the illness wore on, an old nurse assumed care of the child, and Sims felt uncomfortable under her apparent scrutiny. "It is well understood," he wrote, "that there is a curious antagonism between old nurses and young doctors. They have an idea that young doctors don't know a great deal, and the old nurses are not very far from right." One night as they watched the baby, the nurse asked him if he shared her opinion that the baby was destined to die. He disagreed, but recorded: "Externally, I was very calm and self-possessed; but internally I was not, for I really did not know what that child would do." The baby died, reinforcing Sims's sense of his own incompetence and of the nurse's superior discernment.

About two weeks later Sims got his second case, a baby of about the same age and size, in nearly the same condition, and afflicted with the same disease. Sims was disheartened: "I was nonplused. I had no authority to consult but Eberle; so I took up Eberle again, and this time I read him backward. I thought I would reverse the treatment I had instituted with [the first] baby." On this occasion Sims had the benefit of consultation with his former preceptor, who predicted that this baby too would die. When it did, Sims took down his shingle because he was so demoralized. "I was determined," he vowed, "to make up my deficiency by hard work; and this was not to come from reading books, but from observation and from diligent attention to the sick."

This was the key. Medical skill was derived not only from books but also from experience. Neither was sufficient alone.[64] As defined by a writer in the 1835 *Boston Medical and Surgical Journal,* there were two types of medical experience, "general or collective experience, and particular or individual experience." The first, he said, was "the experience of all the great and talented physicians who have gone before us, and of some living ones also." It was this kind of experience that was "recorded in the books, and has now become the common property of all physicians who have talents and industry sufficient to enable them to avail themselves of so large a mass of valuable knowledge." The other sort of medical experience was "the experience of each individual practitioner." He thought it "absurd" and "ridiculous . . . for a man to set up his individual experience against that of thousands as much favored as himself!"[65]

Other orthodox practitioners concurred. The advantages inherent in a "preliminary, strict, and virtuous education," said one, inculcated the first principles of reasoning, essential to guide the practitioner and to enable him to avoid empiricism.[66] Fortified by knowledge, added Yale medical professor Worthington Hooker in his 1849 *Physician and Patient,* the "shrewd and judicious" doctor would be singularly well equipped to decipher "the various and Protean shapes of disease, . . . in all their complications." But because the manifestations of disease were more "mingled and confused" than "the distinct [ways] with which they are necessarily described in books and lectures," there could be no substitute for bedside experience.[67]

Knowledge, then, could not simply be equated with book learning, but rather constituted education tempered by experience. The importance of the proper mixture could not be overemphasized, for this lay at the center of medical legitimacy. Samuel Thomson threatened the orthodox consensus by rejecting outright the utility of formal medical education. He was likewise an offender against the "moral view of the subject." Medicine, said one regular, was "not a trade" but was "a *profession* made by its members, that is, a declaration, an assertion, that the candidate possesses knowledge, skill, and integrity, sufficient to entitle him to confidence." The issue was obvious once put in these terms. "If he is not worthy of this confidence, he is guilty of a deception which jeopards the health and lives of his employers."[68]

A couple of years earlier the *Boston Medical and Surgical Journal* had satirized Thomsonian credentials by reprinting a letter from the popular *Journal of Health,* which its orthodox editors had drawn from a weekly Baltimore paper, *The Wreath.*[69] They intended to demonstrate the "consummate impudence and self-satisfied ignorance of steam practitioners." The missive, signed Christopher Costive and addressed to Timothy Thump, was written after an eleven-week sojourn in Baltimore, where Christopher explained he was "lerning the *Steam Doctoring Business.*" Soon his training would be finished. "Now you will hardley believe mee," wrote Christopher, "when I tell you that in three weeks more I shall get a certificate from my Boss—No, thats what I used to call Jim Vulcan, my old master, and a professional man calls his boss a praeceptor." He bragged to his friend that he "[would] bee astonished to see what wonderfull doctoring this *Steam Business* is; its shure to kill or cure right off, and dont keep people in misery: besides, it is so easily larned; in about three months a person can larn to cure aney disease, and . . . it dont cost so much as the old kind of doctoring."

In an age without standardized medical training, many practitioners exhibited some of Christopher Costive's qualities: legitimation through a short term of study; an obvious lack of learning; and an orientation to the economics of medical practice. However, defenders of a higher ideal were most troubled by Christopher Costive's casual transferral to medicine—a *profession*—the expectations and attitudes more appropriate to a trade. These issues were crucial to growing numbers of orthodox physicians who were trying to establish medicine as a profession. They shared overarching goals common to any professionalizing group: to preempt a specialized body of knowledge; to institutionalize education, training, and certification; and to legitimate the fledgling profession's claims by legal and popular acceptance. In order to be successful, orthodox physicians had to neutralize, absorb, or otherwise control fringe elements such as the Thomsonians.

Professional standards were difficult to establish and to maintain during the antebellum period. They crumbled under attack not only from those outside orthodox ranks but also from within. Nor were all irregular practitioners of humble origins and modest education. Noted botanist Gideon Lincecum, for example, sporadically practiced regular medicine from economic necessity when living in Tuscaloosa, Alabama, in 1818.[70] A dozen years later, having moved to the Tuscumbia area, he shifted to full-time practice. Lincecum became disillusioned with "man-killing" orthodox remedies during the 1832 cholera epidemic, and he began studying botanic medicine with a locally renowned Indian healer. Tempted to abandon regular medicine, Lincecum told his patients that he "was tired of a sham practice, that our medical system was too uncertain, and that it failed too often." They impatiently reminded him that "'people must die'" and insisted he resume his former practice: "'You will never find a system that will cure all your cases. Go to work again, we are satisfied with your practice.'"

About this time, he remembered, Thomson's *Guide to Health* was being distributed at twenty dollars per copy. Contemptuous of "the bragging and prating amongst the steam doctors," Lincecum "verily thought it to be the most perfect tomfoolery [he] had ever heard in all [his] life." Humiliating Thomsonians was easy: "I would often quiz those steam doctors with questions in anatomy and physiology, and confuse them till they would almost weep for vexation."

Soon afterward the scion of a wealthy country family was searching for someone to treat major illnesses among the clan's slaves during his impending absence. The family, reported the landowner to Lincecum, "'[had] discussed the merits and character of all of [their] doctor acquaintances.'" They were well aware, he told Lincecum, of "'all the fool talk and ugly words you have displayed in your game making about the steam doctors.'" Still, the clan had decided to approach Lincecum and ask him to "'study the Thomsonian System and practice it in our families during the time we are engaged in the land speculations.'" Their proposition was precise. "'We don't ask you,'" clarified the patriarch, "'to practice it except in our families, but we demand that you employ no other medicines in them. Such is our confidence in the Thomsonian remedies that we are fully willing to trust them in all cases of sickness; and if you will say that you will undertake it for us we will furnish you with a set of books and you can use what medicines we have on hand while they last.'"

Lincecum first registered incredulity, but he met with a ready response: "'Shut your foolish mouth,' said the old man. 'You are struggling with a big family, and we want to help you. We don't want to mortify your feelings by making appropriations for your benefit. But we have a piece of work which we know you can do with benefit to us and credit to yourself, for which we are able and very willing to thoroughly remunerate you. Take these books and make yourself ready as soon as you can.'" The doctor capitulated and for the ensuing two years treated according to whatever system each patient requested. He finally condemned regular medicine after a two-year-old died as a result of orthodox dosing.

Lincecum's story is instructive, not merely because Lincecum recognized the inadequacies of regular medicine, for large numbers of his lay and professional contemporaries shared those views. What is more interesting is how Lincecum responded to his predicament and the manner in which he began Thomsonian practice. Two aspects of his conduct deserve particular mention. First, his pandering to popular taste fulfilled the prophecy of orthodox doctors who were alarmed to see how many lay Americans fully expected to participate in disease treatment, the doctor's sphere. Lay interference in matters beyond their trained comprehension, these physicians worried, inevitably contributed to the denigration of learned knowledge—and thereby "Truth, which exists independent of us."[71] In addition, Lincecum's unabashed materialism and its impact on his medical actions were antithetical to the learned ideal of the physician's character. The landowner's appeal to his financial plight was regrettable, but that Lincecum should have responded to bribery was abhorrent.[72] Because medicine was a profession, its practices and standards should have been immune from popular demands as well as pecuniary considerations.

Thomsonians and the Doctor-Patient Relationship

But Lincecum's story, like that of Christopher Costive, is revealing in another, equally important but seldom recognized way. Each illustrates the fact that Thomson's followers were seldom as radical as he was. Like these men, most writers of Thomsonian health guides assumed that a physician would continue to direct treatment. Thomson was not alone in his vision that every person could be his or her own physician, but his view lost support as time passed.

Thomson indeed advocated total renunciation of learned medicine in favor of healing based on common sense and experience. He also flaunted his lack of learning, which many of his followers pinpointed as the primary source of the regulars' hostility toward him. "If the wise and learned only were to make discoveries," explained Samuel Robinson in his 1829 *Course of Fifteen Lectures,* "it could be borne" by the orthodox. Thomson, however, represented the exact opposite, "the illiterate, the mere ploughboy, . . . the peasant." The regulars simply found it galling, continued Robinson, that a man "who had spent his life among the clods of the valley—and himself but little superior to the dust he walked on—that he should pretend to make discoveries in the science of medicine; and *invent forms,* and *medicines,* and *rules,* to enlighten its exclusive and profound professors." It was, the Thomsonian writer concluded, almost beyond endurance for "men, *proud* of their high attainments."[73]

Thomson's defenders believed that their leader's lack of formal education and medical training had provided him with a unique opportunity. Thomson possessed, gloated Simon Abbott in his 1844 *The Southern Botanic Physician,* "a mind entirely uninfluenced by all authority, unmoved and unobstructed by anything which had gone before him." This gave him a crucial advantage over those educated in schools, permeated and regulated as they inevitably were by "the authority of books and professors. It is impossible," argued Abbott, "for the most independent mind to perfectly retain its freedom; it will insensibly bow to the opinions of some celebrated or splendid authority." He conceded that eventually "some superior souls are enabled to cast off the shackles of education; but they are the fewest number of that mighty host which walk forth from the schools of the world to propagate the errors of their predecessors." It seemed clear to Abbott and other followers that Thomson, so specially endowed, was particularly favored in his crusade. Trumpeted Abbott, "Heaven sent him forth to work; fortified his mind, girt up his loins, and cleared his way; and it is but just to add, that the smile of approving Heaven has most evidently blessed and accompanied his practice."[74]

Thomson's popularizers embraced their leader's puking, purging, and steaming regimen, and they celebrated his freedom from educated authority.[75] Some seemed even more radical than Thomson. Benjamin Colby, author of the 1844 *A Guide to Health,* fully agreed about the importance of spreading knowledge so that people could take care of themselves and avoid mistreatment at the hands of learned and ignorant quacks. His commitment extended further, however, for "if every man [were] his own physician, the interest of physician and patient would be identified." Colby believed he had found the vehicle for achieving this union; as a follower of Fourier as well as Thomson, he was trying to promote both medical self-help and utopian socialism.[76]

Few manual writers, however, were as extreme as Thomson. Most, including Colby, grounded their own work in the learned medical tradition, and they did not question the fundamental authority of the doctor. They did not attack the structure of the health-care relationship, but the therapies used.[77] "The Thomsonians," as Sumner Stebbins accurately summarized their position, "disclaim all knowledge upon the subject of medicine, which is not derived from Thomson himself." But this was not the full story, claimed the critic. In an astute—and damaging—observation, Stebbins pointed out that "they sometimes endeavor to fortify their system, by showing that Cullen, Brown, and the venerable Dr. Rush, held similar views."[78] Indeed, except for the difference in therapeutics, Thomsonian manuals are strikingly similar to those written by regulars. In describing diseases, Thomsonians usually cite the same European and American authorities as regulars and with about the same frequency. Benjamin Rush was a particular favorite, his stature and expertise likened to Thomson's by virtually every writer of Thomsonian health guides. Benjamin Colby even emblazoned an often-quoted, and apt, injunction of Rush's on the title page of his 1844 *Guide to Health:* "Let reason and common sense be our guide; strip the profession of medicine of every thing that looks like mystery."[79]

In addition to discussing Benjamin Rush at length, these writers demonstrated their familiarity with other learned medical authorities by referring frequently to orthodox doctors and their ideas. Among other things, acquaintance with the orthodox canon—and its disputes—facilitated criticizing regular practices. As Samuel Robinson summarized, "Let it be remembered, I have not made an attack upon the Faculty; they, themselves, have alternately made it on each other. I have merely introduced passages from their own writings for the sake of argument and illustration. They have all admitted the *uncertainty* of medical practice, and its great susceptibility to improvement and reduction."[80]

Thomsonians had more specific warnings about what to expect from orthodox medicine. In his 1837 *Family Guide to Health,* John Brown eloquently conveyed the consequences of regular treatment. With orthodox therapy, he conceded, a "man may be rescued from the grasp of death, and raised from the bed of languishing." But was it really worth the trouble? Brown answered no, convinced that "to be left to drag out a miserable existence, in consequence of the means used to preserve life, [was] an evil of the highest magnitude." He realized that such a person would still be alive, but he thought this "scarcely a blessing; for, deprived of the enjoyment of health, and . . . retaining the seeds of disease [and] premature decay, pain and misery become the companions of his bosom, and he may be said to endure, rather than to enjoy, a *living death.*" Some readers probably found this characterization too accurate, given the consequences of some of the day's heroic therapies.[81]

The solution for most Thomsonians, however, was a change in therapy, not the abolition of the doctor. Given the uncertainty of medicine, Thomsonians resented the confidence people vested in regular practitioners and their remedies. Regular physicians, Dr. L. Sperry bemoaned in 1843, were "looked upon with wonder, admiration, and as almost super-human."[82] Elias Smith, first a trusted assistant and then a bitter enemy of Thomson, concurred. Most people, he said in his 1837 *American Physician,* were amazingly ignorant about medicine. Wrote Smith, "They conclude the doctor knows, and content themselves to remain in ignorance, and do as the doctor says, even when they think his directions are unreasonable and contrary to nature." Smith had some specific examples: "If the doctor says, 'The outside must be blistered to cure the inside,' they consent. . . . If the doctor says, 'burn a hole in the arm or leg and keep it sore with a pea, or a piece of wood,' they consent. . . . If the doctor says 'bleed often,' they consent."[83]

Samuel B. Emmons joined the chorus of protesters. Though Emmons stopped short of labeling himself a Thomsonian practitioner, his 1836 *'Every Man His Own Physician'* relied heavily on Thomsonian works and remedies. Whatever his precise medical classification, the root-and-herb doctor told an instructive anecdote featuring an old-fashioned Connecticut physician, "whose skill had never been doubted" until two years earlier when a new doctor had settled in his town. The newcomer was well attended and well paid. "He had," said Emmons, "diplomas and recommendations from medical colleges, was dressed in the most fashionable style, wore a ruffled shirt, rode in his carriage, was remarkably polite, and in fact there was nothing like the new doctor."[84] The older man, by contrast, "made use of nothing but simple means to cure the sick, dressed no better than other people, rode on horseback, and when not employed in practice, worked on his farm."

Soon an epidemic hit the town. The young physician's patients died; more and more people went to the older practitioner, who "went to work with his old-fashioned mode of treatment, depending on his own experience, and the knowledge he had of the constitutions and habits of the people." The sickness abated, but the young man remained perplexed about his failures, having "gone precisely by the directions laid down in the books." The lesson he failed to grasp was that book learning alone, which Emmons thought constituted "fashionable" medical practice, was insufficient to combat disease.

Together with feeling irritated amazement at popular credulity, Thomsonians saw themselves as horrified witnesses to the destruction of "the grand principle of freedom." In the prevailing therapeutic milieu, Simon Abbott charged in 1844, the patient "is reduced to the condition of the slave; when he must in profound ignorance receive with implicit faith whatever is offered to him."[85] Concluded Daniel H. Whitney in his 1834 *Family Physician,* this was insupportable in America, "the paradise of freedom."[86]

Thomsonians, believing liberty endangered, attached themselves to a wide variety of popular political and social reforms during the 1830s and 1840s. Thomson himself was a fervent supporter of Andrew Jackson, as was Elias Smith, who included Jackson's farewell address in the 1837 edition of his *American Physician.* Smith added a commentary to praise and defend Jackson, whom he thought "worthy of a place in every man's *library,* in every man's *understanding, memory,* and *affections*" and the embodiment of "*Republicanism* in principle, in experiment of more than fifty years." It was clear to Smith that Jackson was carrying on the important work begun by Washington and that both ranked as "great among the republicans of the old school."[87]

As Smith's remarks suggest, Thomsonians often portrayed themselves as embarked on a crusade with very high stakes. By rescuing medicine from the doctors, they saw themselves as completing the great revolution, begun with the Reformation, that had freed government from the lawyers and despots, and religion from the priests. That revolution had continued with the American Revolution, but much remained to be done to secure for the average citizen his or her rights in government as well as in medicine.

The Thomsonian Legacy

What should be done? First, Thomsonian authors, like other contemporary writers of home health guides, sought to equip people to respond to emergency situations or minor illnesses. As Elias Smith explained, "By reading and understanding the medicines here described, [people] may so far become their own physicians, as to prepare medicines and in the first stages of disease, so apply them as to obtain a cure without the aid of any physician whatever."[88]

But Smith was not visualizing a society without doctors. Rather, he anticipated substituting *botanic* physicians for regular ones. The New York Thomsonian Society recognized and supported this distinction. From its founding in 1835, it had two grades of membership, one for nonprofessionals and one for professionals. John Thomson, one of Samuel Thomson's sons, clarified the status of owners of "family rights" in his 1840 testimony before the New York state legislature, then considering the repeal of licensing laws: "We do not consider them fit, as general practitioners; they have merely the right to compound their own medicines, and practice in their own families, and have no right or business to practice on community[;] they are not presumed to be acquainted with disease or medicine, and should not be tolerated to practice, or to collect their pay for their services; community is in danger from these unskillful practitioners."[89] This was Elias Smith's view as well, and he estimated that "three to six months spent with an experienced botanic physician, will enable a man to attend to the sick, to their advantage in all common cases."[90]

An educated *citizenry* as well as an educated *medical profession* was, then, crucial for the larger number of Thomsonians. It was this issue over which Alva Curtis and his followers split from Thomson in 1838, establishing their own Botanico-Medical School and Infirmary in Columbus, Ohio. The eclectic followers of Wooster Beach, at the Worthington Medical School, in Worthington, Ohio, wrote scathingly of Curtis's school but agreed that Thomson had grown intolerably narrow-minded. "The tendency and aim of the Thomsonian system," they charged, was "a total subversion of all medical science and a substitution of a limited patent system of practice, founded upon ignorance, prejudices, and dogmas of a single individual." Thus for Thomsonians to call themselves *"medical revolutionists"* was appropriate. But they balked at other labels. "For such individuals to be styled *medical reformers,* whether they themselves or others, is slanderous, and calculated grossly to deceive and misguide the public mind."[91]

Many writers of Thomsonian manuals recognized the ultimate inadequacy of educating professionals and nonprofessionals about disease treatment, alone or in tandem. Both were necessary, they agreed. People had to be taught about medical matters to enable them to respond intelligently to illness and accident, and botanic practitioners had to be trained in order to ensure better therapeutic management in disease. But there was a growing awareness of a more fundamental area of popular ignorance: disease *prevention.* In addition, this appeared to be a more sensible area to tackle, for, as Abbott explained in 1844: "Towards [prevention], the means are generally in our power, little else being required than strict temperance in all things; but towards [cure], the means are uncertain and perplexed, and for the knowledge of them, the greatest portion of mankind must apply to others, of whose skill and judgment they are in great measure ignorant."[92] Thomson, however, had completely neglected prevention. His *Narrative* combined autobiographical details with case histories, while his *Guide to Health* listed treatments for disease.

To facilitate popular attention to preventive living, writers of Thomsonian health guides increasingly covered rules for healthy living. For some, this entailed providing information about anatomy and physiology. J. E. Carter emphasized the importance of learning about physiology in his 1837 *Botanic Physician*. He argued that anatomical details would "encumber the mind with a mass of useless lumber tinseled with a show of classical lore," but that physiological knowledge would help people keep bodily functions in good working order.[93] Morris Mattson and Daniel Whitney took the opposite approach. Both Mattson's 1845 *American Vegetable Practice* and Whitney's 1834 *Family Physician* included sections on anatomy, and Whitney provided four plates to make his dense written explanation clearer. Neither expected that their readers would try to acquire "minute" anatomical knowledge, as Whitney said, but both thought general knowledge would be very useful.[94] True to their leader's principles, none of the authors felt that any sort of book learning could be more important than practical experience and acquaintance with the botanic materia medica.[95]

Though few Thomsonian writers during the antebellum period gave information about anatomy and physiology, many did provide instruction about preventing disease. J. E. Carter devoted an entire section to the "Art of Preserving Health," but most authors sprinkled suggestions about preventive living throughout their texts on disease treatment.[96] Benjamin Colby's revisions for the 1846 edition of his *New Guide to Health* underscored the individual's responsibility for maintaining health. "So long as we . . . transgress nature's laws," he summarized, "so long we must suffer the consequences; which are pain, debility, and untimely death, in spite of physicians, regular or irregular, homoeopathic, hydropathic, or Thomsonian even."[97]

The medical profession had initially reacted to Thomsonianism by trying to use licensing laws to discredit Thomsonian practitioners or to deprive them of the right to practice. Gradually, they realized that popular education was the only weapon likely to be effective in the battle against sectarianism. Stebbins again captured the essence of the matter: "Neither Thomsonianism, nor Mormonism, nor witchcraft, nor any other kind of foolery, can be put down by legislative enactments, by fines, or imprisonments, and they should not be if they could. Such laws infringe the inalienable rights of the citizen. They force, they exasperate, but they do not convince the mind. The wide diffusion of useful knowledge can alone dispel such gross delusions. Universal Education,—the colossus of light, reason and liberty—aided by the artillery of a free press, is the proper antidote."[98]

Moreover, by the late 1830s and early 1840s, as Thomsonianism was beginning to fade, the regulars were revising their ideas about what constituted "useful" medical knowledge suitable for popular consumption. Their goal remained that of diffusing information, "the great lever, which moves the machinery of the world."[99] Greater and greater numbers of orthodox physicians, however, questioned the wisdom of publishing domestic guides that focused primarily on disease management. Thomsonians had revealed and exploited inherent imprecisions in prevailing ideas about the proper political and social order. Learned physicians shuddered at Thomson's zest for every citizen's being his or her own physician. Such leveling of distinctions, they were convinced, represented not consummate republicanism but rampant, dangerous democratic excess.

Orthodox physicians continued to write and to endorse popular health publications, including domestic guides. The emphasis, however, gradually shifted from disease *management* to disease *prevention*. Such popular works took on new importance, as the next chapter explains, in the face of the bankruptcy of institutional, organizational, and legislative responses to sectarianism in the middle third of the nineteenth century.

Toward a Literature of Prevention

4

The number of state and local medical societies grew steadily from the 1780s through the Civil War. They appeared before 1800 in most former colonies and after the turn of the century spread to the Midwest and through the South. Medical societies promoted scientific activities and regulated members' conduct by establishing fee bills and codes of ethics. Their major concern during the mid-nineteenth century, however, was licensing, which was intended to accredit qualified practitioners and to exclude those deemed illegitimate. By 1830 thirteen of the twenty-four states had passed licensing legislation. Though the statutes varied slightly from state to state, unlicensed practitioners in all states could be fined and jailed, and they were not allowed to sue for nonpayment of fees.

Licensing laws appeared at a time when champions of democracy viewed regulatory efforts as monopolistic and elitist. Under the onslaught of widespread public opposition, the laws were notoriously ineffective and virtually unenforceable. Thus a little more than a decade later, nearly every state had repealed its penalties on unlicensed practitioners. Alabama and Ohio were first in 1833, followed by Mississippi in 1834, Georgia and Massachusetts in 1835, Maine in 1837, South Carolina in 1838, Maryland and Vermont in 1839, Connecticut in 1843, and New York in 1844. Licensing laws remained in effect until 1852 in Louisiana, and they were never repealed in New Jersey.[1]

As the licensing authority of state medical societies was revoked or eroded, orthodox physicians moved defensively to distinguish themselves from unqualified healers. It was a daunting task, complicated by the egalitarian temper of the times and by significant professional discord. Institutional and organizational responses to this situation—the creation of voluntary medical associations and the mid-century formation of the American Medical Association—have been well chronicled by historians of medicine. Another equally important reaction, however, has been neglected: the campaign to educate Americans about health and legitimate medical practice. By the mid-nineteenth century learned doctors were exhibiting growing ambivalence about their customary vehicles of instruction, the domestic health guides. Their dissatisfaction arose in part from the manuals' emphasis on treatment, which these physicians thought encouraged nonprofessionals to be too involved in trying to cure diseases. They also felt that household guides did not offer adequate guidelines about how to distinguish legitimate from illegitimate practitioners.

One response to orthodox criticisms was to modify the guides so that they underscored lay responsibility for prevention and discouraged lay participation in treatment. Increasingly, however, established doctors promoted different forms of popular instruction, particularly lectures, guides to healthy living, and school texts. Whatever the vehicle, the publicists had two central messages. First, disease could be *prevented,* and it was each individual's duty to understand this concept and to live according to the laws of physiology and hygiene. Second, if disease did strike, nonprofessionals should defer to orthodox physicians for proper diagnosis and treatment; only in emergencies should lay people act more independently.[2]

Mid-nineteenth-century popular medical education was either initiated directly by doctors or undertaken by lay people with professional support. From the physicians' perspective, this was a precarious alliance. They were constantly on guard to discredit popularizers of Thomson's ilk, who they felt did not observe the fine line between instructing the population about health and invading the physician's realm. Not all transgressors were lay people; orthodox doctors also criticized their own brethren, most notably some authors of domestic manuals, for assigning too much responsibility to nonprofessionals in medical matters. Imbued with the perfectionistic impulse characteristic of many antebellum Americans, popular health writers were seeking to achieve societal well-being through appeals to individual conscience rather than by calls to political action. Orthodox practitioners applauded efforts to instill preventive concepts but were critical of those who failed to bar nonprofessionals from all but the most rudimentary of medical duties.

The Battle Against Quackery

Without a doubt, quackery was the enemy, but what did this mean? Regulars tended to label all practitioners except themselves quacks, a defini-

RULES FOR LIFE.

1. LOVE, fear, and reverence the God of nations, and keep his commandments.

2. Never steal or beg, lie or swear.

3. Let your pledged word and agreements be sacred and faithfully executed.

4. Pay a debt of one penny as promptly as of one dollar; and, above all, never be pestered with dunners, sheriffs, or suits at law.

5. Advertise your business, so that every man, woman, and child may know you; and be particular to always pay the printer.

6. Plan your business right; then execute with indomitable perseverance and despatch.

7. Be charitable to the poor, merciful to the dependents—hopeful and benevolent.

8. Speak well of thy enemy, but have no dealing with him; and thus you will heap coals of fire on his head.

9. Have all your agreements in writing, and your bills receipted when paid.

10. Calculate your business well, and be sure that you start right; then, do not constantly worry about it, but be patient and calm for success.

11. Marry first love, and marry early.

12. Eat and drink with the brain as well as the mouth.

13. Labor for the education of your children, and the christianization of the world.

14. Avoid extravagant dinners, livery, and laziness—as being both offensive to God, and destructive to human happiness.

15. Do not let extravagant notions of living prevent your marrying.

16. Never fall out with Labor—for he is your best companion, be you rich or poor; and strong muscles and mind will not forsake you.

17. Retire early and rise early, and have no fellowship with the sluggard.

18. Save money against the day of want, for it is one of the best earthly friends; but as it is slippery as an eel, hold fast upon it.

19. Never be bought or sold by the gold of despots.

20. Be a true and faithful Republican, standing fast for equal rights, and ever ready to defend the constitution, hook and line, bob and sinker, both in war and peace.

21. Allow no European nation to interfere in our national or domestic concerns.

22. Be a man, a mouse, or a long-tailed rat; no matter what, only that your colors may be known.

The greatest dinners ever feasted on by man are provided by the American people, viz.: Republicanism, large territories, unbounded oceans, lofty mountains, equal rights, religion, food, clothing, air, light, low taxation, and wealth for all. Such are the dinners of Americans; but they are more than can be digested by the stomachs of the tyrants of despotism.

In *The People's Medical Lighthouse* (New York, 1856), Harmon Knox Root presented an amalgam of popular medical information, extrapolating from it specific behavioral instructions, or "Rules for Life," p. [471].

tion that implied the existence of meaningful and obvious distinctions. In reality, the situation was far more complex and less clear-cut. Regulars were right in charging that many sectarian and lay healers were only marginally qualified to practice medicine, but the point is misleading in the absence of two other facts: first, many sectarian and lay healers had received preparation equal or superior to that of many regulars; and second, many regulars were no better qualified than the "quacks" they denounced.[3] Orthodox physicians, then, faced an embarrassing and vexing dilemma that was to endure throughout the century. Many recognized that any successful—or even credible—effort to exclude quacks from medical practice would have to go hand in hand with internal reforms.

As historians have documented, low entrance and matriculation standards at American medical schools meant that even the students who received diplomas were not necessarily qualified to practice. Many were illiterate, ill-mannered, and unethical. Harvard University President Charles Eliot's remark in the 1870s could have described graduates in earlier decades: "An American physician may be, and often is, a coarse and uncultivated person, devoid of intellectual interests outside of his calling, and quite unable to either speak or write his mother tongue with accuracy."[4] Among the professions, many viewed medicine as the one of last resort. Grumbled one doctor, "It is very well understood among college boys that after a man has failed in scholarship, failed in writing, failed in speaking, failed in every purpose for which he entered college; after he has dropped down from class to class; after he has been kicked out of college, there is *one* unfailing city of refuge—the profession of medicine."[5] Steven Smith, a medical student in the late 1840s and then a prominent physician, more succinctly summarized mid-nineteenth-century public opinion: "A boy who proved to be unfit for anything else must become a Doctor."[6]

Given the abysmal state of regular medical education and practice, some observers predicted that orthodox physicians would not emerge victorious over quackery. The challenge was heightened, they said, by the fact that people had always been credulous and always would be; thus quackery had not only "existed from the earliest periods," but it would "continue to exist as long as human beings are found upon the earth."[7]

Others, like Yale medical professor Worthington Hooker, were more sanguine. He agreed that quackery existed in "endless" forms and "in all ages and in all countries[,] . . . among the savage or the civilized, the rude or the refined, the illiterate or the learned." But Hooker had tremendous faith in the power of knowledge, and he devoted much of his life to popular medical education. Two of his lifelong objectives were interrelated, and both were evident in his 1849 *Physician and Patient*. The first was to teach people about the "fantastic and ever-changing" ways in which quackery manifested itself. The second goal was to spell out what capabilities physicians had and upon what resources they could draw. Unfortunately, wrote Hooker, part of this educational effort had to be spent on "expos[ing] many of the tricks and manoeuvres" used by a certain class of physicians, "who, pursuing medicine as a *trade* instead of a profession, study the science of patient-getting to the neglect of the science of patient-curing." This could be in large part remedied if "the rules of an honorable professional intercourse" were to "come to be properly understood and appreciated by the public." Hooker hoped that spreading knowledge about the differences between illegitimate and legitimate practice would create informed judgment and more realistic expectations among his readers.[8]

Most orthodox physicians were, like Hooker, cautiously hopeful. If people could be shown the error of their ways, they would improve. Since "an intelligent community" would not support illegitimate practice, then the key to destroying quackery must be popular medical education.[9] Georgia doctors had incorporated such beliefs in their 1828 code of ethics, because they felt that popular ignorance about medical matters presented "strong inducements to empirics and illegitimate pretenders, to impose on their credulity." As a result many citizens "employ[ed] the illiterate braggadocio in preference to the regular physician." The only way to improve the situation, they argued, was to make "some acquaintance with the outline of the medical sciences . . . part of an academic education[.]"[10]

Roughly a decade later, the New Haven County Medical Society found itself in partial accord with its southern colleagues. The New Haven report, printed in an 1837 issue of the *Boston Medical and Surgical Journal*, tied the success of quackery directly to "the general want of information regarding the nature of disease, the operation of remedies, and the powers of the human system." They thought the situation was exacerbated by the persisting belief that medicine was an occult science, that medical skill was an inherent talent rather than an acquired expertise. Though they acknowledged educational inadequacies, their solution rested on legislation: "*it is the right and duty of government to protect the people in every possible way against any trade, or craft, or profession, in which the public has peculiar interest, and the temptations to defraud and deceive are great.*"[11]

But they were increasingly in the minority on this point, deserted by colleagues who recognized the futility of trying to suppress or destroy quackery by legal means alone. One was Lunsford P. Yandell, professor of chemistry and pharmacy in the Louisville Medical Institute. In addressing the twelfth annual meeting of the Medical Society of Tennessee in 1841, Yandell maintained that the social context had to be the major factor in deciding what actions to take against quackery. In mid-nineteenth-century America, he argued, this meant that the law could not be relied upon to check or uproot quackery. Even if restrictive laws were passed, Yandell pointed out that they "would be enforced only when they were in accordance with public sentiment. Opposed to it, or in advance of it, they would be a dead letter." Instead of relying on the law, Yandell advocated improving medical practice. Quackery would flourish, explained the professor, "so long as our systems of cure remain discordant and our remedies uncertain, so long as there continue to be maladies that defy the resources of enlightened art." To him the path was clear, but Yandell conceded that many people thought that the task he proposed "[was] above all human power—that there must remain, to the end of time, imperfections in the healing art—diseases which no remedies can reach." Yandell was more optimistic, confident that the medical profession would improve medical practice, thereby guaranteeing the eventual demise of quackery.[12]

The members of New York's Medical Society of Albany County also wrestled with this subject, and their unanimously adopted report of 1844 brought historical perspective to bear on the rationale for using legislation as a tool.[13] In the past, they recognized, lawmakers had always believed that restrictive laws were appropriate and necessary to guarantee medical competency and to protect the public from "the ignorant and unprincipled." To meet this legislative end, legislators and county medical societies had worked together to set standards, organize qualified practitioners, and exercise general supervisory authority over the practice of medicine. The purpose of these actions had been to protect the public from quacks and to promote prudent individual behavior. Yet many people still consulted unqualified practitioners; they were guilty of "gross imprudence," protected by law "against imposition, but not against a foolish choice."

Dismayed by "this sad spectacle of human credulity and folly," legislators had tried to bar all but regulars from practice by enacting prohibitory laws. Prohibitory laws assumed "that it would be . . . absurd to have recourse for medical aid to an ignorant person, when it is possible to procure the services of an educated physician." Those who would "abandon a medical attendant of tried skill and character, for any juggling mountebank . . . must be treated as incompetent to manage their own concerns." Unlike restrictive laws, which were intended to encourage individuals to act sensibly, prohibitory laws aimed to *compel* them to do so. But enactment did not guarantee compliance, and enforcement was virtually impossible. Moreover, restrictive laws often helped irregular practitioners, who were quick to accuse the regulars of "persecution" and "greedy [monopoly]."

The fundamental dilemma lay in adjudicating between professional responsibility and individual liberty. The Albany County doctors recognized the tyranny inherent in restraining choice. No matter how "absurd the opinions and conduct" of people who consulted quacks appeared to be to orthodox physicians, that did not give the regulars sufficient reason or authority "to impose on them our ideas of wisdom." The most legislation could hope to achieve "[was] to give to all the means of knowing the character of those to whom they may apply, and thus enable them to act with a full knowledge of the circumstances, and leave the rest to each man's own wisdom and prudence." Restrictive legislation thus seemed inadvisable, and they advocated instead "enlightening the public as to [quackery's] dangers." The burden would then be on the regulars as they tried to promote "the dignity and respectability of our profession . . . by an increase of individual zeal and a more cordial co-operation." In other words, orthodox practitioners should improve themselves rather than try directly to annihilate quacks; demonstration of obvious superiority would win popular support.[14]

How, then, were people to recognize a good doctor? Nicholas Romayne, an influential practitioner and a president of the New York state medical society, had thought it would be largely self-evident. As he said in 1810, "When Practitioners of Medicine are diligent and judicious in the exercise of their profession, they manifest to men of any discernment, their superior skill and success in the cure of diseases; and will show in a striking point of view, the difference between the well educated Physician and Surgeon, and the mere pretender to professional knowledge."[15]

But as orthodox physicians answered this question in the middle decades of the century, they unwittingly revealed that the differences between legitimate and illegitimate healers were far from clear. A *London Lancet* excerpt that appeared in the 1841 *Boston Medical and Surgical Journal* stressed the importance of punctuality, "a ternary composed of conscientiousness, benevolence and firmness." Everyone, said the article, "can judge of punctuality, but all cannot judge of medical knowledge; their judgment will, therefore, be decided by that which they can appreciate."[16] Punctuality perhaps strikes the twentieth-century reader as a curious criterion by which to identify a good doctor, but it would not have seemed unusual to a mid-nineteenth-century citizen. Nor would urbanity, which Stephen J. W. Tabor emphasized in an 1844 letter to the same journal. "The physician," wrote Tabor, "should not only be acquainted with the diversified and protean forms of disease, and with all that relates to his own peculiar art, but he should also be versed in what appertains to courtesy and to good manners."[17] Credentials based on character and conduct were equally or more important in this period than formal medical training.[18]

Silas Holmes advised Americans to use analogical reasoning to evaluate practitioners, for "a medical man well informed on other subjects, and capable of reasoning correctly on [them]" was apt also to be "well informed on medicine." Recognizing the imperfections of medical practitioners, Holmes had two suggestions for "elevating" the medical profession and broadening public support: to make certain that doctors *and* the public were better educated. The aim of public education would not be to make every person his or her own doctor, but would be to familiarize people with the structure of their bodies, various diseases to which they were subject, and treatments for those diseases. Holmes thought that this information should be disseminated by orthodox physicians themselves, using the press and courses in anatomy and physiology.[19]

Charles B. Coventry, professor of obstetrics and medical jurisprudence at Geneva Medical College, made similar suggestions. As he said in his 1842 valedictory address, it was obvious to doctors that "no man is born a physician, but to acquire this knowledge is the labour of years of unremitting toil." But the public did not understand this, and it was essential to educate Americans, both about practitioners and about their bodies. Once people had been taught how their bodies worked, perhaps they would hesitate to trust "persons entirely ignorant of its several parts, when a single error may cost them their lives." There would be other benefits of "the general diffusion of this knowledge." Not only would it "guard against quackery and empiricism out of the profession," but "it would qualify the community to judge as to the actual and comparative merits of members of the profession." Thus he urged graduates to seize "every opportunity of giving popular lectures on anatomy, physiology and hygiene."[20]

Alabama physician John S. Wilson argued from the same perspective.[21] Improving medical education was crucial, maintained the doctor, as was educating citizens *through the popular channels of intelligence.* Wilson worried that orthodox physicians were not tackling their educational campaign in the right way. Though all the medical journals contained articles on the evils of quackery, he questioned how great an impact these pieces had on popular practices. Wrote Wilson, "These disclosures never reach the *people,* and so far as their influence on them is concerned, they had as well be published in Hebrew, as in a medical journal." He suggested using newspapers and "that happy device of Quackery—'a *Medical Almanac.*'"

Reevaluating Domestic Health Guides

Wilson took his own advice, selecting women as his primary target audience.[22] But Wilson was mistaken about the paucity of popular health materials; indeed, during this period there was an unprecedented proliferation. Medical sectarians generated health tracts and sponsored lectures and periodicals. Orthodox physicians did the same, seeking to defend themselves, to eradicate quackery, and to influence domestic practices. Reform-minded lay people also contributed advice in the form of newspaper and magazine articles, lectures, and books.

Household health guides, anchored still by William Buchan's *Domestic Medicine,* continued to be a popular vehicle for disseminating medical information. Yet orthodox physicians were becoming increasingly doubtful of the domestic handbook's utility, as their receptivity to different versions of Buchan's manual demonstrated. The thrust and character of Buchan's original text survived to an amazing degree, despite the periodic revisions made after the author's 1805 death, by his son, A. P. Buchan, member of the Royal College of Physicians of London. What changed was orthodox reaction, as was mirrored in a newly defensive posture evident in *Domestic Medicine* from the mid-1820s.[23]

Buchan found himself under attack from "a certain low class of self-appointed practitioners, who call themselves of *the faculty*"; these people had charged that his work "serve[d] only to encourage the fatal practice of domestic quackery." This was a complete misrepresentation, complained Buchan, since "the obvious tendency" of his work was to educate people about their health "and thus to guard them against the bad effects of ignorance and rashness on their own part, and of impudence and deceit on the part of others." Moreover, he had aimed to reduce popular reliance on medicine, a goal championed by other orthodox practitioners. As for actual cases of illness, his book posed no threat to the medical establishment, for he had advised "that those who are ignorant of physic . . . confine themselves to regimen alone, and leave the medical treatment of their complaints to persons of better information."[24]

As Buchan intimated, the social climate had changed and regular doctors no longer saw domestic health guides as fitting tools for popular education. Though "family physicians" continued to appear, orthodox support for them began to wane. Criticism was isolated and sporadic in the 1820s, but an important early foe was the *New-England Journal of Medicine,* precursor of the *Boston Medical and Surgical Journal.* One of its reviewers, discussing elite physician Usher Parsons's 1820 *Sailors' Physician,* spelled out criteria of acceptability that were to become increasingly prevalent.[25] The reviewer commended Parsons's work, for it "[stood] on totally different ground" from most popular health guides, which "[were] in spirit and in effect pieces of quackery, calculated to diffuse among those who are in the habit of consulting them, a mass of ill-defined, half-comprehended, narrow ideas and prejudices, excessively embarrassing to the regular practitioner in his intercourse with them." Readers, the critic hastened to add, should not construe these comments as signs of opposition "to the universal diffusion of medical knowledge," because "nothing could be more conducive to the best interests of the profession." However, it was important that "it . . . be the right kind of knowledge—a knowledge of the general and fundamental principles of the science and not of its technological details with respect to particular diseases." Previously published health manuals did not meet this standard. "Few things have contributed so much to the making of habitual invalids," summarized the critic, "as Buchan's Domestic Medicine and other works of the same notorious character."

Parsons's guide, on the other hand, provided the right kind of information for public consumption, because it aimed to help only those people who otherwise would not be able to obtain professional advice. Aware that this meant that the physician's role would inevitably be usurped by a lay person using an advice book, the reviewer did not find this troubling. Parsons's guide would be used, the critic thought, only in situations where the choice was between the *Sailors' Physician* and no orthodox advice at all. For this reason the reviewer warned that it would be dangerous to wait until "a case of disease occurred to turn to the book, and ransack its contents till something was found corresponding to the symptoms . . . observed." Instead, mariners should familiarize themselves with the volume, so that they would be prepared to act quickly and sensibly in the rush of emergencies. The writer was confident that any "judicious and intelligent master of a vessel, who should carefully and attentively study a book of this kind, would, no doubt, especially in the milder cases of disease, be able to render essential service to his crew." Parsons's work, concluded the reviewer, was excellent, for it was "brief and perspicuous," well suited for its intended readership because it "does not run out into those details, nor include those varieties which could only be embarrassing to individuals who are deficient in a medical education."

Though it is difficult to understand why Parsons's guide met the standards of medical propriety when similar volumes did not, subsequent reviews in the same journal help clarify the professional attitude to household health guides. Among them was a brief treatment of Robert Thomas's 1822 *The Way to Preserve Good Health,* drawn from the *London Medical Repository.* Despite his professional stature, Thomas met with contempt, accused with having oversimplified his subject.[26] The following year Thomas's *A Treatise on Domestic Medicine,* as revised in 1822 by prominent New York physician David Hosack, elicited a scathing review, this time coupled with a denunciation of the genre.[27] The reviewer charged Thomas with misjudgment in having made minute symptomatic differentiations in a work for the nonprofessional reader. As he queried, "Do not physicians themselves find that it is impossible to draw those accurate lines of distinction in real life, which are laid down so clearly in systematic works?" Though he agreed that it was a good idea to educate people about medical topics, the reviewer argued that "treatises on Domestic Medicine are not the engines by which this is to be effected." Why? The answer was obvious to this writer: "They disseminate the wrong kind of information." Domestic manuals, wrote the critic, did provide "a few petty details" about disease symptoms and treatment, but this information was worthless: they "teach none of the great principles on which the phenomena of both health and disease proceed, without which these details are not better than the jargon of an unknown tongue."

These books created far-reaching problems for regular practitioners because they "communicat[ed] a quantity of crude half digested ideas upon medical subjects, to many individuals, who immediately fancy themselves qualified to judge and criticise the opinions and conduct of their medical advisers." Assertive patients were often trying, complained the reviewer, largely because "they conceive themselves as authorized to require a reason and an explanation for whatever is going forward." This left the practitioner in an untenable position: "What is more embarrassing than to be expected to make a case clear to one who is not capable, from want of knowledge, of comprehending it? What more vexatious than to be required to do this, when you are in doubt yourself—where every medical man would be so too; and yet where the expression of that doubt would be to forfeit at once the confidence and good will of your patient or his friends?"

Many patients were not only assertive, the reviewer continued, but were also arrogant enough to diagnose and prescribe for themselves and others. The meddling spirit inculcated by reading household health guides was extremely dangerous in the absence of a medical education. Because of "the interferences of this race of knowing ones," doctors often were not summoned until disease had "advanced too far to be checked by remedies." Though this was only one of the countless negative results of lay presumptuousness in medicine, the reviewer thought that its importance should not be underestimated. "There is no such thing," he stated flatly, "as getting over the evil consequences produced by a delay in the application of the proper treatment."

More than two decades later, orthodox practitioners were waging the same battle. Physician Walter Channing blamed "the popular literature of the profession" for diminishing "the ancient reverence in which medicine was held."[28] The Harvard professor of obstetrics and medical jurisprudence objected to "works on the diseases of children, of females, of mothers, on the management of consumption, syphilis, etc. They are written by physicians, have glossaries for explaining medical terms, descriptions or definitions of diseases, with recipes in English to suit." Such works "are designed to show what should be done in slight diseases, or in the beginnings of the graver." Though marketed for the profession as well as for the public, this was a charade. For the nonprofessional, said Channing, "they must be worse than useless, seeing that the public in this regard, and for such purpose, is not educated at all." Their designated audiences, in fact, were "mothers, and nursery maids, since the man of the house has nothing to do with this domestic literature."

The core of Channing's opposition lay in the fact that "these popular works suppose that the persons referred to understand the distinction between diseases, the *diagnosis;* and the disease given, they have only to turn to the treatment." This was "absurd and injurious," even with the caveat to send for the physician if the case grew worse. How, asked Channing, could anyone believe that nonprofessionals could be appropriately discriminating? Moreover, awareness of the situation did not necessarily ensure timely or proper action; too often people did not "send for the physician till his office is useless, or . . . the case . . . so complicated by what has been done, that it is by no means easy to say what may be safely done next." Even when summoned, the doctor faced an aggravating situation: "What can be more annoying than to be met at the chamber door of a patient by a friend, a female friend, with book in hand, welcoming us by reading the history of the disease, and then telling us of remedies and results, adding that calomel and bleeding were now necessary, but she really was unwilling to meddle with mineral poisons, or with edged tools." In Channing's opinion, orthodox physicians should simply refuse to consult with such domestic practitioners.

Channing thought it would be impossible to "exaggerate the trouble or the harm produced" by domestic health manuals. "The effort has of late been to make medicine popular," Channing grumbled, "to unfold its mysteries, and unconsciously to make every man, woman, and child, too, his, her, or its own doctor." Rather than spreading useful knowledge, the books added "injurious activity to ignorance." Channing went so far as to say that the books by orthodox physicians caused more damage in this purportedly educational effort than the ones written by quacks.

For evidence, maintained the doctor, "look at the popular education. The schools are filled with books on anatomy, physiology, hygiene, physical education, chemistry, botany, and what not." In addition, there were "popular lecturers, men and women, who give regular courses on anatomy, and physiology, and means of preserving health." This had not been the case fifty years earlier. Then there had been Willich and Buchan, Channing remembered, "but they were not then parlor books." Medical colleges had offered anatomical lectures, "but we did not make anatomy a tea-table topic." Half a century before, wearing "a false tooth was made a question of morality, since it was considered a mode of obtaining goods under false pretences. And dyspepsia was eschewed from the common talk, as it involved particulars which might not be discussed to ears polite." The contrast with contemporary behavior was nearly mind-boggling. "Now teeth are talked about, as is the weather. Dentists have their friends, almost their parties. Men have bowels, loose, or costive, and women have *spines of the back*." Angrily he asked, "Is it to be wondered at that medicine should have lost something of its earlier veneration, now that it is taught in the nursery, and lies so naked upon the very surface of society?"

Many doctors shared some of Channing's reservations about domestic manuals, but few exhibited his ire. Indeed, a large number continued to applaud general guides for nonprofessional use. When Reynell Coates's *Popular Medicine* appeared in 1838, a reviewer feared its title destined to draw suspicion from a medical profession "who have had just occasion to be disgusted with treatises on domestic medicine, medical advisers, etc." Billed as a "family adviser," *Popular Medicine* boasted "outlines of anatomy, physiology, and hygiene, with such hints on the practice of physic, surgery, and the diseases of women and children, as may prove useful in families when regular physicians cannot be procured." More particularly, Coates designed his book as "a companion and guide for intelligent principals of manufactories, plantations, and boarding-schools, heads of families, masters of vessels, missionaries, or travellers." Regardless of its wide scope, said the reviewer, the volume contained "a large fund of anatomical, physiological and practical truth." Orthodox physicians should also praise the Coates book for helping spread correct medical knowledge and combat "the strong holds of quackery and empiricism, in their thousand Protean forms."[29]

Coates, one of the founders of the Medical College of Philadelphia, spent much of his life writing and speaking on health and medical issues. Among his books was one of the earliest popular physiology textbooks; perhaps this is the reason that he devoted the first third of *Popular Medicine* to an overview of anatomy, physiology, and hygiene. Only then did he discuss disease treatment, starting with first-aid for accidents and other emergencies. Coates frequently distinguished between the action appropriate for a domestic as opposed to a professional practitioner. Unlike some authors of family health guides, he wrote, he did not want his readers to believe that "by a few hours' study, and an occasional reference to a book, they could supersede the necessity of advice from those whose lives and observations are devoted exclusively to the study of disease." Thus, after giving explicit directions for manual treatment of prolapsed anus, Coates halted, having reached the end of the details he thought could be safely given to a well-informed domestic practitioner. Likewise, relief or cure of more severe cases might call for surgery, "but these require high skill, and the very description of them would be unintelligible to most of our readers." Curvature of the spine, on the other hand, needed to have a superior surgeon from the outset, and "madness only could induce the tampering of unprofessional hands with cases of such a character." His instructions about fractures were "merely temporary, . . . designed to procure the patient as much freedom from pain, and security from deformity, as can be obtained by simple contrivances every where at hand, and applied by persons without surgical knowledge." Eye diseases, especially chronic ones, typically "[would] endure to wait until the best advice can be obtained." At the same time, he apologized for discussing palsy. "It is a difficult business, requiring no particular promptitude," he admitted, "and professional advice on the subject may always be obtained in time for all useful purposes."

Some disorders were not amenable to hard-and-fast rules. With inflammation, for instance, Coates wrote, "It becomes more important that even the domestic practitioner should take a broad view of the subject. . . . His general knowledge and practical good sense must often be permitted to modify even his application of these directions." Thus after providing "ample remarks on Inflammation, in general," Coates then "trust[ed] mainly to the intelligence of the reader, in applying the principles and directions to particular cases."[30] Despite his concern about limiting domestic involvement in treating diseases, Coates recognized that there were many situations in which the only practical course was to give each citizen the latitude to act according to his or her own judgment.

Coates's book obviously displayed many of the elements common to its predecessors within the genre of household health guides. It was equally compatible, however, with the growing view that the nonprofessional should limit his role in disease treatment to nursing and emergency care. Many popular writers and lecturers were hammering home the same points. They not only agreed that lay people should relinquish responsibility for disease treatment, but they also advocated that nonprofessionals shoulder the burden for health maintenance. Regular doctors welcomed the publicists' assumption of this role, but monitored them carefully to ensure that they did not overstep their bounds. Yet the line between respectability and fanaticism or quackery was not always clear-cut, as the fortunes of Sylvester Graham and William Andrus Alcott illustrate. It is useful to reconstruct orthodox reactions to these two well-known health reformers, for the reasons for their shifting fortunes illuminate the perceived distinctions between professionals and nonprofessionals.

Clarifying Professional Standards: The Case of Sylvester Graham

Sylvester Graham's crusade has traditionally been introduced as one of history's colorful sideshow attractions. Until recently, historians largely ignored Graham's moments at center stage, except to offer amused tributes to the fanatic whose name now adorns the graham cracker.[31] The first serious effort to reassess Graham came in the 1930s when Richard Shryock assigned him a leading role in nineteenth-century popular health reform.[32] In the past ten years Stephen Nissenbaum and James Whorton have vindicated Shryock's evaluation, and Graham's image as a crackpot vegetarian has been largely supplanted by his status as a pioneer in a continuing health reform movement.[33]

Born in Connecticut in 1792, Graham was the last of seventeen children and the son and grandson of ministers. He was two when his father died, and his mother's inability to care for the children sentenced young Sylvester to a nomadic childhood with different families. By his late teens he suffered periodic bouts of physical illness, emotional exhaustion, and depression. The early 1820s brought increasing involvement in temperance work, which Graham soon combined with ministerial training. In 1826 the young man received his license to preach, soon thereafter becoming an ordained evangelist and a traveling agent for the Pennsylvania Temperance Society. A captivating speaker, Graham, reported a newspaper in 1830, had "astonished and delighted the numerous and crowded audiences which have heard his lectures. Judges, Lawyers, Physicians, and Clergymen as well as the more unlearned, all degrees of society have listened to him, with equal interest and satisfaction."[34]

Unlike other temperance zealots, Graham did not focus on the addictive properties of alcohol or even on "intemperance" generally. He was most interested in the impact of alcohol on normal physiological processes. Alcohol, he said, was an irritant that overstimulated the body, leading to moral as well as physiological injury. Though Graham insisted that he drew these ideas entirely from his own physiological observations, a more accurate lineage would trace them to French physiological theory—particularly Xavier Bichat's vitalism and François Broussais's theory of pathology—together with Benjamin Rush's linkage of "artificial" stimulation with debility. Graham retained this framework as he expanded his horizons beyond the physiology of drinking. By 1831 he billed himself as a lecturer on a far more inclusive subject, "The Science of Human Life," and soon he had added to his repertoire the cholera epidemic, sexual chastity, vegetable diet, and the virtues of bran bread. For the rest of the decade he spoke on these subjects throughout the Atlantic states, New England, and upstate New York. Graham's lectures on cholera, sexuality, and bread-making appeared in print between 1832 and 1837, each going through a number of editions. In 1839 he published his major work, *Lectures on the Science of Human Life,* in two volumes totaling more than twelve hundred pages.[35]

By this time, however, Graham had become a controversial figure, so much so that in the mid-1830s he was attacked by mobs on at least three occasions. Nissenbaum has attributed this to the growing celebrity of his ideas and to his contentious and abrasive personality. Nissenbaum speculates in passing that another factor may have been his dismissal as a charlatan by several respectable medical publications, most notably the *Boston Medical and Surgical Journal.* This point deserves further attention, for it is seldom remembered that the medical establishment welcomed Sylvester Graham when he first appeared on the health reform scene in the early 1830s. Indeed, he seemed the embodiment of hopes expressed by an 1831 reviewer of a couple of Harpers' health publications, who had queried: "Why, among the thousand forms in which the community are solicited to preserve that greatest of all earthly blessings, health, do we not find *popular lectures* given on dietetics, and the means of avoiding disease[?]"[36]

The initial reaction to Graham in the pages of the *Boston Medical and Surgical Journal* augured well. In 1835 one of its correspondents registered amazement at the ridicule that learned doctors had heaped on the young man. Having heard the health reformer lecture on "The Science of Life," the listener could detect no heresy in Graham's teachings. Graham, he said, had "presented nothing extravagant—nothing that was not positively correct in relation to life, health and disease." In fact, continued the correspondent, rather than "being the originator of a new system, totally opposed to those facts in the science of life, already extensively promulgated and practised upon by all well educated physicians, he simply exhibited himself to be a fearless, independent, benevolent expounder of this difficult science, which he seems to be endeavoring to make plain to the comprehension of all classes of intelligent, reflecting people." The vilification to which Graham had been subjected seemed unwarranted, for his propositions were "based upon known physiological laws." Moreover, continued the writer, "his language and his illustrations were in strict accordance . . . with the best medical authors." Were Graham to follow the course set out in his introductory lecture, "the medical profession, above all others, will be benefited and dignified by it, and the world at large must ultimately be bettered by the influence of the knowledge he is disseminating." Despite its favorable tone, the notice ended by reserving judgment on whether Graham was destined to "sink himself in the mazes of designing quackery" or whether he could continue to rely on this prestigious volume for support.[37] Subscribers could judge for themselves, since the volume also contained extracts from Graham's lectures on "the science of human life" and "the vitality of the blood."[38]

The sentiments Graham expressed in the excerpts from *The Science of Human Life* would have been congenial to most orthodox readers.[39] People, he complained, "do not believe that there are any fixed laws of life, by the proper observance of which, man can, with any certainty, avoid disease and preserve health, and prolong his bodily existence." This was entirely wrong, but the view had persisted among Americans because "most or all of their opinions are the results of *feeling,* or what they miscall experience, rather than of deep reasoning and philosophical investigation." These beliefs were extremely difficult to eradicate, since "every person knows from his own *feelings* and *experience,* precisely what kind of constitution he has—and what agrees and what disagrees with it." Graham's aim, like Benjamin Rush's half a century earlier, was not "to convince [people] that they have no *feelings,* nor that they do not know when, and how much they feel[,]" but was instead "to convince them that the kind and degree of their feeling by no means teach them what causes it, nor the principles upon which its existence depends."

Graham illustrated his point with an example drawn from everyday life: the lady who cured her headaches with tea, "'the sovereignest remedy in the world' for headache." Because it was a sensible assumption that the lady best knew her own feelings, it seemed a "gross . . . insult to her understanding . . . to attempt to convince her that tea is a poison, and that her use of it is a principal cause of her headache." Indeed, Graham conceded that "she knows best how her own headache *feels,* and that she knows it is relieved by a cup of tea." But this constituted only a superficial understanding of the situation, as he stressed with a barrage of questions:

But does she know either the remote or immediate cause of her headache? Does she know the vital properties and powers and functional relations of the organs of her body; and does she accurately understand the healthy and the diseased affections and sympathies of those organs? Does she know the qualities of the tea in relation to the vital properties and functional powers of her system? Does she know the direct and the ultimate effects of the tea on her system?—how it produces the pleasurable feelings, and how it removes the pain of her head? And does she know whether the very effects of the tea, by which the paroxysms of her headache are relieved, are not the principal source of her headache, and the main cause of the frequency and violence of the paroxysms?

Graham's final thrust left no doubt about his position: "If not, what are her feelings and experiences worth, to herself or others, as rules of life, by which she or any one can judge of the fitness of her habits to the laws of life and health?" He had his answer ready: "not a farthing!" Even that was a swollen valuation, for "they are worse than nothing—mere delusions by which we are decoyed from step to step along the specious labyrinths of sensuality and suffering." People could not use feelings as a reliable indicator of anything unless they understood "physiologically *how* or *why* they feel" and "the relation of their feelings to the powers and laws of vitality, and to the condition and functions of the living organs[.]"

These were not provocative statements. In fact, they reinforced orthodox teaching about the inadequacy of individual experience alone as a healing credential. Nonetheless, almost immediately after his debut in the *Boston Medical and Surgical Journal,* Graham found himself embroiled in controversy. The health reformer had only himself to blame for initiating the acerbic bickering, and it resulted in his eventual expulsion from the periodical's pages. The sniping started when Graham criticized New Hampshire physician Luther V. Bell, winner of the 1835 Boylston Medical Committee's prize for his essay advocating a mixed diet for New England laborers.[40] Bell's piece opened with what Graham interpreted as a salvo intended for him: the statement that the essay aimed to counter the "schemes of Pythagorean or Utopian dreamers." Even though Bell did not specify whom he meant, the phrase clearly did allude to contemporary vegetarians. Human anatomy, Bell wrote in reversal of the vegetarian's usual argument, did not dictate people's eating habits; because human beings possessed the God-given faculty of reason, their natural diet consisted of any food that their reason could adapt to their bodies.[41]

This was anathema to vegetarians like Graham, who reminded people that reason could be abused. Graham extended this logic to conclude that every human was "*naturally* a fruit and vegetable eating animal." As he argued with Bell, Graham took pains to express respect for the medical profession, but he also pointed out some orthodox shortcomings. In doing so he used language that seemed arrogant and ill-mannered, and in turn raised questions about the sincerity of his praise. Graham's central criticism was that learned doctors, like other humans, tended "to cling to established institutions, and to reverence hereditary usages[.]" This meant that doctors too often upheld and defended traditional beliefs without questioning their truth. If Bell, for instance, "before writing his prize dissertation, instead of ransacking Cyclopoedias and other volumes of printed matter, had done as I have done . . . and carefully observed, and diligently inquired, and honestly sought after the truth rather than to support any theory or hypothesis, he would certainly have been led to a different conclusion." Here the health reformer begins to delineate a different and less innocuous medical position. By setting up individual experience as the superior path to truth, he is now contesting not only the primacy but the utility of formal education. Graham's attack, replete with unsubstantiated criticisms, sparked a wave of controversy; before it ended, journal contributors were debating whether Grahamism caused insanity.[42]

Bell himself responded first. He began by disclaiming prior knowledge of Graham except as an itinerant lecturer of sorts, adding patronizingly that only Graham's "inordinate conceit" could have led him to believe that he was the subject of the essay. Sarcasm dripping from every word, Bell thanked "this *modest, lucid,* and *scientific* reviewer, for not scalping me nor tomahawking me, as he says he might so easily have done, as well as . . . for his magnanimity in not bearing away the prize."[43] A correspondent identified simply as "Beta" sided with Bell and characterized

Graham's attack as "mere swaggering," repeated but unproven declarations of prowess. To Beta, Graham's boasting of "matchless assurance" of the "'length and breadth'" of the field under question was actually only *"prodigious effrontery."* Graham had benefited the community by promulgating some sound physiological principles, but his dietary ideas now seemed visionary or harmful. Moreover, Graham had been rude, guilty of comportment not befitting a medical man. "But whatever Mr. G.'s merits may be as a lecturer, or *will be* as an author," he concluded, "I am persuaded he is entirely out of his element in a medical Journal."[44]

Subsequent articles underscored the importance of meeting the standard of professional decorum. Correspondent "A" feebly parried Beta's charges point by point, first conceding displeasure "with the *manner* in which Mr. Graham defended himself." What others had taken for Graham's "brass," correspondent A explained, was in fact compensatory behavior for his shyness. Here, in fact, was the source of Graham's uniqueness: he was "at one and the same time, an original thinker, and a simple, plain, matter-of-fact man."[45]

Even Graham tried to clear himself of the charge that he had been "offensive or disrespectful." Ostensibly aware that "personal abuse and vituperation" were not considered appropriate weapons, Graham was so busy accusing Bell of poor conduct that he was evidently blind to his own transgressions on that score. Nor did he think he was overreacting by concluding that Bell's remarks about vegetable diet were aimed at him. The only two other possibilities, he felt, were physician R. D. Mussey, professor of anatomy and surgery at Dartmouth College, and minister Edward H. Hitchcock, professor of chemistry and natural history at Amherst. Not only did Graham think they were less well known, but he was confident that "a young gentleman of good education, and of Dr. Bell's just claims to good breeding" would never have "designedly used such indecorous and even insolent language towards one of his own profession." Graham also found it hard to believe that he was "so humble and obscure" that Bell had never heard of him. On the contrary, Graham knew that "[his] name [had] been sounded all over the United States, and almost universally with odium and ridicule, as the name of *the* individual who advocates abstinence from flesh-eating, and a diet of vegetables, bran-bread, etc." Thus "no man can travel by stage or steamboat, or go into any part of our country . . . and begin to advocate a vegetable diet, or even sit down at a table and abstain from flesh, tea, coffee, etc. without being immediately asked—and in no flattering manner—'What! are you a Grahamite?'"[46]

The health reformer felt victimized by misrepresentation. It was unjust to portray "'the Graham system'" as "simply a diet of *bran bread and water*." As Graham reminded *Journal* readers, he shared the mission of the "regular and scientific physician": "enlightening the people in the knowledge of their own nature, and destroying their confidence in the wholesale mode of patent drugging . . . ; and by endeavoring to draw a broad line of demarcation between the true physician and the quack—to sustain the former, and . . . to annihilate all quackery." He thus implored the regulars to "treat me as a man, honest in my errors, . . . and honestly and candidly point out those errors to me." The prevailing mode of "personal obloquy and ridicule and reviling and slander" would not promote truth, honor orthodox practitioners, or injure Sylvester Graham.[47]

Graham's defenders in this forum disappeared as fast as his detractors multiplied. A correspondent identified simply as "W.★ W.★" agreed with Beta that the tenor of Graham's remarks resembled the newspaper puffs of quacks promoting their infallible remedies.[48] Not resting content with this charge, W.★ W.★ set out to prove that Graham himself was a quack. One certain sign for this writer was that Graham had succumbed to the requirements of popularity. Having thus relinquished any meaningful standard of conduct, it would be foolish to expect professional behavior from him. "*Living*, as he does," wrote W.★ W.★, "by popular declamation, and seeking *first* applause and money, he must needs sacrifice everything to *effect*—he must leave nothing in doubt—all must be absolute, universal, infallible—and the darker any point is, the more he must asseverate, dogmatize and denounce."

The vehicle Graham had chosen, contended W.★ W.★, was "'blurting' warfare against the favorite stimulants of mankind." Yet W.★ W.★ could see no sound scientific proof except "that tea and coffee and flesh are not *his* favorite stimulants." W.★ W.★ went even further. "[Graham's] pretended science of life," he charged, "is chiefly the science of [his] own idiosyncracies." Different individuals, W.★ W.★ reasoned, had varying capacities for accommodating any given stimulant. "To maintain that the favorite stimuli of unnumbered millions are, *per se,* poisonous, and repugnant to the vital sensibilities, is flat nonsense." Moderation in food and drink was the key, and, since each individual was different, it was up to each person to decide what constituted moderation. The conclusion was obvious. Graham was "a rank empiric" whose remedies were nothing but "nostrums, grand—absolute—universal." But even W.★ W.★ had to concede that "to do him justice, he is more useful, less dangerous, earns his 'gains' more honestly, than most of those pretenders," and that his remedies were likely to benefit many invalids.

"R" was the next to enter the fray, supporting Graham; again the central questions concerned standards of conduct and character. Critical of W.★ W.★'s "low, scurrilous and dishonest manner, of personal abuse and slander and falsehood," this correspondent was appalled at W.★ W.★'s "cowardly impudence" in anonymously attacking a person whom he had never even heard lecture. "The prevailing and almost the only complaint against Mr. Graham's lectures in Boston," he maintained, "has been that they are too severely scientific and abstruse." Even an eminent writer, Dr. John C. Warren, "[had] declared Mr. G.'s lectures too scientific for a popular audience." Contrast this, he sputtered, with "your impudent correspondent, in utter ignorance, but with a pretension to knowledge (which in a moral point of view amounts to downright and wilful falsehood)," who "asserts that Mr. G. produces his effect on his ignorant audience by mere declamation and assurance." R found W.★ W.★ guilty "of shameless calumny and barefaced falsehood." In a community where "sacredness of personal character is the very palladium of social peace and prosperity," it seemed impossible to think highly "of that individual who thus presumes to assassinate, in public, the character of one of whom he is entirely ignorant!"[49]

But the weight of medical opinion bore inexorably down. M. L. North did adopt a neutral stance, pleading for statements from people who had followed Graham's dietary advice. Disinterested observers could then test reliable case histories, complete with names, places, and dates, for authenticity; on this basis theoretical positions could be verified or found wanting.[50] Graham also tried to silence his critics by qualifying some of the sweeping statements attributed to him. "To suppose that any regimen or mode of treatment can save every individual, whatever may be the kind or stage of the disease, is egregiously unreasonable," granted Graham in one effort.[51]

No one listened. Undaunted, W.★ W.★ resumed his crusade. "Grahamism . . . may be defined," he said, as "the empirical recommendation and use of a vegetable and water diet." Lest there be a mistake, he further specified that "an empirical recommendation is one that is *indiscriminate, incautious,* and *extravagant,*" and would undoubtedly "do much mischief." Orthodox physicians, of course, recommended vegetable diet in some cases, but they did not, like Graham, "prescribe one eternal *Lent* for the human race." In short, concluded W.★ W.★, using a common shorthand reference to quackery, vegetable diet "is the *ism* of Mr. Graham."[52]

By this time, though, there were skirmishes on another front: whether or not Grahamism caused insanity. An anonymous correspondent, later identified by Graham as Dr. Lee of the Insane Hospital at Charlestown, opened this Pandora's box by suggesting that some mental illnesses might be traced to the adoption of vegetarianism.[53] Graham responded to Lee's charges at great length, but the *Journal*'s editors finally closed their pages to the still-raging controversy between Graham and his opponents. Graham was allowed the last word, one final attempt to win favor: "I have nothing to do with medicine—deal in no secret remedies—but in all cases where medical treatment is necessary in those who come to me, I send them to the physician. I am a public lecturer on the Science of Human Life."[54]

Graham's protestations were to no avail, because he had already been irrevocably saddled with a reputation not unlike that of Samuel Thomson. Despite an auspicious beginning, Graham, hurt by his unmitigated dogmatism, perceived boorishness, and apparent conceit, plummeted from medical legitimacy to crackpot status. One of his contemporaries came close to sharing the same fate.

Missionary of Health: William A. Alcott

The epithet of "Grahamism" was commonly applied to William Andrus Alcott's work as well. Though Alcott found the popular association ignominious, there was ample room for confusion. Like Graham, Alcott lectured widely on right living, including the importance of a vegetable diet. Yet Alcott had a broader perspective, and he more successfully elaborated and popularized a complete and balanced hygienic philosophy. Alcott was also a much more prolific author than Graham, and, by the time of his death in 1859, had to his credit more than a hundred volumes of books and journals on self-improvement. Whether about health, religion, or education, Alcott's books, like Graham's, explored different facets of what he saw as a single entity. Alcott's writing was decidedly more accessible, devoid of Graham's obscure technicalities and sprinkled with familiar language and examples.[55]

Born in Connecticut in 1798, Alcott was descended through both parents from pioneers. In delicate health for most of his growing-up years, he floundered until he opted in 1816 for teaching, his life's work. By the late 1820s he was contributing regularly to educational journals, and soon thereafter he moved to Boston, the scene of tremendous educational ferment. In 1832 his *Essay on the Construction of Schoolhouses* won a competition sponsored by the American Institute of Instruction. The outlines of Alcott's philosophy were clear in this piece, which stressed the impact that a school's structures and furniture had on students' health and their

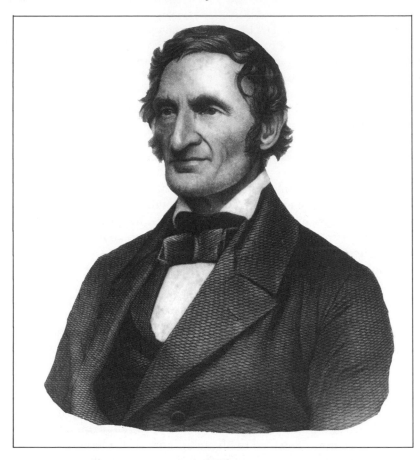

Portrait of William A. Alcott, indefatigable educator and author of how-to-live books, from the frontispiece of his *Lectures on Life and Health* (Boston, 1853).

ability to learn. He buttressed his points with arguments about the economic costs of preventible illness, a note increasingly heard among public health reformers.

During this period Alcott also worked with William Channing Woodbridge, editor of the *American Annals of Education* and the most famous American popularizer of the ideas of Johann Pestalozzi, the early nineteenth-century Swiss educator who advocated making the child's nature the principal criterion around which educational programs were designed. Many of the Pestalozzian emphases appealed to Alcott: cultivating reasoning powers instead of relying on rote memorization; managing children with friendly understanding instead of rigid discipline; and especially developing well-rounded individuals whose physical, moral, and intellectual faculties would operate in harmony with one another. The new educational ideas stressed imparting knowledge about bodily structure and function as an integral part of the quest toward full realization of the human potential. These ideas were to be essential elements in Alcott's strategy of hygienic reform.

That strategy did not evolve solely from his teaching experiences, however. By the mid-1820s Alcott's classroom duties had proven onerous enough to precipitate a physical decline he diagnosed as consumption; he responded by enrolling in Yale to study medicine. He received his degree in 1826, but Alcott marked the real culmination of his studies as his return to health, which he celebrated with a July fifth "declaration of independence with regard to those earthly props [medicines] on which I had so long been wont to lean." Alcott also pledged unflagging "dependence on God, and on his natural and moral enactments." From this point on, he rejoiced, "I was emancipated from slavery to external forms, especially medicated forms." Nature, he was convinced, was the only true physician, and human medical art was not only inferior but was usually harmful.[56]

Despite Alcott's credentials, when his *Vegetable Diet* was reviewed in an 1838 issue of the *Boston Medical and Surgical Journal,* its proper evaluation eluded the writer. As the title trumpeted, the book had been "sanctioned by medical men," and the reviewer acknowledged that Alcott had presented medical testimonials supporting a vegetable diet and advising against eating meat. Yet, as the reviewer pointed out, medical opinion was far from united on the subject; in fact, the works Alcott cited in support of a vegetable diet also contained passages recommending meat eating. The reviewer did not press the point, conceding that Alcott's crusade might be beneficial in a country where too much meat was ordinarily consumed.[57]

The subject was considered at greater length in five issues of the following volume. An anonymous correspondent praised Alcott as the "industrious," "worthy and intelligent" author of several books, "some . . . of considerable merit, designed to improve the health and morals of the community." Through this commendable work, he continued, Alcott had helped diffuse physiological knowledge, show its educational applications, and combat medical imposture and charlatanism. But on the subject of dietetics, wrote this contributor, "He is evidently beside himself. As often as he touches it his mind runs riot." The anatomical argument in which Alcott and Graham invested so much did not convince this writer, who thought it more logical to assume that a person's reason allowed him or her to adapt many foods for individual use. "Were animal food as poisonous, as noxious to health and life, as the bran-bread gentlemen would persuade us to believe, why was not the universal yankee-nation long ago extinct?" queried the correspondent. The facts seemed to argue in favor of the opposite conclusion: that these meat-eating citizens had "better health, longer life, more robust bodies, and a little shrewder minds." How, he wondered, could this be reconciled "with . . . practical illustrations of the effects of bran-bread and dried apples, . . . the cases of half a dozen gaunt, wry-faced, lantern-jawed, ghostly-looking invalids, who . . . are so many walking proofs (those that are able to walk)?"[58]

More to the point, it was those who were sick, not those who were well, who had to pay special attention to food. For the healthy, he argued, appetite was "a safe and competent guide." The "hardy yeomanry" were "not the class of those who run after mountebank lecturers on health for advice." They did not need to listen to "cranium-cracked dyspeptics, or their vaunted system of living. They have within themselves a sure guide . . . which never misleads them or jeopards their safety."

This contributor conceded that some people might thrive on a vegetable diet, but he thought such a dietary change for the masses "would be productive of great evil." Not only were Alcott's ideas "false" and of "injurious tendency," but they also "serve[d] to agitate, unnecessarily, the public mind." This was because they turned everyone's "attention . . . to their health, and they become anxious to know what they shall eat and what they shall drink." This anxiety often led to a harmful preoccupation, where people became so fixated on themselves that they began to "be over scrupulous and whimsical about their food, and drink, and whatever concerns their bodies." A sick person should never be encouraged "to [think] about his own complaints; and the surest way to make a well man sick is to alarm him about his health, to set him to watching his stomach and quarrelling with his food." For these reasons the writer had no doubt that most "of the books and periodicals . . . published within the last dozen years on health, . . . addressed to the public," were outright "nuisances," having "caused and aggravated, beyond calculation, the class of complaints which they were intended to prevent and remove." The contributor thought that the authors were generally "misguided men" who lacked sufficient knowledge to offer competent advice. To be sure, some of the writers were "medical men; but they have generally been mere M.D.'s—physicians without practice and without knowledge." Though he did not place Alcott in the camp of offenders, he obviously found his advice questionable.[59]

The editors published the health reformer's response. Like Graham, Alcott protested that he had been misrepresented. He objected to the "perpetual misnomer" of bran-bread advocacy and the fact that the author had unfairly "interlarded" his essay with "old, hackneyed, newspaper epithets." The remainder of Alcott's article addressed misquotations and misconstructions ranging from bad grammar to the number of years he had been compiling the book to the inevitable confusion with Grahamism. The defense was far from substantive.[60]

The following year he tried again. Opening with an attempt to dissociate himself from Grahamites and Thomsonians, Alcott tried to clarify his mission. He dreamed, he said, of carrying out "the great object of Christianity—TO MAKE MANKIND BETTER." Previous "instructors and elevators of mankind," he believed, had "made a serious mistake, in not endeavoring to elevate, in due proportion, their *whole* nature. They have hoped to raise man, *intellectually* and *morally*, . . . without doing much for him *physically.*" Furthermore, "the most aimed at has been *correction;* few, indeed, have done much in the way of *prevention.*"[61]

As this passage suggests, vegetable diet was less the centerpiece than a cornerstone of Alcott's philosophy, which melded morality and physiology. Aptly labeled "Christian physiology" by James Whorton, this guiding philosophy made individual perfection an indispensable vehicle for societal redemption. The prolific Alcott exemplified the first generation of health reformers. Like crusaders for other causes, health reformers promulgated advice that was an amalgam of evangelical beliefs tempered by Enlightenment ideas. For them, a growing faith in science was not only compatible with a familiar religious framework, but scientific and religious explanations were in fact mutually enhancing. They asserted that the laws of nature, ordained by God, could be discovered by rational individuals. Once Americans understood these principles and acted accordingly, they would achieve personal and societal perfection. Alcott's philosophy of living fueled an outpouring of advice books, published and often reissued from the 1830s though the 1850s. In these popular works, each directed at a specific audience, Alcott sought to interpret God's laws by defining people's duties to themselves, their families, and their communities.[62] The medical profession, suspicious of his vegetarian tracts, lauded these books as extremely useful.[63]

The Young Wife, for instance, went through twenty editions in roughly as many years after it appeared in the mid-1830s.[64] In it Alcott expressed themes on which he was to embroider for the rest of his life. Education—its meaning, its importance, its duties, and its effects—served as one of Alcott's central and unifying concepts. He focused on adult education here, reserving children's education for discussion in *The Young Mother.* The first task was to define education, which was much more than "mere instruction in knowledge." Alcott used the term "in its largest sense, as implying and including everything which forms character for this world or the world to come." This was "the great office of woman," whose role in "mere instruction" was subordinate to her responsibility for "the formation of character, physical, intellectual, social, moral, and religious—its formation, both for time and for eternity." By this definition, virtually every aspect of living fell under the rubric of education—and therefore within Alcott's bailiwick.[65]

Nothing was too insignificant to warrant attention, for often neglect in trifling matters courted disaster in larger ones. Tight clothing, for instance, horrified Alcott because "the mischief which ensue[d]" extended beyond the offender "to generations that come after her." The damage assumed tragic proportions. "If," postulated the health reformer, "in the progress of the world's history, she should have thousands of descendants, not one of them, to the remotest periods of time, would be precisely what he might have been, had she conformed more strictly to the natural laws—the laws of the human constitution."

With stakes of this magnitude, any detail could undermine or facilitate obedience to the laws of right living. Thus character traits were as important as physical vigor or intellectual development, and all were intimately related. As a result, each chapter, whether it treated delicacy or sobriety or some other subject, was a new showcase for healthy living, with behavioral advice interwoven throughout the text. It was for this reason, explained Alcott, "that I so frequently suffer one chapter to run into and trench upon another. Such is the connection which I plainly perceive between health and morals, that I scarcely know how to separate them."

"Health" and "Attending to the Sick" got their own chapters, since Alcott believed them necessary parts of female education. But he did not discuss disease treatment; nor did he even provide detailed information about how to maintain health, arguing that to do so properly would take volumes.[66] More importantly, it would be inappropriate. People who learned rules by rote were not as well equipped to apply them in daily living as were those who understood the underlying principles. Alcott therefore argued that wives should be knowledgeable about anatomy, physiology, and chemistry, and as encouragement he recommended specific books. William Paley's *Natural Theology* he judged the best starting point, after which he suggested George Combe's *Constitution of Man,* "rejecting, if you choose, the phrenological part." Next on the list came Sir William Lawrence's *Lectures on Physiology, Zoology, and the Natural History of Man.* After this, Andrew Combe's *Principles of Physiology* would be appropriate, followed "by some of the more complete and scientific works on physiology." Only after having built this firm foundation should the young wife study books on health, among which he specified James Johnson's *Economy of Health,* Anthony F. M. Willich's *Lectures on Diet and Regimen,* and Robley Dunglison's *Elements of Hygiene.* Not until this point might the young wife "with entire safety, study the nature or cure of disease, either infantile or adult." But Alcott thought that lay people should limit their study of medicine, because he believed that it was not "a part of human duty, except as a matter of curiosity, and with a view to prevention." He agreed it might be helpful to "look over such a work as Buchan's *Domestic Medicine,*" but "not to render every one 'his own doctor.'"[67]

How appropriate was this advice for the wife once she became a mother? At that point more opportunities for ministering to the sick would surely arise. To what extent was treatment her responsibility? Alcott had answers for these questions as well. In the mid-1830s he published *The Young Mother; or Management of Children in Regard to Health.*[68] The volume met an eager readership. Issued in an edition of two thousand copies in May 1836, by July of that year there were three thousand more ready for the bookstores. By 1839 it was in its seventh stereotyped edition, and in 1855 the twentieth stereotyped edition appeared. Orthodox doctors also warmly welcomed Alcott's seventy-five-cent book. As the reviewer in the *Boston Medical and Surgical Journal* explained, Alcott had not tried to be original or brilliant. The book's "excellence," the critic judged, "consists in its being a safe, intelligible and full directory to young families and *nurses.*" This would meet a tremendous need, especially since Alcott had gauged his presentation to his audience, "avoiding technicalities, and . . . making his work really popular."[69]

Alcott described the ideal nursery, particularly its ventilation, but he devoted most of his energy to discussing the proper physical care of children. He granted that there were prejudices against dwelling on these topics, but they had arisen, he insisted, "not so much because the Scriptures have charged us not to be over 'anxious' on the subject" but because the healthiest people were reputed to be those who paid the least attention to their health. Just the opposite was true, claimed Alcott. The healthiest people were those who carefully observed the laws of health, for they had good "HABITS."

Again he emphasized self-denial and self-government in smaller matters as an aid to physical and moral rectitude in larger things. The use of confectionary was a perfect example. "The GREAT evils of confectionary . . . are of three kinds," Alcott lectured, "PHYSICAL, MENTAL and MORAL." Grimly, he predicted that young people who indulged in "confectionary, [were] on the high road to gluttony, drunkenness, or debauchery; perhaps to all three." Wandering from the path of right living seemed particularly grievous to Alcott, who firmly believed that every infant was born healthy, consonant with Divine intentions. "Civilized society has placed the human race in artificial circumstances," he lamented, and he wanted to guide people back to correct habits and behavior. The potential reward was literally immeasurable: "I regard man as susceptible of endless progression."[70]

Much of this responsibility for improvement rested with the mother, the "arbiter of the present and eternal destiny of her child." But the mother should not act independently. Instead, she should rely on higher authority, specifically the physician, whose instructions she should uphold in every way. At times Alcott elevated fathers to the same level as doctors, relegating "unthinking nurses or mothers" to a more subservient position. In some situations, he explained, "It requires all the resolution which a father, uninterrupted, can summon to his aid, to administer a dose or perform a task, on which he knows the existence of his child may be depending." If mothers and nurses then bombarded the father with "thoughtless entreaties . . . , it makes his condition most distressing. Mothers, in such cases, ought to encourage rather than remonstrate. They who *do not,* are guilty of cruelty, and—perhaps—of infanticide."[71]

As before, Alcott had specific recommendations for reading. He especially favored physician William P. Dewees's *A Treatise on the Physical and Medical Treatment of Children,* five editions of which had appeared in nine years. Like other writers on child management, Alcott reinforced his recommendations with copious references to accepted medical authorities; he depended on older writers such as Buchan, Cadogan, Locke, and Willich, as well as more recent ones such as Buffon, Dunglison, and Beaumont. But there were no prescriptions, a policy in keeping with his stress on prevention over cure. The closest Alcott came to treatment advice was to point out "a few certain signs and symptoms by which [parents and nurses] may know a child's health to be declining, even before he appears to be sick."[72] The mother, like the wife, should educate herself about bodily conditions, but she should refrain from interfering with treatment, the physician's prerogative. Preventing illness was her responsibility.

For the unmarried or childless woman, Alcott presented similar advice in another comprehensive volume, *The Young Woman's Guide to Excellence*.[73] After an introductory chapter on "Female Responsibilities," Alcott followed a familiar pattern by using successive chapters to discuss desirable traits and interspersing among them capsules on exercise, rest and sleep, health and beauty, neatness and cleanliness, dress and ornament, dosing and drugging, and taking care of the sick. Once again the health reformer advocated studying anatomy, physiology, and hygiene, which he deemed indispensable for any young woman to "do her utmost in the work of self-education." There had been much progress with both sexes through lectures and books "on the structure, laws and relations of their bodily constitution." Nonetheless, every young woman should study these subjects for herself, beginning perhaps with two of Catharine Maria Sedgwick's moralistic tales, *The Poor Rich Man and the Rich Poor Man* and *Means and Ends: or Self-Training*. The works of the Combes should come next, followed by other popular physiology and hygiene texts, among them his own elementary primer, *The House I Live In*. Alcott's remaining recommendations testify to the interlocking importance of religion and physiology in his philosophy of living: John Mason, *Self-Knowledge;* James Burgh, *Dignity of Human Nature;* Isaac Watts, *Improvement of the Mind;* Amelia A. Opie, *Detractions and Scandal;* Francis Wayland, *Elements of Moral Science;* and Thomas H. Skinner, *Religion of the Bible*.[74]

As had his other volumes, Alcott's *Young Woman's Guide* emphasized that breaches in physical conduct were also moral transgressions. To illustrate the connection, Alcott asked whether "there is any moral character in the error, if it be one, of sitting up an hour later than usual, and then making it up by sleeping an hour after the arrival of day-light;— whether it is not a matter of *propriety,* merely, rather than a question of positive right or wrong in the sight of Heaven." For the answer, he referred readers to his chapter on conscientiousness, where he had stated unequivocally that no action was too insignificant to be exempt from this stringent moral code. Everything, *"whatever we do,"* was to be done "to the glory of God[.]" Given this, "where is the line to be drawn between those actions which are too small or too trifling to be worthy of having any right or wrong attached to them, and those which are not?"[75]

In that same chapter, Alcott had maintained that what was most important was "to meet the approbation of an internal monitor." Diligence in this matter was crucial, because it seemed obvious "that the individual who habitually disregards the voice speaking within, on a particular subject, [would] be likely, ere long, to extend the same habit of disregard to something else." Proper childhood training was essential. Self-approbation was the only invariable yardstick, and those in whom it was inculcated would act for the glory of God, always cognizant that "there is a right and wrong in every thing." From that stance, it was an easy matter for Alcott to go one step further: "We should remember that it is not only sinful to do wrong, but that it is also sinful to *omit to do right.*" Individuals then had a duty not only to themselves and to God but also to society to live properly; conversely, they did not have the right to do otherwise.[76]

Moral progress and physical improvement were inextricably joined. Indeed, preached Alcott, "Mere physical improvement—or even physical perfection, were it attainable—would hardly be worth the pains, if it were anything more than a means to an end." The most zealous and conscientious student of health could hardly count herself blessed if her knowledge only increased her "efficiency in the service of the world, the flesh and the devil." When mankind fell with Adam and Eve, the physical fall had been almost as great as the moral one. Logically, then, restoration could come only with "obedience to those laws by the transgression of which it came." Obedience to God's laws would benefit absolutely everyone, for "no person, in any employment whatever, is so healthy as to exclude all possibility of further improvement. It is not yet known how healthy an individual may become."[77]

The Young House-keeper, which also appeared in the late 1830s, conveyed the same message. "Whatever views may be suggested by the title, this book is really and truly a work on Physical Education," explained Alcott. He compared it with *The Young Mother,* for it had the same "principal end and aim, the physical improvement of the community." He sought to transform housekeepers into "thinking beings" rather than "mere pieces of mechanism; or, what is little better, the mere creatures of habit or slaves of custom." Though it shared the objectives of *The Young Mother,* it was "a separate and entirely different volume," being "almost wholly confined to the nature and preparation of food."[78] Used in conjunction with one another, Alcott's books offered virtually all-inclusive guidance for American women.

Alcott also wrote advice books for young men. When the second edition of *The Young Man's Guide* appeared in 1834, the notice in the *Boston Medical and Surgical Journal* urged physicians to promote "the general diffusion among the young men of our country, of a work that must contribute greatly to the *preservation* of their health, as well as to their general improvement, success, and usefulness."[79]

Since many character traits were desirable to everyone, Alcott covered some of the same material in his guides for men as he did in his books for women. Thus, *Familiar Letters to Young Men,* the companion piece to *The Young Man's Guide,* provided sections on self-respect and self-reverence, self-knowledge, self-dependence, self-education, and the love and spirit of progress. Alcott also warned of the dangers of excitement, and he discussed purity, pleasure-seeking, civic and conjugal duties, and religion. New topics concerned employment, including how to start a business and how to make money. Physiology was important to men as well, and its definition sounded familiar: "all such knowledge as pertains to the physical education and management of human beings." As Alcott had informed women, he explained to men that preventive living, not self-treatment, was the goal. To this end Alcott thought young men should attend lectures, either those illustrated by manikins or those that covered the laws of health more generally. Of the former types, he recommended the ones given by Weiting, Darling, Cutter, and Wright. He thought that the best of the general lectures were conducted by Mussey, the Fowlers, Gove, and Alcott himself. Nor was the reading list a surprise, featuring works by the Combes, Sweetser, the Fowlers, Graham, and Alcott.[80]

In a new twist, Alcott advised young men to study phrenology after learning about physiology. Though doubtful "that every thing which is called Phrenology is worthy of . . . confidence," he thought that the mental faculties constituted an important branch of physiology. It was neither necessary nor desirable to become "adepts in this science," but he encouraged young men to acquire "a practical general knowledge of the subject," preferably by reading the works of the Combes and the Fowlers. He disagreed with people who roundly condemned phrenological ideas as "visionary," believing many of them to be "soundly sensible." The point of studying phrenology, even more than physiology, was to "make every thing practical. Apply the subject to your own personal improvement, either immediately or prospectively." Wherever there seemed "a deficiency in your mental, moral, or corporeal structure, seek to supply it in the best manner."[81]

Corresponding to *The Young Wife,* in 1835 Alcott published *The Young Husband.*[82] There he stressed the male spouse's various duties as a social, intellectual, and moral agent to his family and community. Again his advice was wide-ranging, and, though he did not shortchange health, he felt free to limit his remarks, due to the full discussions in his other books. Once again, however, Alcott emphasized his belief that people could be healthy if they conducted themselves properly. Though following physical laws was important, Alcott also reminded his readers that morality was equally critical. Proclaimed Alcott, "To be healthy, we need to be holy." It was crucial, he continued, to "understand the whole intention of Christianity[.]" This entailed realizing "that the salvation and sanctification of man includes his whole being—body, soul, and spirit— . . . and that, until man is in this respect fully redeemed, the whole object of his divine mission to our earth will not be accomplished[.]"

Legions joined Alcott and Graham in proclaiming the indissoluble links between physical and moral health. If all individuals in society could attain bodily and spiritual salvation, social redemption would be achieved as well. Legal safeguards about medical practice would be superfluous if Americans lived according to correct principles, such as those promulgated in William Alcott's advice manuals. Vexing questions of medical legitimacy would also vanish or recede because citizens would be capable of recognizing qualified healers and because they would be more likely to respect the physician's sphere.

An Outpouring of Health Advice

Guidebooks for young men and women proliferated during this period, and they typically promoted healthy and temperate living as the building blocks for happiness and success. In 1848 Frank Ferguson's pocket-sized *The Young Man,* for instance, included a chapter on "Regular Hours" and one on "Temperance."[83] Peter Parley's 1836 *Every Day Book for Youth* briefly covered exercise, cleanliness, and diet. The point, as the best-selling author indicated a few years later in *What To Do and How To Do It,* was to cultivate the reason which God had bestowed on humans. Unlike man, animals were guided entirely by instinct. As a result, "we do not send animals to school, and give them books, for God is their teacher." The situation was different for people, who were "to be educated, instructed, and by a gradual progress, elevated to that high destiny for which they are qualified. Instruction is the means by which we are to be taught our duty, and by which we may accomplish the end for which we were created." But instruction alone was insufficient "unless we listen to it, and obey its teachings. We must not only *know* what is good and right, but we must pursue and *do* what is good and right."[84]

T. S. Arthur's *Advice to Young Men on Their Duties and Conduct in Life,* published in 1847, offered a chapter called "Health." Arthur, best known

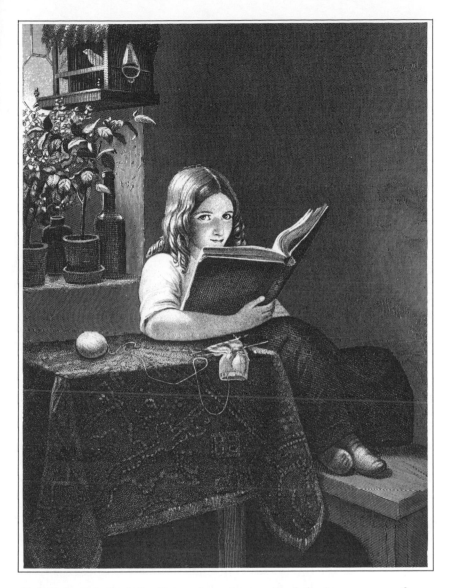

Godey's Lady's Book for December 1855 stressed the importance of children's "Reading from a 'Sense of Duty'" in both its frontispiece illustration and an accompanying story.

for his enormously popular temperance classic, the 1854 *Ten Nights in a Barroom and What I Saw There,* began by stressing that "late hours, irregular habits, and want of attention to diet" were errors common to young men. These actions "gradually, but at first imperceptibly, undermine the health, and lay the foundation for various forms of disease in after life." This was serious: "As health is the indispensable prerequisite to a proper discharge of the duties of life, every man is under obligation to society not to do any thing, which, by producing a diseased condition of the body, renders him unfit to attend efficiently to his work or office. . . . No man stands alone in society, or can be independent of others. Each forms a part of the great social body, and must faithfully and diligently do what he can for the common good."[85]

A more religious phrasing of this same view came in 1855 from E. H. Chapin's *Duties of Young Men.* His first lecture, "Self-Duties," had as its cardinal rule *"a careful preservation of the health."* Chapin preached the importance of living according to God's will: "Live that you may not in any way weaken your ability to do good to yourselves or to others."[86]

Sometimes writers went beyond rules for healthy living and advised on sickroom conduct. One example is the unknown author of *The Well-Bred Boy and Girl,* who devoted one chapter of the 1850 text to "The Sick Chamber."[87] The chapter was written from the vantage point of Alfred, a little boy who awoke one day, "hot and uncomfortable" and plagued with "a bad headache." Judging him to be quite ill, Alfred's mother sent for the doctor, who wanted to examine his tongue and throat and "to ask him a great many questions." The youngster was recalcitrant, for he "felt sick and heavy, and did not like very much to be disturbed; but his mother told him that the doctor could not do any thing for him unless he could carefully examine him, and see what was the matter." Convinced, Alfred "opened his mouth as wide as he could. . . . He told the doctor exactly how he felt, not describing his feelings as any worse than they really were, that he might be pitied a great deal, nor telling of them as if they were not so bad, that he might escape taking medicine, but the exact truth."

Soon the doctor told Alfred he had the measles, which was "troublesome . . . , but not often . . . dangerous." As the disease progressed, Alfred tried to bear the pain as well as he could. He rested quietly and "took exactly what his mother and the doctor thought would be best for him." Alfred's conduct remained exemplary. If he had to take foul-tasting medicine, "he did not stop to think about it, and look at it, and shudder, and turn away; this, he knew, would make it much more difficult for him to get it down; but he opened his mouth wide, gave one good manly swallow, and it was all over." As he improved, he was served "gruel, and broth, and some things . . . he did not love very well." In response to his complaints, "his mother told him it was better for his stomach than his usual food." Responding to this reasoning, Alfred "tried to think it tasted good; he knew it had been fixed on purpose for him, and he tried to make the best of it, and found it tasted, on the whole, rather better than he expected." By his compliant behavior, "he spared himself and those about him a great deal of pain," and he quickly recovered his health. His sickness reminded him of "what a great blessing health is" and made him more sympathetic to other sufferers. It is hard to imagine that many of Alfred's flesh-and-blood contemporaries were so angelic, but to encourage imitators, writers promulgated criteria about how to be an ideal patient.[88]

Similarly didactic health stories featuring child and adult characters were often found in the women's magazines and annual gift books that were so popular in antebellum America. There was also more practical written advice available to middle-class citizens. Magazines as diverse as *DeBow's Review,* the *North American Review,* the *Southern Literary Messenger,* and *Peterson's Magazine* included articles on public and private health matters.[89] Periodical literature, however, rarely touched life's most intimate aspects. For advice about sexuality, Americans after about 1830 could turn to a burgeoning advice literature, much of it semilicit. Sylvester Graham was an important figure here, using lectures and books to urge the sexual restraint that was integral, with his dietary ideas, to what Nissenbaum has called his "physiology of subsistence."[90] William A. Alcott was a self-proclaimed expert in this area as well. His *Physiology of Marriage,* first published in 1855, reached twenty-seven thousand copies by 1866 and went through at least seven editions.[91] They were joined by many others who feared the immediate and long-term effects of "the solitary vice" (masturbation) and sought to inform the population about the importance of sexual hygiene.[92] Nonetheless, explicit anatomical and physiological details about sexuality tended to be beyond the scope of antebellum authors on sexual hygiene, as they were for their counterparts writing anatomy and physiology schoolbooks.

Cookbooks also advised about health, primarily by offering dietary suggestions for both healthy and sick people. One of the most popular was Sarah Josepha Hale's 1839 *The Good Housekeeper, or the Way to Live Well and To Be Well While We Live.* The first edition had sold two thousand copies in one month, bragged Hale as she readied the second edition for publication later that same year; by its 1840 third printing she was claiming its production to have already reached three thousand. The fifty-cent volume contained "directions for choosing and preparing food, in regard to health, economy, and taste." The laudatory review in *Godey's Lady's Book* pointed out as well that her health precepts had been "compiled from Dr. Andrew Combe's most valuable work."[93]

Indeed, Hale was another significant figure in health popularization, enormously influential through her editorship of *Godey's*. Her editorial career began in 1828 with the first issue of the *Ladies Magazine* and continued forty years beyond its 1837 merger with *Godey's Lady's Book*. Under her direction the magazine's circulation increased from roughly ten thousand in 1837 to a reported one hundred fifty thousand by 1860. From her editor's chair Hale was a tireless champion of exercise, fresh air, proper diet, and sensible dress. Articles on health appeared on virtually every subject in virtually every number. Thus readers could learn about hygienic rules, calisthenics, the causes of consumption, health and beauty, diet, useful medical books, and related topics.[94]

The 1853 *Ladies' Indispensable Assistant* and similar volumes of miscellany resembled contemporary women's magazines in the wide range of information they packed between their covers. This one did seem to offer almost everything, including "the very best directions for the behavior and etiquette of ladies and gentlemen, ladies' toilette table, [and] directions for managing canary birds." It also printed recipes intended to "[form] a complete system of family medicine [and enable] each person to become his or her own physician." The majority of its pages, however, presented recipes comprising "one of the best systems of cookery ever published," a sure guide to maintaining or regaining health.[95]

Cookery was but one part of household management, and guides to "domestic economy" appeared during this period as well. They too included advice about healthy living. Lydia Maria Child's best-selling *American Frugal Housewife* was published in 1832 and was in its twelfth edition seven years later, but Catharine Beecher's *Treatise on Domestic Economy* was even more popular. Published in 1841, Beecher's *Treatise* was in its fourth printing within two years, and it was reprinted nearly every year from 1841 to 1856. Together with a supplementary receipt book, reprinted fourteen times between its 1841 appearance and the 1869 publication of *The American Woman's Home,* Beecher's texts virtually dominated the market. Beecher's *Treatise* pulled together in one volume practical material related to homemaking that previously had been available only in disparate locations. Thus she not only discussed plumbing and housebuilding, but she also probed matters of health, diet, hygiene, and general well-being. Unlike Child's volume, which gave treatments for common ailments and injuries, Beecher placed her advice within the larger framework of anatomy and physiology.[96]

Beecher's approach foreshadowed a new thrust in the dissemination of health information to Americans. Orthodox doctors, waging war against quackery, continued to support the efforts of health popularizers as long as they did not try to undermine or usurp the physician's role in treatment. Regardless of the very real importance of the diffusion of the kinds of health information discussed in this chapter, the regulars became increasingly convinced that its provision alone was ultimately inadequate to the task of guaranteeing a healthy population. With only general behavioral guidelines, even the well-intentioned and committed individual might easily lose his or her moorings. During the mid-nineteenth century, growing numbers of people supported what they saw as the necessary and ideal complement: school texts in anatomy, physiology, and hygiene. As William Alcott lectured parents in 1853: "You are bound to see that anatomy, physiology and hygiene are taught—not in that profoundly scientific way which is desirable and even indispensable in the professional schools, but in a plain and popular manner—in all the schools of the land."[97] Education in the schoolroom would not only complement and reinforce the work of parents and other adults, but it would constitute another powerful alternative to political action to achieve the good society. This battle and its warriors next demand our attention.

5 The Pedagogical Crusade

"It may be an easy thing to make a republic, but it is a very laborious thing to make republicans."[1] The words belonged to Horace Mann, the person whose name was virtually synonymous with the mid-nineteenth-century public school movement. *"The common school,"* Mann announced in 1841, *"is the greatest discovery ever made by man."* John Griscom agreed. In addition to his public health activities, Griscom served as town super-intendent and trustee of public schools in Burlington, Massachusetts. "The prosperity of the common, district, or public school," Griscom proclaimed in 1847, was "the surest test of the enlightenment of any district,—of any country. It is the thermometer of civilization."[2]

What made the common school so special? After all, many other edu-cational opportunities existed: household education, charity schools, town-sponsored classes, church-supported ventures, and quasi-public academies. These same mid-century years saw the birth of infant schools, high schools, and schools for special groups, such as the feeble-minded or blind. The most important feature of the common school, however, was that it was supposed to be open to everyone. It would, its promoters claimed, properly educate children by systematically spreading knowl-edge, nurturing virtue, and cultivating learning. Among the results they anticipated were social harmony and enhanced morality, both of which were deemed to be crucial for the future of the republic. Writing fifty years after Benjamin Rush, Mann recognized that the Revolution was still incomplete because of its very nature: "Revolutions working down among the primordial elements of human character; taking away ascen-dancy from faculties which have long been in subjection;—such revolu-

140

tions cannot be accomplished by one convulsive effort, though every fibre in the nation should be strained to the endeavor." The political upheaval of the 1770s had freed the colonists, but liberty had also removed many historical restraints to human passions. Post-Revolutionary leaders feared that unless morality checked passion and physical force, the blessings of liberty would be worse than the evils of tyranny.[3]

As part of his work as secretary of the Massachusetts Board of Education from 1837 to 1848, Mann achieved some of the goals articulated by William A. Alcott and other health reformers. Dismayed in 1842 to discover how few Massachusetts students were being taught physiology, Mann contended that the subject should "claim rightful precedence," for it was "an exposition of the laws of health and life." Knowledge of physiology would show people how to keep their bodies in "a state of vigor, usefulness, and enjoyment[,]" which would increase their "ability to perform the arduous duties and to bear the inevitable burdens of life."[4]

As Mann continued the crusade in subsequent lectures, essays, and annual reports, support for his position gradually grew. In April 1850 the state legislature passed a law requiring that physiology and hygiene be taught in Massachusetts schools and that candidates to teach these subjects be examined for competence. Implementation was problematical and slow, and the introduction of physiology textbooks lagged behind that of more traditional subjects, such as reading, grammar, arithmetic, geography, history, and spelling. Nonetheless, in Massachusetts and gradually in other states, a commitment to offering physiological instruction in the schools did begin to take hold.[5] A similar trend was evident in the nation's academies and colleges.[6]

Citizens of this generation witnessed the first concerted attempt to disseminate knowledge about disease prevention and health promotion, downplaying or omitting altogether information about disease treatment. Imbued with the perfectionism and pietism prevalent at mid-century, regular doctors and a few nonprofessional writers defined their crusade as much in terms of moral as physical redemption.[7] The appearance of this literature also coincided with growing awareness among Americans of the pathbreaking work being done in France by Pierre Louis and the Paris School. Using observation and statistical methods on large hospital populations, French clinicians documented the inefficacy of much of the orthodox materia medica. Americans greeted the French findings with much ambivalence and debated their implications for medical theory and practice. Some physicians followed Harvard professor Jacob Bigelow's lead when he conceded in 1835 that some diseases were "self-limiting" and that in such cases the doctor should not interfere with the healing powers of nature. Many doctors, however, were not only skeptical of the Paris School's claims, but they were also hostile. One reason for this hostility was that though the Paris School's methods and findings helped eradicate harmful practices, the fact that they so avoided experimentation meant that they could propose very few therapies or explanations to substitute for what they discredited. Some Americans did advocate using experimentation to fill the therapeutic and intellectual vacuum, but they had little success until German experimental methods became influential after the Civil War.[8]

In this situation popular physiologists played a pioneering role that scholars have previously underrated.[9] They anticipated and showcased what their postbellum counterparts were to capitalize upon decades later: that burgeoning knowledge of anatomy and physiology *could* and *should* be used as a strong foundation for the study and teaching of hygiene.[10] Especially in a time of acknowledged therapeutic uncertainty, the study of prevention, they argued, was essential. First the French and later the German findings dovetailed with the prevailing climate of social reform in America to give the crusaders for hygienic living significant medical credibility and cultural authority. As this group of writers turned to schools as the vehicle for enlightening Americans about proper living, they simultaneously contributed to the more and more precise delineation of nonprofessional and professional roles in health and medicine. In so doing, the crusaders introduced and developed a new type of health literature, the school text for anatomy, physiology, and hygiene. These books provided increasingly systematic treatment of body structures (anatomy), functions (physiology), and derivative rules for proper living (hygiene). With this knowledge, health popularizers enthused, nonprofessionals could realistically assume responsibility for prevention.

Faust *Catechisms* as Transitional Texts

In 1797 physician Elihu Hubbard Smith, one of the "Hartford Wits" and a founder of the New York *Medical Repository,* wrote his sister, Mary S. Mumford, and suggested that she read "Dr. Faust's 'Catechism of Health'; a work designed for children, but more proper for parents, & those who have the immediate charge of children." He had read the book himself in December 1795, recording in his diary that "with some exceptions, it is a good book. Much of it is excellent." The Germans, he thought, should be commended. "More of their men of learning & genius have turned their attention to the composition of their initial books—for the aid of children—& the unlearned."[11]

According to Charles Carpenter, Bernhard G. Faust's *Catechism* was probably the earliest physiology text used in America, since an adaptation from the German appeared in Boston and Philadelphia in 1795.[12] It is true that Faust claimed that his book was for schoolchildren and that he used a catechismal format that would have been familiar to youngsters. But it is misleading to classify Faust's *Catechism* as even an embryonic form of the soon-to-emerge physiology, anatomy, and hygiene textbook. Rather, Faust's book had much more in common with *existing* written traditions of health education, particularly the longevity text, with its emphasis on providing general guidelines for the proper way to live. Faust's *Catechism* also shared features of contemporaneous domestic health guides, for it gave instructions about what to do in the event of illness. Later, derivative editions bore no greater similarity to the nascent physiology text nor were they addressed primarily to children. But they were increasingly explicit about parental responsibilities for child care, revealing and reinforcing the larger cultural trends discussed especially in chapters 2 and 4.

Religion shaped Faust's view of sickness and health. As the eminent German physician explained in the 1795 translation, neither earthly nor heavenly happiness was possible without good health, for sickness ran counter to God's will. He thought most people sinned because they knew little about the human body, so he sought to educate by presenting more than four hundred sets of questions and answers, recapitulating important points in occasional illustrations and frequent "Observations" and "Addresses to Children."[13]

The first section, "Of Health," constituted nearly three-fourths of the tome. Faust admitted that fifteen of his twenty-one chapters "regard grown-up persons as much as children," and the range of subjects included the non-naturals, alcoholic beverages, tobacco, beauty, and even lightning and thunder. A lengthy passage summarized Faust's central message by spelling out the characteristics of the "truly happy" person who "enjoys terrestrial bliss" and could, "anticipating the joys of eternal felicity, brave all the horrors of death." That individual would have been born to and educated by "healthy, strong, sensible, and industrious parents." Blessed from infancy with a clean and well-ventilated home, the child would have been taught by his or her parents to be clean, temperate, neat, persistent, and industrious. The adult citizen, Faust concluded, would be exemplary: he would "[work] six days out of seven for the maintenance of a wife and children," and he would "[fear] God, [love] mankind, and [do] justice."[14]

The remainder of Faust's work, "Of Diseases," distilled information contained in domestic health guides and especially emphasized prevention and nursing. When stricken, people should remain "tranquil and composed" and immediately consult a learned physician, surgeon, or apothecary. Under no circumstances, warned Faust, should anyone rely on quacks, domestic medicines, secret nostrums, universal medications, or witchcraft. To ensure successful treatment once the doctor had arrived, it was the patient's responsibility to give the doctor an exact and accurate account of everything that had happened from the beginning of the illness through the time of the doctor's arrival. If it were impossible for a doctor to see and speak to the patient himself, "some intelligent person" should draw up an "exact and circumstantial statement of his case" to be sent to the physician. Once medicines had been prescribed, the patient should take those medicines "faithfully, regularly, in due time, and in the dose prescribed."[15]

Like those writing household health guides, Faust also had advice for the invalid's attendants. "A patient," he explained, "is a poor, helpless creature, oppressed by anxiety and pains," and therefore should be treated "with the greatest tenderness, kindness, and affection." Faust offered precise guidelines about every aspect of the sick chamber and then discussed briefly the principal therapeutic agents of heroic medicine: bleeding, clysters, purgatives, and blisters. General instructions followed on how to treat wounds, contusions, ulcers, scalds, and sore nipples. Faust gave little attention to contagious diseases other than smallpox, which he thought "as bad as the plague!" He hoped that omitting the encyclopedic disease information commonly available in home health guides would discourage nonprofessionals from treating disease. Instead, he tried to encourage proper living by discussing prevention; when disease did strike, the appropriate role for the lay person was nursing.

Faust's book was innovative in two important ways: its purported audience—schoolchildren—and its use of the catechismal format. Yet Faust also addressed his remarks to parents, and the information he imparted had much in common with older written traditions of health literature, the longevity text and the domestic health guide. Given its stress on building model citizens, it is not surprising that it got a warm reception from Americans interested in creating and sustaining a strong republic. Despite Charles Carpenter's claim, Faust's *Catechism* did not break new ground by covering anatomy, physiology, and hygiene. Nor did later versions of the book, though they remained congenial to the republican temperament.

In 1810 an anonymous derivative, *A New Guide to Health,* appeared in Newburyport, Massachusetts. Compiled and adapted from Faust's *Cate-*

chism by Edinburgh physician James Gregory, it boasted enhancements drawn from works of eminent practitioners, particularly Anthony F. M. Willich's *Lectures on Diet and Regimen* and James Parkinson's *Medical Admonitions*. Despite its more learned tone, the book still sought to appeal to a broad audience, especially families and schools. The author stressed that the catechismal format had great advantages for a schoolbook, because "the frequent, and seemingly needless repetitions" would help readers remember and apply what they read. The intention was neither "to convert School-masters into Doctors," nor to make children "adepts in medical knowledge." The point was to spell out how to maintain health and prevent disease, particularly through "Temperance, Prudence, and Cleanliness."[16]

The author obviously envisioned parents as an integral part of his audience. How parents handled their infants and children, he said, determined whether "a good or bad constitution is formed." A good constitution was all-important, not only for the child's later "health and usefulness . . . but likewise [for] the safety and prosperity of the state." Thus the introduction, based on work by Anthony F. M. Willich and new to the 1810 text, gave explicit instructions about childhood diet, clothing, exercise, sleep, ventilation, and cleanliness.[17] Only the catechismal format and the author's stated intentions distinguish this advice from that found in guides for the proper management of children.

Yet the anonymous 1810 *New Guide to Health* was also very similar to Faust's 1795 *Catechism*. Though the illustrations and many of Faust's "Observations" and "Admonitions" are missing, the volume's overall meaning is unchanged, and the language is in many cases exactly or nearly the same. Even the new material, much of it related to medicine and disease treatment, seems quite familiar.[18] Despite the modifications made in the 1810 version, it remains a hybrid of two genres, the longevity text and the household health manual.

Much the same is true of William Mavor's 1819 version of *The Catechism of Health*. Mavor was a popularizer, a British writer who wrote a number of school texts, including biographies of famous Britons and a best-selling English grammar. Mavor removed the Scriptural passages used copiously in earlier editions, though he still favored using a religious framework to interpret matters of life and well-being.[19] In fact, though Mavor's edition was substantially shorter than its 1810 predecessor, its thrust was nearly identical, primarily because its questions and answers were more broadly conceived.[20] This edition of *The Catechism of Health* did more strenuously promote the importance of childrearing, suggesting that parents remained an important constituency for the book. Mavor thought that it would be "wise and humane in governments" to ensure dissemination of proper knowledge about childrearing, for "every nation should be considered as one great family, of whom the rulers are the head, or parents." Even though Mavor believed that parents usually had good intentions for their children, he felt that they too often acted out of ignorance or superstition. Educating parents, he wrote, would not entail "usurp[ing] the province of the physician," but would equip them and their children to carry out their own duty: preserving health. This edition, then, still conveyed advice about proper living in a vein reminiscent of the longevity text, but, like guidebooks for mothers, it gave even greater priority to spreading knowledge about childrearing.[21]

The 1831 *Catechism of Health* was yet more unabashed about seeking parental readers, particularly mothers. It appeared under the aegis of Henry Porter, the Philadelphia publisher of the *Journal of Health,* the *Journal of Law,* and the *Family Library of Health.* Labeling it the "ladies' edition," Porter said it encompassed "plain and simple rules for the preservation of the health and vigour of the constitution from infancy to old age."[22] There were no biblical verses embellishing Porter's *Catechism,* and there were fewer and more indirect references to Divine intentions and agency. Like previous editions, this one taught that it was largely within each person's control to be healthy, since most diseases resulted from an individual's "own ignorance, folly, vice, or imprudence." Being attentive to health was also a moral obligation, Porter emphasized, because the reason for each person's existence was "to engage in certain active and necessary employments." Since "the want of health" was obviously incapacitating, "the care necessary to preserve the body from disease must necessarily be numbered among the duties of indispensable obligation."

Porter provided minute advice on every subject, whether it was the frequency of foot washing according to season, or the proper garments for children, piece by piece. Though Porter's topical arrangement differed substantially from earlier editions, the subjects he covered in his first division corresponded closely to those treated in earlier texts. The most pronounced shift was Porter's advocacy of a vegetable diet, which he argued would make people "more strong and robust," not "weak and stunted" as critics charged. This stance was not surprising, given Porter's publishing connections with health reform.[23]

It was in the second division of his book that Porter deviated most from the design used in previous editions. Porter did not discuss diseases, medicines, or doctors, but instead set himself the task of mapping out exactly how "the day should be spent under ordinary circumstances, . . .

to ensure the health of the body, and . . . the tranquillity of the mind." The ensuing discussion centered on different periods of the day and the meals normally consumed during them.[24]

Regardless of differences in design and content between Porter's *Catechism* and the Faust *Catechism* from which it was derived, Porter's book bore no greater resemblance to an anatomy and physiology text. Moreover, because Porter, unlike Faust, omitted information about disease treatment and medicine, his 1831 version was in fact a detailed guide to healthy living.

Not everyone, however, viewed this as an unadulterated blessing. Indeed, its appearance, together with that of Porter's popular *Journal of Health*, provoked lengthy consideration in the *Western Medical and Physical Journal*.[25] The reviewer used the device of "a venerable female friend" to articulate and counter the central objections made to the entire genre of popular health literature. The "fair *quintagenarian*" featured in the article railed against the outpouring of health books, which she thought encouraged people to be excessively preoccupied with their health. As she phrased it, "The tendency of the whole, is to subject to artificial rules, that which can be safely confided only to the instincts, appetites, and experience, of each individual." The healthiest people, she insisted, were the ones who paid the least amount of attention to their well-being. Health, she believed, was the "natural" result of a person's "industrious pursuit" of those objects for which he or she was created. The quintagenarian did not deny that an individual might "have excellent health, while observing the minute and multiplied precepts of the Journal and Catechism, but it by no means follows, that he would not have been equally well, if these entertaining books had never been written." It was her contention that "such works, like treatises on domestic economy, can but embody the experience of the world, in reference to which each individual might safely be left to appropriate to himself, such a portion as his peculiar situation might require." The disgruntled woman's final objection was "that to 'live, move, and have our being, beneath a written code of hygienic laws, is to be subjected to a new dominion, in addition to those which society had already imposed.'"

The reviewer conceded the quintagenarian's point that "much depends on a good natural constitution, and still more on exposure and hard labor in the open air." Beyond this, he wrote, the woman's analysis and expectations were naive, because she assumed that everyone had inherited a solid constitution and enjoyed a decent standard of living. But this was far from the case. Especially for people who lived in the artificial and stressful atmosphere of cities, "some organs are overworked, others languish in sloth; this is kept in perpetual irritation, that in stagnation and torpor; the temptations to improper indulgences of every kind, are greatly multiplied; the appetites are bribed and pampered; the dominion of fashion is mad and tyrannical." The results could be frightening: "new infirmities and diseases unknown in the country, are generated; children are born with frail constitutions; and their native tendencies to disease, await but the action of slight exciting causes, to rouse them into fatal energy." Given this reality, the reviewer saw two possible choices: passively succumb to illness and premature death; or actively seek health and longevity. Popular health literature would help those who wanted to join the battle against disease and for health.

The writer praised the *Catechism* as "strictly didactic, and totally divested of all references to authorities, and of every extraneous embellishment." The book was, in fact, "a rigid elementary and practical treatise on hygiene," designed "to sustain the attention of the reader, and render the various subjects intelligible to the humblest capacity." The reviewer thought it was "a valuable family book" and a subject that all young people should be required to study.

This endorsement notwithstanding, there were other Americans who would have agreed at least in part with the unhappy quintagenarian. Unlike her, they needed no convincing about the benefits conferred on society by "books on the art of health," some form of which had, after all, been in existence for centuries. Like her, however, they would have agreed that obeying hygienic rules as described in such volumes would be "artificial" and unreliable. Her solution was to cease publishing such books; theirs was to broaden the context in which the laws of hygiene were discussed. The result was a new type of health literature that sought to educate nonprofessionals about hygiene by teaching them basic anatomy and physiology.

"Rational Hygiene"

Many people undertook the task of educating mid-nineteenth-century American students, both elementary and more advanced, about proper living. Some used variations on the question-and-answer format, but over time their books resembled Faust's work less and less because they gave as much space to anatomy and physiology as to hygiene. This change in approach grew out of the conviction that a person's ability to live correctly was directly related to how much that person understood about the underlying rationale for behavioral rules. Thus anatomy, physiology, and hygiene were fundamentally inseparable, a message underlined by Amariah Brigham's important *Remarks on the Influence of Mental Cultivation and Mental Excitement upon Health*. Published in Hartford in 1832, it quickly went through four printings in America and three in England. The young doctor believed that Americans had the capacity "to become the most vigorous and powerful race of human beings, both in mind and in body, that the world has ever known." To accomplish this, Brigham urged repeatedly, it was essential that "the whole man should be improved," body as well as mind.[26]

Brigham's maxim for living was *"mens sana in corpore sano,"* said a reviewer in the *Western Medical and Surgical Journal*. This he applied to every aspect of existence. "If any organ or faculty, either of the body or mind, be neglected," summarized the reviewer, "it falls into debility and disorder and never fails to react on the others and limit their perfectibility."[27] In order to ensure the requisite attentiveness, Brigham argued that "all plans of education" should be founded on anatomical and physiological study. The "general neglect" of these subjects was both an "extraordinary" and "most lamentable evil."[28]

The similarity of Brigham's views to those of phrenologists is striking. Following in the footsteps of Johann Gaspar Spurzheim and Franz Joseph Gall, European phrenologists constructed elaborate theories to explain the interrelations of anatomy, physiology, and well-being, which included morality.[29] The American version of phrenology was more practical, increasingly divorced from its theoretical underpinnings and billed as a literal guide to living.[30] As John Davies has documented, phrenology had an astonishing impact on mid-nineteenth-century American workers in education, medicine, mental health, and many other fields. Congenial with the perfectionistic and pietistic temper of mid-nineteenth-century America, phrenology posited the infinite perfectibility of human beings; if an individual were only cognizant of his or her inherent propensities for good or ill, he or she would then possess a personalized blueprint for improvement. Phrenological ideas—specifically the linkage of physical, mental, and moral qualities and the stress on human perfectibility—filtered through American thought.[31]

Andrew Combe, a Fellow of Edinburgh's Royal Society of Physicians, enjoyed enormous popularity as a phrenologist, eclipsed only by that of his brother George, best known for his 1828 *Constitution of Man*. Andrew Combe's 1834 *Principles of Physiology* was an influential European precursor of a type of physiology text that became increasingly common in mid-nineteenth-century America. Published in a stereotype edition in Harper's Family Library series in 1836, Combe's title promised that these physiological principles would be "applied to the preservation of health, and to the improvement of physical and mental education." Physiology was in Combe's view nearly all-encompassing, since "in its widest sense" it embraced the study, maintenance, and interactions of bodily functions and processes. The object of studying physiology was "to secure for the organ the best health, and for the function the highest efficiency." This definition had significant implications for the conduct of life, for "a true system of physiology" was "the proper basis, not only of a sound moral and intellectual education, and of a rational hygiene," but it was also "the basis of every thing having for its object the physical and mental health and improvement of man."[32]

Combe echoed writers of orthodox health guides in denying any desire to teach nonprofessionals about medicine or disease treatment. Like those writers, he wanted to spread the kind of information that would allow individuals to maximize their physical and mental abilities. This knowledge would also help people avoid many illnesses and facilitate the recovery process when sickness did strike. Most fundamentally, understanding and following physiological principles would "fit each individual for the particular sphere in which the Creator intended it to exist."

Combe's overall purposes, then, were strikingly similar to those who wrote domestic health manuals. But his execution deviated sharply from that used both in household guides and the Faust texts. Combe systematically and thoroughly presented information about anatomy and physiology, deriving from that hygienic principles. Selective rather than exhaustive in coverage, he examined the "most influential . . . and . . . least familiarly known" body systems. Thus Combe included chapters on the anatomy and physiology of the skin, muscles, bones, respiration, and nervous system. Some systems—circulation, the senses, reproduction—he omitted entirely, while "others of essential consequence . . . , such as . . . digestion" he thought warranted only brief mention. Including the former, he argued, would have added unjustifiably to the welter of detail, while incorporating the latter would have been redundant, since treatises on digestion already existed.[33]

Most of the structures and functions Combe described were complicated, and he used some everyday examples to make the explanations easier to understand. Combe reminded his readers, for example, that coughing expelled foreign objects from the lungs "just as peas are discharged by boys with much force through short tubes by a sudden effort of blowing." Speaking of the skin's sebaceous glands, he likened one's size to "a millet seed." His most extended analogy simplified muscular action by comparing it to the working of a ship, which proved helpful at the end of a lengthy and technical passage.[34]

Combe, however, used few such comparisons in *Principles of Physiology,* a work intended for advanced rather than elementary audiences. Most of his text is scientific and theoretical, buttressed with information drawn from eminent medical authorities and clarified by a few illustrations. For example, Combe's description of muscular action is scientific, though he also concedes that muscles "are familiar to every one as constituting the red fleshy part of meat." Information on the skeleton is likewise given in scientific language, including the proper Latin names of bones. Combe's discussion of the backbone combines familiar and technical language. "The spine, vertebral column, or back-bone . . . ," he begins straightfor-wardly, "which supports all the other parts, is a very remarkable piece of mechanism. It is composed in all of twenty-four separate bones called *vertebrae,* from the Latin word *vertere* to turn, as the body turns upon them as on a pivot." From this point, the description becomes more complicated as Combe further distinguishes among the cervical, dorsal, and lumbar vertebrae, all of which rest on the sacrum. Further explana-tion, while certainly not beyond comprehension, is less easily accessible:

While the smooth or rounded forepart or *body* of the vertebrae affords support to the superincumbent parts, the projecting ridge behind, and rugged processes at the sides, combine with it to form a large tube or canal, extending from the top to the bottom of the column in which the spinal marrow is contained and protected. Between each of the vertebrae a thick compressible cushion of cartilage and liga-ment is interposed, which serves the triple purpose of uniting the bones to each other, of diminishing and diffusing the shock in walking or leaping, and of ad-mitting a greater extent of motion than if the bones were in more immediate contact.[35]

Despite Combe's technical presentation, he melded science and re-ligion.[36] The skin's structure, enthused Combe, "like that of every other part of the animal frame, displays the most striking proofs of the tran-scendent wisdom and beneficence of its great Creator." It was important to understand each part because God's plan mandated that "every part has a use or function peculiar to itself." Thus the structure of the cuticle, Combe explained, was "in admirable harmony with its uses," which in-cluded protection, touch, perspiration, absorption, and body heat. Be-havior that interfered with the skin's work should therefore be avoided or at least curtailed.[37]

Combe's purpose in covering the anatomy and physiology of the cuti-cle and other parts was to disseminate knowledge that could be prac-tically applied. Since bodily parts and functions were so inextricably interrelated, wrote the phrenologist, any transgression, regardless of its seeming insignificance, was harmful. The reverse was also true: an action that benefited one part would benefit all others.[38] Obviously, then, uninformed people were in constant peril because they would not be able to understand the consequences of their behavior. Unfortunately, few people seemed interested in learning about their bodies. Healthy people tended "to look upon the effects of air, food, exercise, and dress as very much matters of chance, subject to no fixed rule, and therefore little worth attending to, except when carried to palpable extremes, or in the cure of disease." This attitude, Combe complained, was counterproductive, because illness usually arose from bad habits that "gradually, and often imperceptibly . . . [ruin] the constitution before danger is dreamed of."

Much temporal harm could be averted simply by following the laws of nature, wrote Combe with assurance, rejecting the widely held idea that disease resulted from circumstances beyond man's knowledge and control, sent by a superintending Providence. After all, he reminded his readers, "The progress of knowledge, and the increasing ascendancy of reason, have already delivered us from many scourges which were regarded by our forefathers as unavoidable dispensations of an inscrutable Providence." Notable examples were plague, smallpox, and ague. For Combe, the only convincing explanation was that disease resulted from "the direct infringement of one or more of the laws or conditions decreed by the Creator to be essential to the well-being and activity of every bodily organ, and the knowledge and observance of which are to a great extent within our own power." Though these laws were "invariable and unchanging," they were not hard-and-fast rules that would guarantee good health if scrupulously followed. Instead, they were general principles, and sensible adherence to them would bring rewards. Moreover, because they were grounded in Divine authority, there should be no question about obedience.[39]

Evidently a large number of Americans were listening to Combe's message. The editors of the *American Medical Intelligencer* thought Combe's work had had a "surprising sale," two American reprints having been issued at their 1837 writing. Combe, they reported, had estimated twenty thousand sold in England and America within two and one-half years of its publication. "Perhaps no other work," they concluded, "has had a greater effect in diffusing a taste for the study of physiology through the community." British reformer Harriet Martineau also remarked on the great American popularity of Combe's *Principles of Physiology* as she traveled through the country in the mid-1830s. Characteristically acerbic, however, she judged Americans still poorly informed and lazy about matters of health and hygiene.[40]

There were many who agreed with Martineau's charges and sought to remedy the situation. The majority of them tried to reach the public through lectures, which had great appeal and authority during this period. Orthodox physicians generally applauded those lecturers, many of them women, who attempted in a serious and decorous manner to educate the public about anatomy and physiology.[41] In 1844 the *Boston Medical and Surgical Journal* praised these "energetic [and] popular teachers." They were "not a calamity, but a direct benefit . . . so long as they simply explain[ed] the mechanism of the human body, in connection with the elements of physiology." Lecturers increasingly used manikins, which simplified and improved their enterprise, not in the least because they replaced corpses for demonstration purposes, thereby substantially reducing the danger of offending or shocking the audience.[42] Some physicians, like the conservative William Workman, were more critical, charging that the public was "often misled, and sometimes corrupted, by the host of itinerant lecturers, 'professors' of 'physiology,' 'phrenology,' and 'psychology.'" What Workman deplored was "their too often indecent exhibitions of manikins and pictures, and . . . their low ribaldry and obscene jests under the guise of science." But Workman agreed that physicians did have an "important mission": to "instruct the people on medical subjects" in order to destroy quackery.[43]

Anatomy and Physiology for Children

Others during this period sought the same goals with different tactics, relying instead on the written word—and, for the first time, trying to educate young people. In the two decades following the publication of Combe's *Principles of Physiology,* nearly two dozen American authors produced popular anatomy and physiology texts. Most of the texts were reprinted several times, and many authors wrote more than one volume. Writers of physiology texts articulated increasingly concrete examples of the interconnections of structure, function, and behavior. Moreover, like the *Catechism of Health* and the *Principles of Physiology,* these volumes won acclaim from the medical profession.

Textbook authors comprised a varied group. Most were orthodox physicians with strong but divergent interests in reform, particularly in the areas of medical education, public health, and popular medicine. Many had formal affiliations with schools, primarily at the college or academy level. Several, including nonphysician Catharine Beecher, were heavily involved in improving educational opportunities for women. Most, if not all, were veteran lecturers, and often their books grew out of or accompanied that work. Certainly, their volumes complemented the nationwide efforts of both male and female lecturers on physiology, who attracted crowds during the middle decades of the nineteenth century.

Given his ideas about "Christian physiology," it comes as no surprise to find William A. Alcott prolific in schoolbook publishing as well. In the same year that Combe's *Principles of Physiology* appeared, the health reformer published *The House I Live In,* much of it reprinted from volume I of his young people's magazine, the *Juvenile Rambler.* The review in the *Boston Medical and Surgical Journal* praised Alcott's effort and chastised any physician who would "sneer at . . . teaching little people even the outskirts of a science . . . considered difficult for their seniors." Instead, argued the reviewer, regulars should support such efforts "to familiarize all classes of persons with the curious structure of their own bodies."[44]

Alcott's book broke new ground. Unlike Combe's *Principles of Physiology* or the Faust catechisms, *The House I Live In* was meant for children only. As a result, it is filled with clear illustrations, simple language, and common examples. Alcott's textbook also highlighted anatomy to an unprecedented extent. To be sure, many household health guides had brief sections on anatomy, but they were actually surveys aimed at adults and meant to aid in treatment. In contrast, guides to healthy living did not typically spell out the anatomical or physiological underpinnings for their hygienic advice. Alcott's book represented the first phase in the American development of a popular preventive literature grounded in anatomy, physiology, *and* hygiene.

Using the motif embodied in the title, Alcott portrayed the body as a modern frame house, two stories in height, featuring a cupola with windows and doors, two pillars, a great post, a number of rooms, furniture, and many functions. In addition to the extended house metaphor, Alcott employed scientific concepts and images, using commonplace comparisons to make them easier to grasp. For example, he likened the shape of "the hollow where the femur is fastened" to "the inside of an eggshell, with the small end broken off." The backbone's twenty-four separate pieces stood "on the top of each other, much like [a] pile of cups and saucers." The foot and its arch could be envisioned as a bridge with two abutments. Some joints he compared to common hinges, whereas others, he explained, "allow the parts that turn on them to move in every direction; but it would be hard to find a door that will open sideways, upwards, downwards, backwards, and forwards, with equal ease." Alcott's explanation of how muscles worked relied heavily on his readers' familiarity with ropes, particularly their properties when wet. In fact, he found it necessary to caution against interpreting his metaphor too literally. Wrote Alcott, "Nobody pretends these 'contrivances' will shrink by wetting them, as *ropes* do, but they will shrink *when we wish to have them.*" Beyond this, he could offer no explanation. "How our *thinking* or *wishing,* or *willing* to have them contract, can *make* them do so, nobody knows. On this point, the wisest philosopher is *almost* as ignorant as a child."[45]

Yet human comprehension was not essential for Alcott, because, like Faust and Combe, he attributed the body's construction to God. Alcott emphasized the pains "the Builder" had taken with the cupola, which encased and protected valuable and easily damaged goods. The result, he judged, was "a thousand times more ingeniously contrived, and wisely constructed, than if I had built it for myself." Even though there was much that people did not understand about their bodies, this did not weaken Alcott's conviction about the larger design. For instance, there were *"four little bones"* near the tympanum of the ear, and "nobody exactly knows for what purpose the Creator intended them." This did not trouble Alcott at all, because he was confident that "every part of [the ear] is useful." Moreover, marveled Alcott, "The Father of the Universe is the *Preserver* as well as the Creator of this 'wondrous frame.'" Look for proof, he wrote, at the joints, which would not function without lubrication. God had anticipated this need, providing *"synovia,* which answers all the [lubricating] purposes of oil or tar, [and] continually oozes out on the inside of the ligaments at the joints, and keeps the ligaments themselves, and the joints, soft and moist." Synovial fluid, Alcott pointed out, was "of just the right quality and quantity when we are in the most perfect health. If we are unwell, there may be too little or too much; or it may be too thick or too thin." It was therefore each person's responsibility to maintain his or her body in conformity with God's intentions.[46]

Alcott helped bridge two types of literature: older texts resembling both longevity guides and domestic manuals in their presentation of health advice, and newer ones that presented similar information in the context of anatomical and physiological knowledge. Much like William Buchan's *Domestic Medicine* had been in its genre, *The House I Live In* was a pioneer in its field. As physiology textbooks themselves evolved in tone, presentation, and content, Alcott's themes and techniques were borrowed, extended, and modified.

Two of Alcott's contemporaries, Jane Taylor and Worthington Hooker, wrote physiology texts aimed at the same very youthful audience. Taylor reverted to the catechismal style of Faust, but the contents of her books more closely resembled Alcott's. Taylor's evident interest in popularizing physiology makes it tempting to postulate a link with health reform. Such suspicions, however, remain speculative in the absence of biographical information.[47]

Taylor's *Primary Lessons in Physiology for Children* was first printed under a shorter title in 1839, and at least four stereotyped editions appeared before the revised version in 1848.[48] Like Alcott's, her book dealt primarily with anatomy rather than physiology or hygiene. Taylor also began with a house image, but she abandoned it in favor of lessons devoted to specific topics, usually different parts of the body. As she explained structures and their importance, Taylor, like Alcott before her, worked with everyday comparisons and familiar language. Thus her definition of the backbone made the one significant scientific term easily accessible. "It is," she wrote, "that which runs from the head down the back, and is made up of twenty-four round pieces, like twenty-four rings piled one above the other. These pieces are called *vertebrae*." Her explanation of how muscles enabled movement was equally prosaic. They functioned, she wrote, "by being lengthened out so as to be much longer at one time, and then again by shrinking up, so as to become much shorter than the natural length—just as we can make shorter or longer a thin piece of India Rubber." The skin, Taylor explained in another graphic portrayal, was "that which covers the body as the bark covers the tree." Nerves she defined as "small parts of the brain [which] run off in every direction through the body." The nervous system, by extension, constituted "those parts of the brain which are in small strings extended through the whole body." Lungs could be imagined as "pieces of soft flesh filled with holes or cells," resembling "a sponge." Yet she could not convey every process so simply to her readers. When discussing food, she candidly admitted ignorance about "[w]hat turns chyle into blood[.] No one has yet found out; neither do we know at what time it turns red."[49]

In 1858 Jane Taylor published another catechismal volume, *Wouldst Known Thyself, or The Outlines of Human Physiology*. "Designed for the use of families and schools," the profusely illustrated pamphlet sold for ten cents. Despite the title, Taylor once more focused primarily on anatomy rather than physiology. This time, however, she stressed hygiene as well, so that structure and behavior receive more attention than function. Her book contained, she boasted, "many useful hints about clothing, diet, exercise, health, and the care of the body generally." It was easy to see how desperately people needed this information "from the simple fact, that neither parents nor children understand a word of physiology, but leave all that relates to their physical training and health to chance and the care of the doctors." She hoped the book would open parents' eyes to

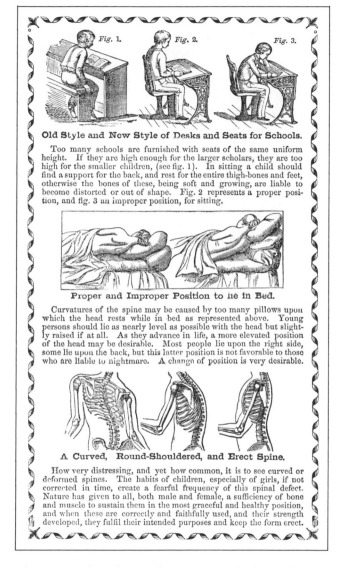

Old Style and New Style of Desks and Seats for Schools.

Too many schools are furnished with seats of the same uniform height. If they are high enough for the larger scholars, they are too high for the smaller children, (see fig. 1). In sitting a child should find a support for the back, and rest for the entire thigh-bones and feet, otherwise the bones of these, being soft and growing, are liable to become distorted or out of shape. Fig. 2 represents a proper position, and fig. 3 an improper position, for sitting.

Proper and Improper Position to lie in Bed.

Curvatures of the spine may be caused by too many pillows upon which the head rests while in bed as represented above. Young persons should lie as nearly level as possible with the head but slightly raised if at all. As they advance in life, a more elevated position of the head may be desirable. Most people lie upon the right side, some lie upon the back, but this latter position is not favorable to those who are liable to nightmare. A change of position is very desirable.

A Curved, Round-Shouldered, and Erect Spine.

How very distressing, and yet how common, it is to see curved or deformed spines. The habits of children, especially of girls, if not corrected in time, create a fearful frequency of this spinal defect. Nature has given to all, both male and female, a sufficiency of bone and muscle to sustain them in the most graceful and healthy position, and when these are correctly and faithfully used, and their strength developed, they fulfil their intended purposes and keep the form erect.

This unnumbered page from Jane Taylor's *Wouldst Know Thyself* (New York, 1858) typifies how authors of elementary anatomy and physiology texts used illustrations to underscore the perils of violating the laws governing bodily structures and functions.

"the wonders of our physical frame, . . . the wisdom and benevolence of the Creator in the adaptation of the parts to their ends," and the health consequences of their "carelessness, neglect, exposure, and indulgence."[50]

Again she used the house metaphor, very nearly quoting herself exactly. As before, Taylor chose not to persist with the analogy, but she did continue to use commonplace expressions rather than scientific terminology. Many of her comparisons were new ones, as was her explanation that skull bones "are united like two saws when the toothed edges are pressed together. To make this comparison more exact, the saw-teeth should be a little crooked, so as to hook into each other." Nor did she use scientific names when describing most of the other bones. The only leg bone she identified, for example, was the "knee-pan," as opposed to the patella. She followed the same practice in discussing the structure of the eye: "The globe, or ball of the eye, has three coats or coverings around it, the same as a ball with three covers, and is placed in a deep bony socket in the skull." The outside covering she called "the 'white of the eye.' It is quite hard," she continued, "and to it are fastened the muscles which move the eye in any direction desired by the will." Next *"spread over the inside of the middle covering of the eye"* could be found "a layer of very dark colored matter, which absorbs and softens the rays of light, after they enter the eye." Taylor gave no scientific appellation for the *"third or innermost covering of the eye,"* characterizing it as "a flattening out or expansion of the nerve which connects the eye with the brain, and . . . the immediate seat of sight."[51]

Taylor also discussed ways in which human beings differed from other animals, a theme which was to be elaborated in later physiologies. Humans, she summarized, possessed a proportionately larger brain, articulate language, reason, imagination, wit, and humor. Most important, though, was that man had "the moral or religious faculty; the faculty which tells man he *ought to do right,* and which gives him pain when he does wrong." This meant that people were "capable of being educated in a career of endless improvement." Animals, she emphasized, did not have the wherewithal to improve their situations: "the first beehive, the first anthill, the first bird's-nest, the first beaver's dam and dwelling-house, the first spider's web, have only been repeated through their countless generations, the last one being not only no more skillfully made than the first, but exactly like it."[52]

It was each person's duty to understand and obey all of God's laws, and physical rules could not be separated from moral laws. "Every family," she advised, "should possess one or more works on Physiology, to consult as they would a 'Family Physician,' and to teach them not only how to preserve health, but how health may be restored, when . . . it has become partially destroyed." Taylor recommended obtaining Edward Jarvis's *Practical Physiology,* William Alcott's *Laws of Health,* and Calvin Cutter's *Anatomy, Physiology and Hygiene.*

Though it was not on her list, Taylor might well have praised Worthington Hooker's *The Child's Book of Nature.* Like her texts and Alcott's, the Yale physician's volume was intended for less advanced pupils than the ones she actually recommended. First published in New York in 1857, Hooker's book had three separately paginated divisions to cover plants, animals, and the elements. The second part most resembles the work of Alcott and Taylor, beginning with Hooker's use of house imagery to describe the body's structure. "The body," he wrote, "is the house or habitation of the soul," a portable structure that could be "easily moved about, just as the soul wishes." For this reason, it had "a great deal of machinery in it." Important for proper functioning were the "little cords" of the soul "called nerves, running to all parts of this machinery, like telegraphic wires." Other types of machinery accomplished other jobs, such as respiration, digestion, and circulation. "The soul resides in the top of this house, the brain. Here, it sends out messages every where by the little cords, and receives message by them. Here it thinks and acts, and some of the time sleeps."[53]

Hooker likewise used unpretentious language and analogies drawn from daily life. Thus, to illustrate the fact that arteries were stronger than veins, Hooker wrote: "You sometimes see the hose of a fire-engine burst when they are working the engine very hard; but, though your heart pumps away sometimes so fast and hard, as when you have been running, not one of all the arteries gives way." To explain why and how the muscles moved, he reminded his readers that "[the mind] does not go out of the brain to them, just as a man goes out of his house among his workmen to tell them what to do." Instead, "there are white cords, called nerves, that go from the brain to all parts of the body, and the mind sends messages by these to the muscles, and they do what the mind tells them to do." Nerves could be imagined, he continued, as "act[ing] like the wires of a telegraph." Beyond this, explanation was more difficult. "This is done by electricity in the telegraphic office, but how the mind does it we do not know."[54]

There were other commonplace examples. Hooker used the increasingly conventional idea of India rubber to illustrate muscular activity, and he suggested examining a drumstick for an even more concrete example. The bones, he said, "are to the body what whalebones are to an umbrella, what timbers are to a house, or what the ribs of leaves are . . . to the leaves." The brain was also rendered in nonscientific terms; it was, explained Hooker, "the central work-shop of your mind; or it is like an engine-room of a factory, where the engine is that [which] keeps the machinery in other parts of the building in motion." Like Alcott and Taylor, Hooker spoke of the eye's construction without using scientific language. "What we call the white of the eye," he began, "is a strong, firm sort of bag. It is filled mostly with a jelly-like substance. . . . Into the open part of this, in front, is fitted a clear window." He continued the description in the same vein, concluding by sounding another theme found in the work of Alcott and Taylor: "No man could make . . . this shape, and have it work like this."[55]

Hooker celebrated God's handiwork throughout this volume. Speaking still of the eye, Hooker proclaimed what "a very wonderful instrument" it was. But God's majesty was evident in other body parts, including the joints which, because of synovial fluid, never required "oil[ing] . . . as men oil machinery." Moreover, human beings were but one example of God's wisdom, which was displayed throughout the animal world. As Hooker reminded his readers, "God has put thousands of [eyes] just as wonderful into the head of the fly that buzzes about you. It is as easy for him to make little eyes as large ones, and he can make a multitude as easily as one." Hooker strongly emphasized comparative anatomy, devoting nearly half his text to the anatomy and physiology of other creatures.[56]

These elementary physiologies, written by inveterate popularizers who tended to be doctors, were supplemented during the middle decades of the nineteenth century by more advanced physiology texts. The higher-level books used plain language and commonplace examples less frequently, employing instead more technical language and detailed engravings to illustrate the minute structures and complicated processes that they described. Authors of the more advanced texts also drew on the Combes' work, and they cited contemporary medical authorities on anatomy and physiology. An important achievement was to provide scientific but accessible demonstration of the inextricable connections between structures and functions on the one hand, and proper behavior, or hygiene, on the other.

Deriving Hygiene from Anatomy and Physiology

Physicians George Hayward and John L. Comstock published two of the earliest textbooks for more advanced students, and both were reprinted frequently,[57] Hayward, an eminent surgeon and pioneer in anesthesiology, served the medical profession in leadership and teaching positions throughout his life. His 1834 *Outlines of Human Physiology* delivered precisely what its title suggested: a summary of physiological knowledge. Like the elementary physiologies, Hayward's book combined an increasingly scientific orientation with a religious sensibility. As might be expected in a more advanced text, however, Hayward seldom used commonplace language or extended examples. Thus there were no metaphors about skeletal construction, joint action, or other bodily parts and functions. But Hayward deftly combined illustrations with the occasional explanatory phrase to clarify the scientific terminology. The cochlea of the ear, he said, received its name from its resemblance to a snail's shell, while the ear's vestibule "is, as its name imports, a sort of porch or entry, which communicates with all the other parts." Both parts were clearly labeled on the accompanying illustration. Hayward handled his discussion of the eye in much the same way, appending to it some general remarks about the physiology of vision.[58] Orthodox physicians praised Hayward's "plain, intelligible manner," as the reviewer in the *American Journal of the Medical Sciences* phrased it.[59] In fact, wrote contributors in the *Boston Medical and Surgical Journal,* the volume was so useful that at least one author, J. F. W. Lane, seemed to have plagiarized Hayward's text.[60]

Outlines of Human Physiology was unusual, however, in both format and content. For each subject, Hayward gave a historical overview of the development of physiological knowledge in that area. As a result, every few pages Hayward conceded the limits of current knowledge about one function after another. But Hayward's text differed in a second, more important way from other popular physiology texts, both elementary and advanced: Hayward's discussion rarely extended beyond physiology. Unlike the other writers, Hayward gave only enough anatomical information for the physiological information to be clear, and he offered no detailed behavioral rules, even in the sections on digestion and respiration, which attracted scores of nineteenth-century advisers. For other popular physiologists, discussing structure and function was the necessary prelude to the most critical subject, behavior. For Hayward, understanding physiology alone was a worthy and sufficient goal in itself, and it was left to the reader to make behavioral inferences.[61]

John L. Comstock's 1836 *Outlines of Physiology* was more representative of the emerging genre of popular anatomy and physiology textbooks for advanced students. Like the authors of elementary physiologies, Comstock used illustrations and questions at the bottom of his pages to reinforce important points. Comstock also took pains to demonstrate his scientific lineage, and he quoted at length from scientific sources—including the Combes, Alcott, and Hayward—where he thought appropriate. Like Hayward, Comstock used an occasional commonplace word to explain a scientific term. The spine, he wrote, "is the great central beam of the whole fabric of the skeleton." The clavicle, he said, received its name "from the Latin *clavis,* which appears to come from *clando,* to shut, this bone resembling in shape an ancient key." He added that it also went by the name of collarbone, which was probably more helpful to his readers. After covering the anatomy of the eye in a similar fashion, he discussed the mechanics of vision, providing the first extended treatment of that subject to appear in a popular physiology text.[62]

As was true of the other popular physiologists, Comstock had no trouble fitting his scientific ideas into a religious framework. In fact, part of the reason for including extended discussions of comparative anatomy and physiology was to reinforce the certainty of God's "Almighty power and Infinite wisdom." For Comstock, interlocking scientific and religious arguments underscored the importance of understanding anatomical and physiological laws so that they could be properly applied to behavior. Of particular interest to Comstock were exercise and sensible dress, to which he devoted a third of his volume.[63]

Physician Reynell Coates's 1840 *Physiology for Schools* combined features found in the texts published by Comstock and Hayward. To an even greater extent than had Comstock, Coates focused on comparative anatomy, an approach designed to "improve the reasoning power" of students and reveal "the universality of the physiological laws that should regulate the health, habits, and morals of man." Though Coates used few commonplace examples, he clarified his explanations by including over fifty illustrations and numerous review questions to highlight key points. Unlike his predecessors, Coates also suggested some simple experiments to help students grasp the structures and functions discussed in the text. Despite his scientific bent, Coates shared his colleagues' overarching religious perspective.[64]

Like Hayward, however, Coates expected his readers to be able to deduce correct behavior from anatomy and physiology. Coates did give some behavioral advice, particularly on dress, but his primary goal was to teach people about structure and function, not behavior. Yet Coates thought hygiene was important enough to include some specific information about behavior in hopes of demonstrating "the practical utility of facts and principles that may seem dull and uninteresting when not thus forcibly impressed." Coates, like most of his colleagues, took this educational crusade very seriously, devoting much of his life to writing for and lecturing to popular audiences.[65]

As other popular physiologists published textbooks, they increasingly spelled out proper behavior, linking rules of conduct to the structures and functions of different bodily organs and systems. Among them was one of the nation's foremost public health pioneers, John H. Griscom. Environmentalist Griscom, author of the pathbreaking 1845 *Sanitary Condition of the Laboring Population of New York*, first trained at the Rutgers Medical College and then received his medical degree from the University of Pennsylvania in 1832.[66] Griscom's 1839 *Animal Mechanism and Physiology* appeared in the same Harper's Family Library series in which Andrew Combe's had been printed. "Designed for the use of families and schools," Griscom's book acknowledged its indebtedness to Combe and adopted his method of covering anatomy, physiology, and hygiene. Like Combe, Griscom occasionally used everyday language to describe bodily structures and processes.

Unlike Combe's, however, most of Griscom's metaphors were mechanistic ones, consistent with his substitution of "animal mechanism" for "anatomy." This signaled, he explained, his decision to write of the human body "as a *machine,* composed of apparatus of various kinds, adjusted to each other in a surpassingly ingenious manner, carrying on their apparently incongruous operations without interruption from each other, and all working together for the attainment of the one great end for which the machine was devised with the most perfect harmony." Thus Griscom compared circulation to a city waterworks system and ventricular action to a bellows.[67]

But Griscom relied most heavily on scientific terminology. Though in footnotes he offered English translations for many Latin names, nearly ninety illustrations clarified Griscom's explanations more. His discussion of the visual apparatus is representative of his method. The accompanying eight illustrations are precisely labeled, and each part is allocated at least one full paragraph to explain its structure, function, location, and characteristics. To a greater extent than any of his American predecessors, Griscom also tried to elucidate vision, including "the nature of light," a highly technical topic involving principles of physics.[68]

Griscom's scientific and particularly chemical bent did not lead him to repudiate religion. Instead, his knowledge of science deepened his conviction that bodily structures and functions were all part of God's master plan. Learning more about the laws of chemistry had allowed Griscom to understand and appreciate many natural processes that had previously been beyond his grasp. Wrote Griscom, "Almost every change wrought in the composition of the material world, if within reach of the chemists, is capable of being understood and defined by him." Many bodily functions, like secretion or joint lubrication, eluded human comprehension but reaffirmed the power and wisdom of God. "To the mechanism of the joints . . . ," asserted Griscom, "we can point in full confidence . . . to establish incontrovertible proof of the existence of an Architect infinitely surpassing man in ingenuity of design and power of execution."[69]

Anatomy and physiology received nearly all of Griscom's attention, but he sprinkled behavioral inferences throughout. The reasons bad air and tight lacing were damaging, he explained, derived logically from the structure and functions of the chest and lungs. A "flexible elastic cage," the chest was designed to expand and contract in concert with the lungs during respiration. Impure air cheated the system by failing to replenish oxygen and overtaxing the lungs as they struggled to rid the body of wastes. Especially in combination with the constant restriction of tight lacing, bad air was "a practice baneful to the health, destructive to the intellect, subversive of the morals—it is *suicidal.*" Griscom also included an entire chapter on physiology and the effects of exercise. There he primarily explored the close connections between circulation and muscular action, and advised regular, moderate exercise to promote health. Again decrying tight lacing, he recommended calisthenics for females.[70]

Animal Mechanism and Physiology was, then, a clearly presented but technically dense exposition of human anatomy and physiology. Griscom went further than authors of other advanced texts in surveying anatomical and physiological principles with an eye to the behavioral rules they mandated. Yet Griscom's mechanistic analogies harkened back in time to increasingly outmoded ways of imagining bodily functioning.

Benjamin N. Comings chose Griscom's book as one of the models for his 1853 *Class-Book of Physiology,* but the resulting text embodied a slightly different and more progressive approach. A physician, Comings was also professor of physiology, chemistry, and natural history at the Connecticut Normal School.[71] Like Griscom, Comings used scientific language and numerous illustrations to explain anatomy and physiology to "schools and families." To make the scientific terminology as accessible as possible to his readers, Comings added a glossary and frequently translated Latin words into their English equivalents or more familiar language. His discussion of the brain, where he used both techniques, is representative. "The human brain," wrote Comings, "consists of two principal portions—the *cerebrum* or large brain, and the *cerebellum* or small brain." Readers could mimic the arrangement of the brain's gray and white matter by "taking two pieces of cloth, laying one upon the other, and collecting them up into folds in a globular shape." Accompanying illustrations depict the different parts of the brain and their relationship to the spinal cord and rest of the nervous system. Comings also recommended experiments to demonstrate more vividly the structures and processes he described. Like Griscom, though, this scientific orientation incorporated rather than excluded religion.[72]

Comings, like his predecessors, seldom spelled out the behavioral implications of the anatomical and physiological principles he discussed. As those writers had, he stressed that well-being and longevity would result only from obedience to "the laws by which [the body] may be preserved in health and vigor." Yet in only a few instances, primarily concerning dress, diet, and ventilation, did he give pointed instructions about behavior. He did add a chapter on the human form and an appendix to summarize rules of health.[73]

Hayward, Comstock, Coates, Griscom, and Comings were pioneers in producing anatomy and physiology textbooks for students in academies and colleges. Following the examples of Combe and others, each in his own style described the body's structures and functions from a scientific perspective that reinforced an overarching religious framework. Though each author helped to promote proper behavior by educating Americans about anatomy and physiology, each to a different extent left his readers with the task of inferring behavioral rules from the welter of anatomical and physiological details provided.

The Anatomy and Physiology Text Comes of Age

The work of these pioneers was significant, but their contributions are overshadowed by those of a triad who individually and together probably had the greatest influence in defining and popularizing the anatomy and physiology text: Edward Jarvis, Calvin Cutter, and Thomas Lambert. Beginning in the 1840s each man published a series of textbooks that remained in print well beyond the Civil War, and Cutter's family took up the banner from him.

Edward Jarvis, an orthodox Massachusetts physician, won fame for his innovative work with statistics and the insane.[74] His eighty-eight-cent *Practical Physiology for the Use of Schools and Families* came out in 1847 and remained in print until after the Civil War. Fifteen thousand copies of it were printed between 1847 and 1855, and the prestigious *American Journal of the Medical Sciences* immediately praised the four-hundred-page volume. But Jarvis realized that the book's length and level of difficulty made it inaccessible to younger children, and by the following spring had reduced the book by two-thirds. Titled *Primary Physiology, for Schools,* ten thousand copies of the shortened text were printed between 1848 and 1853.[75] The editors of the *Boston Medical and Surgical Journal* lauded the abbreviated version and its author. Jarvis, they wrote, was "a pattern of industry, . . . always doing or writing something for the promotion of the health, comfort and longevity of the present and coming generations." Deeming the new volume "handy" and essential, they thought it "contain[ed] the pith and marrow of a physiological library, adapted to the comprehension of those for whom it was written." Others must have agreed with this assessment, for *Primary Physiology* and a third volume, *Physiology and the Laws of Health,* were still in print in the mid-1870s.[76]

As had other popular physiologists, Jarvis began his *Primary Physiology* by defining anatomy and physiology, justifying their study as necessary "in order to understand the uses of our organs, the extent of their powers, and the purposes to which they may be applied." Like his predecessors, Jarvis believed that correct living was each individual's duty and that everyone had to learn about the principal bodily processes and organs. Otherwise, he asked, how could individuals have the informed awareness necessary to abide by the rules for right living? Superficial understanding could not provide sufficient incentive or knowledge to obey. To illustrate his point, Jarvis declared that "the sole object of the saliva is to moisten the mouth when it is still, and to wet the food when it is eaten." From this seemingly insignificant fact, many rules for proper behavior could be derived. "To excite the glands, and to increase the flow of this fluid for any other purpose, by chewing tobacco, or any matter excepting food, or by the offensive habit of spitting, is unnatural as well as disgusting." This perspective also highlighted the importance of the mouth as the site of mastication. The stomach, "merely a soft and fleshy bag," was not equipped to "do the proper work of the teeth upon the food." Since it was not designed "to crush hard substances or divide large morsels," the stomach that received poorly chewed items faced "a long and painful labor." Jarvis specified the implications with respect to food choice, which he said had to be made in "reference to its quantity and quality, to the frequency and the hours of eating, to the constitution, temperament, health, habits, and age of the person, to the season of the year, and to many other circumstances."[77]

Jarvis repeated this pattern, extrapolating from "the leading elementary principles of anatomy and physiology" to outline "their most obvious applications to the ordinary exposures and habits of life." For instance, the structure and functions of the lungs meant that it was important for buildings to be well-ventilated. Dirt hindered cutaneous processes, which led Jarvis to recommend clean clothes and bathing; for the latter he gave precise guidelines as to duration, water temperature, and time of day. Regular exercise and erect posture were essential for good muscle tone and overall bodily health. Jarvis's fairly systematic derivation of hygienic principles from anatomy and physiology—despite its essential simplicity—set the course that later physiologies adapted and modified.[78]

Like his colleagues, Jarvis sometimes avoided scientific words altogether, as in his discussion of the brain, but more frequently he used scientific terminology. Yet he did so in such a way as to translate technical words into familiar terms. The esophagus, for example, could be remembered as the gullet, and the lungs were called the *"lights"* in lower animals. Jarvis vividly characterized the stomach as an "oblong, soft, and fleshy bag," and he added that "the structure of [its] three coats is familiarly shown by examining a piece of tripe, which is a preparation of the cow's stomach." The muscular coat of the stomach, he continued, "is composed of stringy fibres, such as compose the lean meat which we see on our tables. These fibres have an active power of contracting or drawing themselves up, and thus diminishing their length, like the earth worm." In another passage, Jarvis wrote about heart valves that had "the same purpose as the valve of a pump-box, which opens to let the water pass upward, but closes and prevents its passage downward." To try to explain the articulation of the ribs and backbone, Jarvis likened it to the way "one part of a gate hinge moves in the other." Simplifying his description of respiration, Jarvis explained that "the chest expands and contracts like the bellows, and receives at each expansion as much air as its increased cavity can admit."[79]

Jarvis, like other authors of physiology texts, did not see his scientific orientation as incompatible with or undermining religious understanding. For him scientific and religious perspectives were mutually enhancing. Thus he praised God for "how fearfully and wonderfully we are made," equally astounded by "how nicely . . . all the works of the benevolent Creator [are] fitted to their intended purposes, and how beautiful are the harmonies between the organs and powers of the living body and external matter." He reminded his readers that part of God's gift to each individual had been the power of reason—and therefore the duty of maintaining health. No one was exempt; concluded Jarvis, "Every human being is . . . responsible for the care of his own health, and the preservation of his own life."[80]

Convinced of the need for his book, Jarvis sought to get it incorporated into school curricula, particularly in the Boston area. He was infuriated when a printing delay for *Primary Physiology* led the school committee to adopt instead a similar book by physician Calvin Cutter.[81] Originally published in 1847, Cutter's *First Book on Anatomy, Physiology, and Hygiene, for Grammar Schools and Families* was similar to Jarvis's. Cutter stressed prevention, knowledge about which should be acquired from a "complete" education that encompassed moral, intellectual, and physical teaching. For fuller explanations Cutter recommended one of his other volumes, among them his four-hundred-fifty-page *Treatise on Anatomy, Physiology and Hygiene*. First issued in 1845, it was intended "for colleges, academies, and families." He also suggested his *Second Book on Anatomy, Physiology and Hygiene*, this one intended for "academies, schools, and families." Another text, *Analytic Anatomy and Hygiene*, was issued in 1849 and twice revised. Several hundred thousand copies of these books were sold in the 1850s and 1860s, and the Cutter family continued to produce popular anatomy and physiology texts beyond the Civil War. In the 1880s, Cutter's son John wrote *Comparative Anatomy, Physiology and Hygiene*, completed while he was professor of physiology and anatomy at the Imperial College of Agriculture in Sapporo, Japan.[82]

The thrust of Cutter's *First Book* was indeed similar to Jarvis's aims in *Primary Physiology*. Like Jarvis, Cutter moved from definitions of anatomy and physiology to arguments about individual responsibility for understanding these subjects as well as hygiene. Cutter felt that this was crucial because "disease is under the control of fixed laws—laws which we are capable of understanding and obeying." However, he proceeded by a much more formal organization, taking the anatomy, physiology, and hygiene of each body system in turn, thus for the first time systematically linked behavioral advice to anatomy and physiology. Readers of the *First Book* could anticipate finding lengthy, detailed behavioral advice about a particular body system or function immediately following its anatomy and physiology. Cutter's textual arrangement exemplified and reinforced his argument that hygiene was inextricably connected with anatomy and physiology.[83]

Cutter used many of the same techniques found in other popular physiologies. Thus he employed commonplace examples to make his discussions more accessible, and he provided eighty-three engravings to help readers understand complicated explanations. Like Jarvis and their colleagues, Cutter attributed body structure and function to Divine intentions. Despite these meaningful similarities, Cutter's book embodied a distinctly more scientific perspective. It was, for instance, filled with proposed experiments, many of which entailed rudimentary anatomical or

378. The CEREBRUM, or larger portion of the brain, is composed of a whitish substance, with an irregular border of gray matter around its edges.

379. The CEREBELLUM is also composed of white and gray matter, but the latter constitutes the largest portion. The white matter is so arranged, that when cut vertically, the appearance of the trunk and branches of a tree (*ar'bor vi'tæ*) is presented.

Fig. 69.

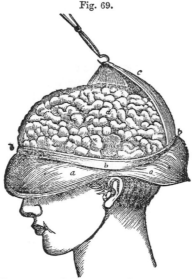

Fig. 69. *a, a*, The scalp turned down. *b, b, b*, The cut edges of the bones of the skull. *c*, The external membrane of the brain suspended by a hook. *d*, The left side of the brain, showing its convolutions.

380. The brain is surrounded by three membranes. The external membrane is thick and firm; the middle membrane is thin, and looks somewhat like a spider's web; the inner membrane consists of a net-work of blood-vessels.

---

378. Describe the cerebrum.   379. Describe the cerebellum.   380. What is said of the membranes of the brain?   What does fig. 69 represent?

Page 128 from Calvin Cutter's *First Book* (New York, etc., [1852]) is representative of his method of combining proper scientific terminology with commonplace language, detailed illustrations, and review questions.

dissecting work. The human spinal column would be better understood, Cutter suspected, if the reader examined one belonging to a dog, cat, or other domestic animal. The construction and working of the joints could be well illustrated by studying a fresh joint of a calf or sheep. Every body part would become more familiar if it were compared to its mate in another animal. Yet not all experiments involved comparative anatomy. Several demonstrated the workings of human veins and arteries, including the action of the pulse. Many aimed to teach scientific principles, such as the composition of the air or how respiration worked. Though Cutter was not the first to recommend experiments, he did include an unprecedented number.[84]

Cutter was also conscientious about using proper scientific terminology. Abhorring "low, vulgar terms," he recommended his "ample Glossary" or a dictionary for words beyond the reader's comprehension. Correct pronunciation of scientific terms was equally desirable, and he made certain that they were "divided into syllables, and the accented syllables designated." Cutter was thorough in his use of proper technical terms, as demonstrated by his treatment of the anatomy and physiology of vision. He labeled each part of the eye with its proper scientific appellation but carefully translated them when necessary into more common terms as well. "The SCLEROTIC coat is firm," he wrote, "and its color white; hence, it is frequently called the 'white of the eye.'" The "transparent" cornea "is shaped like the crystal of a watch," and the two-sided crystalline humor could, if boiled, "be separated into layers like those of an onion." Unlike Jarvis, Cutter covered the eye's physiology as well, using drawings and the laws of physics to explain vision. As in other sections, however, it was hygiene that was of paramount importance; understanding structure and function would make it possible to correct behavior.[85]

Cutter's *First Book* still had several features typical of the domestic health guide. Achieving and maintaining health should be every citizen's goal, but Cutter thought it was equally important to know "what *should be done,* and what *should not be done*" in the event of illness. The initial stages of disease were particularly important, for if the treatment then adopted were not "proper and judicious," the patient's "sufferings . . . are increased, and life, to a greater or less degree, is jeopardized." Accordingly, Cutter devoted five of his one hundred ninety-one pages to directions for "removal of disease," and a six-page appendix covered poisons and their antidotes. The physician, Cutter stressed, should have authority over the patient, but Cutter also provided guidelines about how to manage a sickroom.[86] This advice, however, included neither prescriptions nor details about specific diseases.

Cutter's other books followed the pattern of his *First Book,* with modifications according to the targeted audience. The 1850 *Treatise,* for example, was designed to teach older students about body structure, function, and derivative behavioral rules. Again Cutter included a glossary to promote the "use of proper scientific terms" rather than "vulgar terms and phrases." Cutter emphasized that he made "no pretensions to new discoveries in physiological science" but had chosen to draw on specified "able," "splendid," and "meritorious" works in the fields of anatomy, physiology, and hygiene. Cutter now boasted more than one hundred fifty engravings to make his text "more intelligible," and he reprinted the information on disease removal and antidotes for common poisons. Though his organization and aims were the same in his *Treatise* as in his *First Book,* Cutter did change his style: he consistently used technical language and gave more detailed explanations about each topic. Accordingly, the presentation was more dense, typically retaining or revising simple comparisons previously used but rarely adding new ones.[87]

Cutter's vision of the body, however, remained firmly rooted in a religious tradition, as his remarks on synovial fluid illustrate. "In this secretion," he asserted, "is manifested the skill and omnipotence of the Great Architect; for no machine of human invention supplies to itself, by its own operations, the necessary lubricating fluid." Even more amazing was that "it is supplied in proper quantities, and applied in the proper place, and at the proper time." Insights from science, including results of experiments, strengthened rather than diminished religious faith.[88]

Physician Thomas S. Lambert, professor of anatomy and physiology at the Pittsfield, Massachusetts, Young Ladies' Institute, also wrote a series of physiology texts. Two appeared in 1850: *Practical Anatomy, Physiology and Pathology; Hygiene and Therapeutics* and *Popular Anatomy and Physiology.* The following year Lambert produced *Pictorial Physiology* "for the youngest class of scholars, . . . to excite in their minds a desire to know themselves, and to study the wisdom and greatness of the Creator." Often bound with *Pictorial Physiology* was another of Lambert's texts, the 1851 *Hygienic Physiology.* Though the titles changed, Lambert textbooks were still in print in the 1870s.[89]

After cursory examination, the editors of the *Boston Medical and Surgical Journal* predicted all three publications would be worthwhile, living up to the reputation Lambert had already established with his other books and lectures. Earlier J. D. Mansfield had fulsomely praised Lambert's *Second Book* in the same journal, having been particularly impressed by its straightforward style, practical bent, and scientific orientation. It was, concluded Mansfield, "up to the present state of anatomical and physiological knowledge." Moreover, wrote Mansfield, the medical profession should appreciate Lambert's educational efforts; this book, like the lectures he had given all over the Eastern and Middle states, always warned against quacks. Mansfield need not have worried about orthodox reception, for the journal's editors had always looked favorably on Lambert's lectures.[90]

Reviewers also raved about Lambert's *Popular Anatomy and Physiology,* among them Mansfield again, who called it the best work of the type he had ever read. "He forgets," explained Mansfield, "all technicalities, except so far as they are absolutely necessary in elucidating his subject." So impressed was he that he thought "no one should be considered as having even a common-school education, who is not familiar with the general principles of anatomy and physiology." The *Boston Medical and Surgical Journal* editors concurred, judging that "the text is correct, the inferences appropriate, and [it is] void of technicalities." Equally laudable, they thought, were its copious illustrations, including four lithographic plates.[91]

"Adapted to the use of students and general readers," *Popular Anatomy* treated each body system in turn except, of course, reproduction. As Mansfield and others had observed, Lambert both stressed orthodox superiority over quacks and delineated lay responsibilities in medical care. Lambert conveyed much of this kind of information in footnotes, as when he warned against "lotions, plasters, and all this class of things so commonly used" for sprains and similar ailments. Another note cautioned that it was "absurd" to think "that one medicine shall cure all diseases having the same symptoms" or "that any [one] medicine or course of treatment shall cure all diseases." It was the *cause* of disease that was important. Thus it would be "folly" to try "'doctoring' signs or symptoms, or administering remedies without great knowledge, the result of study and experience, and especially without a knowledge of the *cause* of the symptoms exhibited."[92]

Not all disease or first-aid information was relegated to footnotes. Textual information on treatment also emphasized the physician's primacy in sickness. Though Lambert recommended surgical aid for dislocated or broken bones, he bowed to expediency and included brief advice on how to manage them. He discussed some diseases because he believed that early diagnosis would greatly improve the patient's prognosis. Among them were "hip disease" and "diseases of the spinal cord," both of which required expert nursing and "a person of real science, skill, judgment, and industrious patience to investigate and apply." Lambert also advised readers to follow the doctor's orders in eye complaints, measles, mumps, smallpox, scarlet fever, and other ailments. Additional first-aid instructions explained what to do in cases of poisoning or gas inhalation. Lambert relied on eminent medical authorities from start to finish, but he also frankly acknowledged the limitations of medical knowledge and expertise.[93]

Lambert's overarching goal, however, was to educate people about anatomy, physiology, and hygiene. His book abounds with scientific terminology and detail, making it extremely theoretical and densely argued. Explanations are accessible primarily because Lambert made liberal use of illustrations and carefully translated scientific language into everyday words. A good example of his technique is Lambert's forty-page chapter on the eye, where he set himself the ambitious task of explaining human vision. Other popular physiologists, particularly John Griscom, had taken stabs at this process, but most had rested content with discussing the most obvious structures of the eye.[94]

Like the other writers, Lambert used commonplace examples to simplify his descriptions of the parts of the eye. Many definitions, in fact, sounded familiar. "[The lens]," said Lambert, "is composed of layers like an onion. . . . The outer layers are almost liquid, the next like jelly in consistence, the middle of the lens being almost like gum-arabic for density." Lambert borrowed other definitions as well, including those for the sclerotic coat, the cornea, and the humors. But Lambert also mentioned many parts that the others had typically omitted. "The tear apparatus" was one, "consist[ing] of a small organ, about the size and form of a sparrow's egg, of a whitish-yellow color." Another part seldom examined was the "ciliary (like the eyelashes) processes" that connect the lens to the choroid; they "do not . . . resemble," said Lambert, "[eyelashes], but more resemble a plaited, narrow ribbon."[95]

Thus Lambert delved much more deeply into the eye's structure than had his predecessors. His discussion was even more unusual in its attempt to explain the mechanism of seeing, which necessarily involved principles of physics. The explanation, both of structure and function, was enhanced by plentiful illustrations—twenty-three in the forty-page chapter—and numerous suggestions for experiments.

Lambert used a similar organization and expressed the same concerns in his 1854 *Hygienic Physiology,* but the later book was more accessible since it was not so theoretically dense or freighted with scientific terminology. Again he emphasized that physiological knowledge would help people recognize quacks and stay healthy. Once more Lambert warned against self-treatment and gave advice about how to identify legitimate practitioners. Still convinced of the wisdom of preparing readers for emergency situations, Lambert covered bleeding, fits, drowning, choking, and poisoning. Nonprofessional action had to be suited to the severity of the case. For both drowning and choking, he explained how to cut into the windpipe if necessary; fits, however, elicited advice to send for "the skilful physician" and to take no further action until his arrival.[96]

As he had done in *Popular Anatomy,* Lambert frequently invoked contemporary medical authorities where appropriate, but he did not try to hide medical ignorance. "How the ends of the nerves terminate in the muscle we no more know than we do how they commence in the brain," he confessed. Along with factual documentation of bodily functioning, Lambert continued to credit God with the body's superb construction and working. From God's design also could be deduced behavioral rules, as Lambert made plain in some remarks about the skull: "When such extraordinary pains have been taken by our Creator to prevent jars of the brain, we should never unnecessarily jump from great heights, nor should we give or receive avoidable blows upon the head."

Scientific experimentation was not incompatible with Lambert's perspective; among his suggestions was one to demonstrate how the lungs worked: "Obtain a pair of uncut lights or lungs of an animal, with a piece of the windpipe attached. With a tube, blow into the pipe and fill all the air-cells, and the lungs will be enlarged and appear beautifully. As soon as the mouth is taken from the pipe the lungs contract instantly, and with considerable force expel the air." Obviously, then, the chest expanded and then diminished with the air flow, and hygienic rules could be inferred. Anything that interfered with the free and easy movement of the chest and abdomen would similarly restrict a person's ability to breathe.[97]

As readers tried to avoid bad habits, they should not go to the opposite extreme and become overly preoccupied with health. Fanaticism would be as harmful as neglect. People should arm themselves with knowledge and be guided by common sense. The key was to develop a sensible, moderate approach to living, especially in matters related to exercise, diet, pure air, and cleanliness. "Regular habits," Lambert summarized in *Popular Anatomy and Physiology,* "in every respect should be formed, and a cheerful, amiable, and active state of mind must be cultivated and preserved." If sickness did intrude, Lambert enjoined, physical and mental rest were essential, "and all the laws of health must be more strictly observed." Do not, he concluded, "oppose nature. If . . . she need[s] assistance, . . . those best qualified by honesty of feeling, natural talent, acquired knowledge, and experience, are the only persons in whom confidence can be placed."[98]

Physiology texts by the time of Lambert's writing were quite different from the earliest elementary schoolbooks of Alcott, Taylor, and Hooker. Following and then elaborating on Andrew Combe's example, American authors gradually moved toward an increasingly standardized textbook that would offer systematic coverage of all body structures and functions. The mid-century period witnessed important strides in this direction, as the pioneering work of popular physiologists brought an unprecedented amount of explicit anatomical and physiological information before the American public. By mid-century, roughly twenty years after the first popular anatomy and physiology text appeared, medical authors were placing growing emphasis on hygiene, the behavioral rules derived from the facts of anatomy and physiology. They were not alone in this enterprise, sharing the task with writers who embarked on the same crusade from a nonprofessional vantage point.

Hygiene to the Fore

Worthington Hooker, bastion of the medical establishment, stressed hygiene in his 1854 *Human Physiology*, "designed for colleges and the higher classes in schools, and for general reading." Like authors of other physiology texts for every level, he used examples taken from everyday living to help explain body structures and functions.[99] Though Hooker emphasized that his book focused on physiology over hygiene and anatomy, he repeatedly drew behavioral or functional conclusions from physiological facts. For example, he described in detail the anatomy and physiology of respiration, covering the functions of the lungs, bronchial tubes, pleura, ribs, and diaphragm. Because the work done by the lungs is so crucial to life, he explained, "extraordinary provisions are made to secure an abundance of room for them under all circumstances." Conclusions about hygiene were inescapable. To begin with, it seemed obvious that it must be harmful to interfere in any way with lung function. If anything hindered chest expansion, blood quality would suffer, which would weaken the system and increase the lungs' susceptibility to disease. Women's clothing was particularly injurious, wrote Hooker, and he demonstrated with drawings contrasting the unfettered form of Venus de Medicis with that of "a lady with an artificially small waist." Having said this much, Hooker abruptly halted: "The subject is an important one; but as this book is not designed to treat of hygiene, I can not go into it further."[100]

Yet again and again the orthodox physician gave hygienic advice in the middle of a physiological discussion, because he thought that physiology and anatomy were the means to a more important end, "the principles and rules of Hygiene." Once people understood how the organs functioned, it would be easy for them to learn "what those circumstances are which favor their due performance, and what those are which interfere with it." Why was this important? Not surprisingly, Hooker's response matched that given by other popular physiologists: the "causes of disease . . . are more or less under our control. Some of them are entirely so. A knowledge of their operation, and an earnest endeavor to remove them, would, therefore, vastly diminish the amount of ill health and disease." Thus it was imperative, declared Hooker, that people awaken from their "blind indifference" and become more attuned to preventive living. Like his colleagues, Hooker looked to schoolroom instruction in physiology to help remove "the prevalent indifference" and reinforce good habits. The *Boston Medical and Surgical Journal* concurred in this judgment and felt that Hooker's *Human Physiology* would be a valuable aid in this work.[101]

In his book, Hooker had little to say about medical treatment, but William A. Alcott took the opposite approach in his profusely illustrated *Lectures on Life and Health; Or, The Laws and Means of Physical Culture.* Published in Boston in 1853, the book, aimed "for the 'million,'" was meant to be the quintessential expression of Alcott's ideas on health.[102] Life expectancy could be lengthened, preached Alcott, because disease did not result from Divine appointment, malevolent agency, or chance occurrence. Rather, it had human origins, arising because of identifiable moral and physical transgressions. As Alcott explained, "God has established certain laws within the organic domain, as well as without it, which are as fixed—as immutable—as those which were given at Sinai." Everyone had the choice between obedience, which would have "its appropriate reward," and disobedience, which would have an "appropriate and irrevocable penalty." In short, "man . . . , under God," is "the artificer of his own health and happiness." Alcott drove home his point with a striking image. Both health and disease, he said, were "products[s] of manufacture, just as truly and certainly, as cloth, paper, or pins." Manufacturing health entailed avoiding harmful behavior as well as taking positive steps, and there were no acceptable excuses for failing to adopt a healthy lifestyle.[103]

Doctors had a special role to play in increasing American life expectancy. "Physicians who are worthy of the name . . . should be philanthropists . . . [and] reformers" at the forefront of the educational effort. Or, as Alcott phrased it elsewhere, "[a physician] must be essentially a missionary of health." Engaged in work as important "as that of the moral or religious teacher," he would have to be always assiduous as he thus "indirectly . . . spread the gospel of the soul."[104]

These remarks were ancillary to Alcott's central purpose of providing the "mechanism and laws" of different systemic functions. He began with digestion, he wrote, "not so much on account of the superior claims of the subject," but because of the centrality of digestion to other bodily functions. Alcott's "mechanism" of digestion began with the ingestion of food and briefly described the various organs involved and their structures. The laws of digestion followed, which, explained Alcott, were primarily "based on structure, and derived from it; and are all in harmony with it." Since structure and function determined proper behavior, Alcott reasoned, people should view food and cooking as "semi-religious concerns," because "for every act, at every age, which weakens their constitution, they are answerable, if not to any human tribunal, at least to a divine." Alcott treated all other body parts and systems in the same manner, and for each drew specific behavioral rules from anatomy and physiology. Without a doubt, people should learn about their bodies, concluded Alcott, for "it is high time for reason, and science, and Christianity to triumph over the customs of ignorance, superstition, and heathenism."[105]

Catharine Beecher echoed Alcott's concerns. Born in Long Island in 1800, Beecher was the eldest daughter of reform-minded Presbyterian minister Lyman Beecher and his wife, Roxana Beecher. Instilled from youth with her father's aspirations and moral fervor, Beecher made her life's crusade the improvement of the American race, particularly women and children. In 1823 she founded the Hartford Female Seminary, later opening other schools for women in Cincinnati and Milwaukee. Particularly in the 1840s, she traveled incessantly to promote her ideas about women's education, which included the necessity of physical exercise and instruction in anatomy and physiology. She also wrote books to publicize her beliefs, cementing her reputation with the 1841 *Treatise on Domestic Economy,* which was adopted for use in Massachusetts public schools within two years of publication. *Letters to the People on Health and Happiness* appeared in 1855, followed the next year by *Physiology and Calisthenics,* her most distilled statement on the subject.[106]

Most schoolbooks on these topics, Beecher charged in *Physiology and Calisthenics,* were "repulsive" and intimidating because they were "so encumbered with terms needed only by professional men"; she, on the other hand, prided herself on using "no technical term . . . when a word in common use will express the same idea." Furthermore, her proffered course was "*short, easy,* and *comprehensive,*" largely because it included only those details "that can be made *practical* in enforcing the laws of

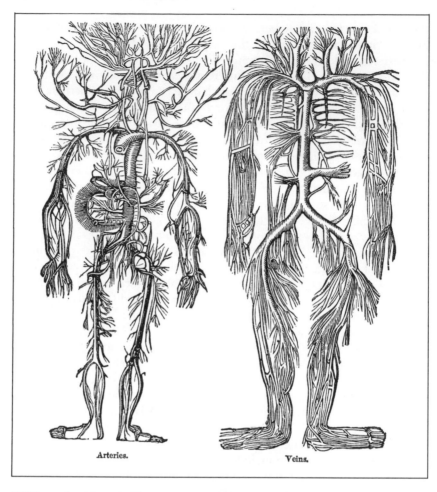

Arteries.   Veins.

William A. Alcott's illustration of the circulatory system in *Laws on Life and Health* (Boston, 1853), p. 173, reinforced his repeated warnings that injury to one part of the body inevitably injured all other parts.

health and life." Beecher also bragged about having produced a work "so popular in form" that it would appeal not only to children but to their parents as well. This, Beecher thought, was crucial, for "the main hope of the adult generation is through the knowledge that may be carried by the children to their homes, and there rendered practical." She anticipated a wide distribution; having successfully "been tested with the humblest class of uneducated persons," the work was equally "fitted to the comprehension of the young and uneducated" and to "the wants of the highest class of minds."[107]

Beecher appended the section on calisthenics to the end of her volume, so that it followed her discussion of physiology, "*the reasons* for all these rules and exercises." There were, she said, "two grand causes of . . . ill health and physical deterioration: . . . first, a want of *knowledge* of the construction of the body and the laws of health; and, next, a want of *thought* and *conscience* on the subject." Something had to be done, for both children and adults seemed to be experiencing increasingly poor health. As Beecher explained, since "feeble and sickly fathers and mothers sel-

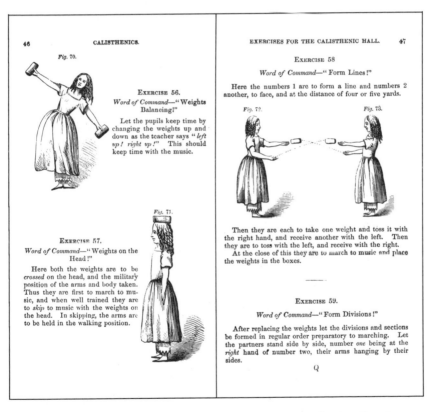

In addition to covering anatomy and physiology, Catharine Beecher included a formal exercise program in her *Physiology and Calisthenics* (New York, 1856). As the illustrations on pp. 46–47 suggest, Beecher targeted women as her primary audience.

dom have strong and healthy children[,] . . . the more parents become unhealthy the more feeble children will be born. And when these feeble children grow up and become parents, they will have a still more puny and degenerate offspring." To avoid national catastrophe, "some great and radical change" seemed imperative. Beecher encouraged her readers to participate in this public and private health reform by attending weekly lectures and lessons, preferably *"illustrated by specimens."* To guarantee that the instruction would be "interesting and lucid," she encouraged using "models, drawings, and manikins," as well as butcher's samples of "the most important bones of the body, the windpipe and lungs of some animal."[108]

Beecher envisioned her text as playing an important role in hastening this reformation, especially among women. The first part of *Physiology and Calisthenics* is devoted to bodily functions, excluding, like the rest of the genre, reproduction, despite its intended female audience. Beecher used a scientific orientation, including occasional suggestions for simple experiments. One proposed soaking a bone in acid to see the results, and another encouraged readers to trace the construction of cartilage, ligament, bone, and muscle in a fowl's leg.[109]

Beecher's descriptions, though clear and concise, were not as technically detailed as those being used by her medical counterparts. In speaking of the eye, for example, she distinguished "the white of the eye," "the middle coat, which is black," and the retina. She also pointed out the eye's three humors: the vitreous humor, which "is the dark portion, . . . fills the largest part of the eyeball [, and] looks like jelly"; the aqueous humor, which "looks like water"; and the crystalline humor, "which is white, hard, and shaped like a *lens*." Accompanying illustrations gave more specific information about nerves, tears, and muscles, but Beecher simply omitted "many other beautiful and curious contrivances about the eye."[110]

To a much greater extent than did her medical contemporaries writing physiology texts, Beecher chose to focus on hygiene, or the rules for living that were derived from physiology. Even in the chapters about structure and function, she repeatedly documented types of behavioral abuse, especially with respect to the thorax, pelvis, and spine. Beecher also used the entire middle part of *Physiology and Calisthenics* to spell out the hygienic rules for each physiological process previously covered. Wrote Beecher, "The rules for the proper treatment of the various organs of the body are called *the laws of health and happiness,*" because God rewards the obedient with health and penalizes the disobedient with illness. Because God intended humans to be happy, they had the God-given gifts of reason, conscience, and experience that made well-being possible. People who failed to use these tools "sin[ned] against both God and [themselves]."[111]

Beecher's object was to help people follow God's commands by explaining the laws of health and specifying what constituted proper and improper behavior. This she did systematically and in detail. Over and over she stressed the necessity of proper nourishment, exercise, pure air, light, and clothing. Always behavior was to be attuned to the designated duties performed by the bodily function under discussion. The lungs, for instance, had "two offices to perform: one is, to prepare the food sent from the stomach by adding the oxygen of the air to the chyle; the other is, the emptying out from the body the carbonic acid and water which are formed in the capillaries by the union of this oxygen with the decayed particles of the body." Since every pair of lungs used one hogshead of air per hour, anything impeding the delivery of this much air to the lungs was to be avoided—whether poorly ventilated and overcrowded rooms, tight clothing, or poor posture—and everything promoting respiration was to be encouraged. But multitudes violated these rules.[112]

Similar principles applied to diet, and Beecher provided a great deal of information about the quality and quantity of food as well as the frequency, speed, and hours of eating. Other topics she treated in the same manner, concluding with a warning: in the short term, the body would compensate for virtually any kind of abuse, so a person's bad habits would not necessarily produce "any immediate or perceptible injury." Obviously, people had to learn about their bodies and the laws that governed them. This campaign would have to include men and women, boys and girls:

> Mankind will never obey the laws of health till they know what they are, and what are the penalties of disobedience. To secure this, they must be made to understand the construction of their bodies, the functions of the different organs, and their modes of healthful action. They must learn the nature of the air they breathe, of the fluids they drink, and of the food they eat and the influence of their habits, customs, and employments on the health of their bodies. When they do understand all this, then reason, conscience, self-love, domestic affection, and religion will all furnish motives to secure obedience to laws that are seen to be wise, and sustained by penalties that, though slow, are inevitable.[113]

Burgeoning Interest in Physical Fitness

What were the results of this proliferation of school texts in anatomy, physiology, and hygiene? How influential were they? It is difficult to measure precisely their impact, either in terms of people's lives or incorporation into school curricula. Though there was clearly demand for their introduction, their acceptance was neither automatic nor universal. Not until after the Civil War do they seem to have met with much success outside of urban areas in the Northeast.[114] The *Western Journal of Medicine and Surgery* offered insight into the situation when an American translation of Frenchman Milne Edward's *Physiology and Animal Magnetism* appeared in 1841.[115] "From the number of these elementary books, which have been published within the last 12 or 15 years," the editors wrote, "it might be supposed that the demand for them has been very great." This was an erroneous assumption. "Each has been to a certain extent, a failure," they claimed. Why was this so? Critics downplayed any defects in the volumes themselves, placing greater weight on "the difficulty of introducing a new study into our academies; especially when it presents no *prima facie* claims to utility, in the vulgar acceptation of that term." Though they did not mention it, prevailing notions of propriety and delicacy often constituted formidable barriers to acceptance.[116] Even anatomical instruction for medical students and physicians met tremendous public opposition during this period, and only a handful of states managed to enact legislation to support such endeavors.[117]

Though exact measurement is elusive, it is obvious that physiology texts revealed and contributed to larger movements advocating healthier personal habits, among them more sensible dress and greater physical exercise.[118] Much of the initial impetus can be traced to the first large nineteenth-century wave of German immigrants; they brought with them to America the *Turnen* system of gymnastics, developed early in the century by Friedrich Ludwig Jahn to build German strength and unity. Americans expressed much interest in the new gymnastics during the late 1820s and early 1830s, but it was not sustained. A physician in 1837 ridiculed the system, saying it was "better adapted to the Spartan youth than to the pallid sons of pampered cits, the dandies of the desk, and the squalid tenants of attics and factories."[119]

Others attested less cynically to the intensity and brevity of the early interest in gymnastics. Unitarian clergyman Edward Everett Hale recalled his fear when taken by his brother to a Boston gymnasium in 1827 or 1828. Years later, all he could remember was his "terror" after he had "climbed up a ladder and cut off [his] retreat." He "had seen the other boys climb between the rounds and slide down the pole which supported the ladder, and [he] wished to do this." Though he "got through the rounds" successfully, he "then was afraid to slide." At this juncture, fortunately, "a competent teacher . . . instructed me in the business, and I won the high courage by which to loosen my feet from the rounds and slide safely down." When he reached home he told of his adventures "with delight, but never repeated the experiment."

Hale evidently demonstrated little athletic prowess in other areas, recording only marginally greater success in learning to ride a horse. Swimming seemed better suited to his abilities and interests, and he spoke enthusiastically about his experiences at the swimming school established along with the gymnasium. Instructional techniques were extremely crude, consisting of shouted directions to the novice, who wore a rope attached under his arms. Slow learners and weaklings, among whom Hale counted himself, "were a whole summer before they could be trusted without the rope." But that did not diminish his pleasure, for "the training was excellent, and from the end of that [ninth] year till now I have been entirely at home in the water."

"The drift for athletics," Hale recorded, at the same time "swept over the Latin School," and the square yard at the rear of the building "was fitted up with a vaulting-horse, parallel bars, and so on." By the time Hale entered the Boston school in 1831, however, "the fad" was "[wearing] itself out," and the equipment was neither repaired nor replaced.[120]

Eminent surgeon John Collins Warren also described the Boston gymnasium, having served as president of the society that organized it. Opening to great success in the mid-1820s, it was frequented, Warren said, by "a great number of gentlemen of the different professions." Moreover, it "acted contagiously on the city and country. Small gymnasiums were established, in connection with most of the schools, academies, and colleges, male and female." Warren found it particularly satisfying that "literary men, who had been perishing in groups for want of air and exercise, could as in Germany and England, be able to maintain their health, without interfering with their mental occupations." Like Hale, though, Warren regretfully acknowledged that "the spirit of physical cultivation has gradually become feeble." There were, to be sure, still some gymnasia, and "the educated part of the community" had become informed about the necessity of physical as well as moral and intellectual education, but he thought physical exercise was no longer allotted the attention it deserved.[121]

Though interest waned, it was rekindled with the post-1848 influx of *Turners*. By the end of the following decade, they had established gymnastic societies, *Turnvereine,* all over the country. New and colorful popularizers appeared, among them George Windship ("the Roxbury

Hercules") and the inimitable Dioclesian Lewis, the father of the "New Gymnastics," which became the national rage in the early 1850s.[122]

There was, as well, some curricular incorporation of anatomical and physiological study. At Amherst the subjects had been sporadically taught before Edward Hitchcock took them over in the 1820s, but he complained that the school "had not a single anatomical model or preparation, not even a skeleton, nor any of the large works on anatomy; and of course the instruction given must be very meagre." Though he had no formal training in anatomy, the author of the 1830 *Dyspepsy, Forestalled and Resisted* taught the course for decades. In 1843, exasperated by the poor teaching aids, Hitchcock used his own money to buy "a seven hundred dollar manikin, with a skeleton, and many other models." If undergraduate William Gardiner Hammond, Jr., was representative, Hitchcock had a receptive audience. In October 1847 Hammond noted the beginning of the then-president's lecture series, recording in his diary: "think these will be interesting; have always fancied the subject."[123]

Women were not overlooked in this educational innovation, and a student at nearby Mount Holyoke called Hitchcock's 1844 lectures "*exceedingly* interesting." Exercise also became part of the curriculum at many female academies. The same Amherst undergraduate, in fact, commented on having seen "some of the young ladies exercise in calisthenics, a species of orthodox *dancing* in which they perambulate a smooth floor in various figures. . . . The whole movement is accompanied by singing, in which noise rather than tune or harmony seems to be the main object."[124] Hammond was not very impressed with this so-called advance in female exercising. Indeed, the opportunities for girls and women did continue to lag behind that for boys and men, but the middle decades of the nineteenth century constituted an important period for female education in America. A number of female seminaries were particularly significant crucibles for change, primarily because of the work of three pioneers. In addition to Catharine Beecher's efforts as outlined above, Emma Willard opened the Troy Female Academy in upstate New York in 1821, and Mary Lyon began Mount Holyoke Seminary in 1837. Each developed systems of physical education for women, and Willard even made physiology a part of the curriculum, despite having to cover up pictures of the human body to satisfy the standards of propriety. Elizabeth Blackwell, the nation's first accredited woman doctor, likewise advocated more exercise for women and denounced tight lacing.[125]

All of these women traveled extensively to promote their ideas. Their campaigns also received energetic, unceasing support from Sarah Josepha Hale, who used *Godey's Lady's Book* to try to improve the health and well-being of American women and children. As part of her campaign, Hale regularly recommended popular medical books, including anatomy and physiology texts. She praised, for instance, John Griscom's *Animal Mechanism and Physiology,* and she endorsed two different editions of Reynell Coates's *Physiology for Schools.* The powerful editor also found George Hayward's *Outlines of Human Physiology* satisfactory, being particularly pleased with Hayward's "propriety and delicacy" in treating subjects about "which both sexes should be instructed." In 1841 she issued a pronouncement on the utility of anatomy and physiology texts. "An acquaintance with anatomy and physiology has now become," wrote Hale, "as it ought long ago to have been, indispensable to every person of any pretensions to a complete—nay, to an ordinary education."[126]

Even if anatomy and physiology texts were not immediately accepted everywhere as legitimate curricular offerings, the influence exerted by their appearance was far from negligible. For most writers, school texts represented only one facet of a larger, more all-inclusive effort to achieve a healthier society. Their outpourings exposed and contributed to a massive mid-century interest in health and medicine. In tandem with phrenological and Pestalozzian ideas about educating the whole individual, emphasis on anatomy, physiology, and hygiene helped direct the nation's attention to the importance of each citizen's physical condition and well-being. The crusaders, then, were victorious, even if not precisely in their own terms.

During the same mid-nineteenth-century decades, there were many other advocates of healthy living. Among the most prolific were hydropathists, homeopathists, and quasi-professional women. Though each in varying ways and to different degrees posed a threat to the medical establishment, orthodox physicians endorsed their efforts to enlighten American citizens about healthy living. It is to this story that we now turn.

6 The Unorthodox Physician

Many kinds of written health information flourished in antebellum America. Domestic health manuals, guides for right living, medical articles in the popular press, and schoolbooks addressed the many-faceted issues of sickness and well-being. Orthodox physicians selectively supported efforts to disseminate health information, opposing works that they thought assigned too much treatment responsibility to nonprofessionals or to improperly qualified healers. They believed Thomsonians erred on both counts. But orthodox physicians did not greet other mid-century sectarians with the implacable opposition with which they had met the root-and-herb healers. The two most powerful medical sects of the period were homeopathy, renowned for its use of infinitesimal doses,[1] and hydropathy, which combined various types of water treatments with a spare regimen.[2] Orthodox physicians did find homeopathy and, to a lesser extent, hydropathy threatening, and those fears certainly spurred and helped shape efforts to strengthen the profession. Sectarian conflict was real and often virulent, so much so that recent historians have tended to view antebellum medical history along sectarian lines, a crucial but incomplete explanatory axis.[3]

Stressing the antipathies blurs significant areas of tacit or explicit consensus. Recasting this evidence throws into relief certain unifying attitudes which in turn highlight the inherent fuzziness of the boundaries of medical legitimacy. For instance, orthodox physicians still insisted that they were the most reputable and qualified healers, but many hydropaths and homeopaths were themselves regularly educated. In addition, some issues transcended boundary disputes, linking practitioners from a variety of different perspectives. This chapter seeks to delve beneath the acrimonious sectarian rhetoric to determine the extent to which there was agreement on crucial issues about health and disease—most notably, the management of illnesses; the importance of preventive living; the proper care of the sick; and the necessity of educating Americans about medical matters. This is not to suggest that all mid-nineteenth-century healers held identical views; their diversity on these particular issues, however, is surprisingly small, and the overall thrust of their ideas is mutually compatible. This will become evident as we contrast the beliefs of leading irregular practitioners—hydropaths, quasi-professional women, and homeopaths—with those of orthodox physicians as presented especially in chapters 3 and 4.[4]

Mid-century sectarians did criticize orthodox medicine and advocate greater self-sufficiency for nonprofessionals in matters related to health and disease. Their rhetoric suggests that the increased autonomy they envisioned for lay people would come at the expense of the doctor's authority—and ultimately of the doctor's very existence.[5] In reality, however, hydropaths and homeopaths supported interrelated goals of critical importance to their orthodox adversaries: redefining professional *and* lay responsibilities for the treatment as well as the prevention of disease. In their view of how disease should be managed, hydropaths and homeopaths assigned physicians the responsibility for directing treatment, which *enhanced* the doctor's authority and *circumscribed* lay participation. Hydropaths and homeopaths reversed these roles in their view of how disease should be prevented. The only sensible division of duties, they thought, was for each individual to assume primary responsibility for staying healthy, and for the doctor to monitor and guide those efforts. The mid-century sectarian contribution to this longstanding orthodox effort should not be underestimated; to an unprecedented extent, hydropaths and homeopaths gave Americans a very practical, well-publicized blueprint for hygienic living, and their followers provided tangible proof of the rewards of adhering to the laws of life and health. Armed with more concrete evidence than ever before, orthodox physicians co-opted desirable sectarian elements and put redoubled energy into the campaign for preventive living. In very different ways and from very different perspectives, mid-century healers helped transform the doctor-patient relationship in directions that would be reinforced and extended in the years after the Civil War.

Experimenting with Sectarian Alternatives

George Templeton Strong was a leading citizen of New York City, a public-spirited lawyer and an architect of the Civil War Sanitary Commission. Yet throughout his life he experimented with medical innovations from every source, motivated in part by the desire to banish the crippling headaches that plagued him. Never gripped by fanaticism, he evaluated each new hope carefully. On 29 June 1844, for instance, the twenty-four-year-old recorded in his diary that he had visited Pike's establishment that morning "to look at some electromagnetic apparatus of his that's reported to be sovereign for sick headache." He and his companion, noted Strong, "shocked ourselves and sent currents of the mysterious fluid marching and countermarching through our several systems with most scientific gravity and perseverence." He decided it was "a very nice and ingenious contrivance," but skepticism lingered about "whether a sick headache will bow before it." Despite his uncertainty about the equipment's actual power, Strong had to concede positive results. "It may have been fancy, or the fine weather, or unaccustomed eupepsia, but I certainly felt extremely fresh, vigorous, and bright after my dose of magnetism." The following afternoon he tried the galvanic apparatus once more, "for the premonitories of a headache." Again he felt better, but this was still insufficient proof for Strong, who reported that "the headache took itself off, but whether I'm to thank Pike for the deliverance must be resolved by future experience." The challenge, Strong thought, would be to see whether the apparatus could "vanquish a well-developed assault of that my fiercest and fellest temporal foe." Strong neglected to record a verdict, and it seems likely that he abandoned electromagnetism in favor of other experiments.[6]

By the following year Strong had shifted tactics, adopting homeopathy against the same enemy. A week before Easter, Strong found himself eagerly anticipating the next visit of Charles J. Hempel, his German teacher for the previous two months. Hempel, a student at the medical college of New York University, would receive his medical degree later that year and would eventually teach at Philadelphia's Homoeopathic Medical College. Strong knew exactly how he would conduct himself as soon as Hempel arrived: "I'll endear myself to him by becoming his first patient and renounce all things on which he lays his veto, and dose myself diligently and obediently with decillionths of belladonna or anything else and give homoeopathy a fair trial, for that allopathy is no match for a sick headache."[7]

By Easter Sunday, Strong had suffered for days from "a frightful headache." Hempel had visited him the night before, and, as Strong explained, "I surrendered myself formally into his keeping, underwent a vigorous cross-examination as to symptoms attendant and symptoms premonitory, and expect my first homoeopathic dose at our next meeting." He did not mince words about what was at stake. "So now we'll see what the children of Hahnemann can do. The old lights—Galen, Hippocrates & Co.—are but blind guides in this matter." Strong stood fully prepared to "renounce allopathy with all my heart and become a zealous convert," if homeopathy could touch his "abominable headaches." Wrote Strong, "Certainly if there be any substitute for the old system, that dispenses with emetics and cathartics and blistering and bleeding and all the horrors anticipation of which makes 'the Doctor's' entry give me such a sinking of spirit, it's worth trying." Two months later Strong was still trying homeopathy as he emerged from a long bout of melancholia. Hempel had recently administered "certain infinitesimals which I swallowed with great gravity—and, 'imagination' or not, I was quite sound the next morning."[8]

In October 1847 Strong turned to homeopathy again, once more hoping to conquer a powerful opponent. Now twenty-seven, Strong penned: "For the last fortnight I've been engaged in the innocent folly of quacking myself homoeopathically, without the slightest serious expectation of success, with reference to this blighting, paralyzing, disgraceful, hideous, unspeakable disease of nervous dejection and instability that has been down upon me like ten thousand tons of granite for the last two years." Once more, homeopathy seemed to have helped: "Today for the first time in all that period I verily believe I've felt perfectly well."[9]

Homeopathy and electromagnetism were only two of the medical alternatives the New York lawyer explored. Like many of his contemporaries, Strong was willing to experiment with virtually anything that held out the promise of relief. Thus he did not overlook mesmerism, spiritualism, or phrenology; hydropathy also won a trial. In the summers of 1856 and 1857, he and his wife visited water-cure establishments, their first destination Wesselhoeft's Hydropathic Asylum, known also as the Brattleboro Water Cure. On 13 August 1856 Strong outlined his experiences: "I tried all the various forms of the Aqua Pumpi treatment: plunge bath, sitz bath, half bath, wave bath, douches of every grade of intensity, and lastly 'packing,' not a pleasant way of spending an hour. The packed patient . . . looks just like the pictures of the gravid female white ant." His characterization of his "hospital or hotel" was vivid and revealing; it combined, he said, "usages appropriate to a German watering-place, an insane asylum, and a penitentiary."[10]

Strong's aggressive quest for effective medical therapies was not uncommon among well-educated, respectable men and women of his time. Historian Francis Parkman was another seeker. Chronically afflicted with various ailments from a young age, Parkman did not rely on regular medicine—despite the fact that his family included three Harvard Medical School graduates, two of whom later taught there. In 1864 he wrote about how doctors conducted themselves during an earlier period of his life:

The Faculty of Medicine were not idle, displaying that exuberance of resource for which that remarkable profession is justly famed. The wisest, indeed, did nothing, commending his patient to time and faith; but the activity of his brethren made full amends for this masterly inaction. One was for tonics, another for a diet of milk; one counselled galvanism, another hydropathy; one scarred him behind the neck with nitric acid, another drew red-hot irons along his spine with a view of enlivening that organ. Opinion was divergent as practice. One assured him of recovery in six years, another thought he would never recover. Another, with grave circumlocution, lest the patient should take fright, informed him that he was the victim of an organic disease of the brain, which must needs despatch him to another world within a twelve-month.

Deciding to devise his own regimen, the author of *The Oregon Trail* depended instead on homeopathy, hydropathy, fresh air, cold water, and exercise.[11]

Kansas pioneer Sarah Jayne Oliver followed a similar program. As her daughter recalled, "'Mother should by rights have been a doctor. Treating the sick was a real gift.'" While looking for means to improve her husband's health, she had learned about homeopathy, which was new at the time. Armed with her box of homeopathic medicines and her considerable diagnostic skill, Sarah Oliver's mother helped her family escape many of the diseases that struck their neighbors. The pioneer women did not rely on homeopathy alone, though. With her husband she visited "'at one of the early-day sanatoriums or 'water-cures' of the East, [and was] inducted into the new and simple forms of diet and the science of water hygiene and cure.'" Thereafter they were "'ardent adherents.'" Sticking to this plan with its simple diet required, judged the daughter, "'something like Spartan qualities . . . in a neighborhood where tables groaned with . . . hot biscuits, salt pork, fried potatoes, and pancakes.'" Yet it was worth the effort, and they believed, "'and rightly so, that the family regimen, directed on these lines, was largely responsible for bringing us all to adulthood in wholeness and vigor.'"[12]

Regularly educated physicians responded with neither complacency nor enthusiasm as people tried other treatment systems. In 1846 one of them, William A. Caruthers, wrote from Savannah to John M. Berrien, an eminent Georgia politician then resident in the nation's capital.[13] The physician reported Berrien's son's recovery from "a complication of bilious and pneumonic disease." This, however, was merely a prelude to what Caruthers wanted more urgently to convey. In the course of his consultations, revealed Caruthers, "I encountered the *Homeopathic* [*sic*] physician . . . attending one of your other children with some affection of the eyes." Shocked and disappointed, his immediate "impulse was to resign the case I had in hand, but then as the child was very ill, I thought should the result be fatal, it might be laid at my door, and that I might be charged with backing out of a dangerous case. Or the new Doctor might attribute whatever untoward symptoms that supervened to my want of skill."

To protect his professional reputation, then, Caruthers resolved "to see the case through," planning at its termination to "have a free and frank communication" with the family patriarch on the subject. "Nothing," he told Berrien, "in the whole course of my professional experience—(now twenty two years) has so disgusted me with my profession as the advent of this new *quackery*. It invades us in a different region from ordinary quackery—it scorns purlieus and subburbs [*sic*], but no sooner have we a patient sick in high life than half a dozen lady missionaries, and sometimes gentlemen, assemble around to preach the new doctrines in medicine, & earnestly recommend the trial of it, in the case in question. *This saps all confidence in the family physician.*"

There was further damage. Employing both homeopathic and regular physicians associated the latter with the former and misled the public. The crowning blow, Caruthers fumed, was the injustice of "joint practice in the same family." Invariably, he complained, "these men are employed in all the slight aches and pains, but the moment a case of responsibility occurs, we are sent for." He detested and resented the consequences: "We have all the pains and sufferings of the profession & none of its pleasures and are debarred of its greatest rewards; confidence and gratitude." Though Caruthers did not mention it, he may also have been worried about the loss of income likely to result from the family's consulting with other practitioners. Homeopathy, Caruthers declared with finality, was "a contemptible humbug," and he found it unthinkable to besmirch himself further by continuing to treat the Berriens "in this sort of conjunction."

Berrien responded immediately, surprised at Caruthers's venom. "In relation to Homeopathy," Berrien wrote, "I know nothing, and therefore believe nothing." His wife's illness, now extending beyond its second year, defined his perspective. Explained the politician, "Her disease has not yet yielded to the prescriptions of the regular physicians who have been consulted, yourself among others. Under these circumstances, she has availed herself of the advice of an individual practising on this new system, confining his attendance to her own case." That choice had not been intended to bar Caruthers from ministering to the family, for Berrien's wife had given "especial direction when she left home, that if any of our children should be sick during her absence, you should be called as usual to attend them." Though Berrien refused to try to "control the wishes" of his children "who had attained to years of discretion," he hoped "further reflection" would "induce [Caruthers] to take a different view of the subject."[14]

As Caruthers's reaction suggests, most orthodox physicians expressed hostility toward practitioners of homeopathy and other "isms and pathies." But this does not capture the full story, for many doctors were more open-minded. In 1843 the *Western Lancet* not surprisingly opposed a bill pending in New York to abolish all legal restrictions in the practice of medicine and surgery.[15] The journal correspondent offered a broad interpretation of the familiar argument stating that legal regulation of medical practice was essential in order to protect the public. Instead of advocating that one system of medicine be legally validated, the *Western Lancet* author proposed that each physician be required to meet certain criteria that he identified as independent of any sect. In his view, every doctor "should be *required by law* to become acquainted with the *elementary* branches of medical science, such as anatomy, physiology, chemistry, pathology, general therapeutics, and the general rules of surgical practice." This knowledge was "indispensable, and he who attempts to grapple with disease without [it], is combatting an enemy, without system, strength or weapons." Establishing these requirements would not entail recognizing any "exclusive system," but would leave "the physician . . . free to select calomel, lobelia, homoeopathy, hydropathy, or other such *modes* of medicine as his fancy might dictate."

Few orthodox practitioners were as welcoming as this writer, because most felt threatened by sectarian success. Criticism of irregular practice clustered around two central objections. First, as an 1848 *Western Lancet* article explained, regulars were outraged at the unrealistic therapeutic claims made by sectarians. People were vulnerable on this score because they so desperately wanted assurance that their illnesses could be cured. Scientific medicine, the *Western Lancet* author insisted rather disingenuously, did not delude on this point. "The certainty of scientific medicine," he argued, "is evinced in the moderation of its pretentions, as well as in the useful ends to which all its resources are directed. To know how to act, when to act, and when to cease from acting, constitute irrefragable proofs that there is an abiding certainty in the premises, and conclusions of scientific medicine."[16]

Many physicians of the period must have been puzzled by the *Western Lancet* statement, for they were very conscious of the imperfections and uncertainties of medicine. Many, like Yale physician Worthington Hooker, thought this awareness made orthodox healers more sensitive practitioners, because it encouraged constant vigilance and flexibility. "The truly judicious physician," wrote Hooker, "is neither bewildered nor precipitate. He takes a rapid view of all the circumstances of the case, and looks carefully at the important and perplexing questions which start up one after another in his mind, and then decides intelligently, coolly, and definitely upon his plan of treatment." Even with painstaking care, the practitioner might make a mistake, but, always on guard for unexpected results, he stood prepared to take corrective action immediately.[17]

The trouble was that the public did not understand "the true powers of medicine," which made citizens more susceptible to quackery.[18] Jacob Bigelow and others tried to delineate what medicine could and could not do, and Bigelow's influential 1835 address, "On Self-Limited Diseases," argued on behalf of an inherent tendency toward recovery in most diseases.[19] Numerous writers conveyed Bigelow's ideas to the public, among them Dan King in *Quackery Unmasked,* an 1858 work for the general reader. Explained King, "Every one ought to know that in all diseases, even the most fatal, there is a tendency towards recovery. . . . The ancients called this 'The *Vis Medicatrix Naturae,*' and we consider it as a recuperative principle indispensable to animal life."[20] The public should measure all medical claims against this backdrop, they suggested, and citizens would be forced to conclude that most sectarian claims were exaggerated.

In addition to criticizing the inflated promises of sectarians, orthodox physicians charged that sectarians were "exclusionists," those who adhered to one medical system and excluded all others. As physician Samuel Henry Dickson put it in an introductory lecture for the 1847–1848 session of the University of New York, he was not troubled "if . . . a well-informed, educated physician, choose upon a comparative examination of the several systems of therapeutics, to follow with narrow tenacity any one of them." He might, he confessed, "wonder at his error and delusion," but that would not warrant "absolute condemnation" of his course. There were others who ostensibly made the same choices but who did elicit his disapproval. Those people, he explained, did not weigh the merits of the different systems but devoted themselves "with an inconsiderate, and therefore by no means innocent enthusiasm, or with a deeply guilty calculation of mere selfish profit, to the unmodified and monotonous employment of any."[21]

Of course, in a very real sense orthodox physicians were exclusionists themselves. This was clear in the commentary of the *Western Lancet* editors, who thought Dickson had gone too far in his openness to irregular practice. They were "astounded, grieved, and mortified" to see that Dickson made no distinctions between legitimate and illegitimate healers: "Hahneman and Broussais, Brown and Thompson, with Priesnitz, are placed upon the same level, and their respective schemes of medical interference are brought upon the same Procrustean bed." Like Broussais and Brown, Benjamin Rush represented all that was good in medicine. A "thoroughly educated, enlightened, [and] benevolent physician," Rush had devoted his life to improving medicine "by enlarging the boundaries of discovery in legitimate medicine." Hahnemann, they sputtered, was the opposite, "a most arrant empiric, who, in all his works, has traduced the regular profession, and vauntingly held himself up as a great discoverer and innovator." They had similar difficulties with Samuel Thomson, "the asinine originator of the thunder and storm practice," and with Vincent Priessnitz, "the ignorant and crafty Silesian peasant, the blind and reckless hydropathist." The conflation of legitimate and illegitimate was dangerous because it was "calculated to depreciate our profession in the eyes of the public, by breaking down all the enclosure by which the regular profession is kept separate from that mixed multitude of pretenders which infest society at large, and which are ever hovering around the borders of that circle within which the lights of legitimate medicine shine."[22]

Many others worried about the public's ability to identify legitimate practitioners among a swarm of illegitimate healers. Though this was in many ways a perennial concern, the mid-nineteenth-century context—with sectarianism rampant—seemed to make its resolution both more vexing and more essential. How, wondered Worthington Hooker, could the nonprofessional possibly distinguish bad from good practice? Given the various medical systems that prevailed, he thought confusion seemed inevitable. What made the situation even more complicated was that there were no remedies that always worked or always failed. "There are," admitted the staunch defender of orthodoxy, "some good points in every system of practice. However bad it may be on the whole, it will do some good in some cases." Despite this acknowledgment, Hooker advocated neither piecemeal nor wholesale adoption of irregular practice. "The truth is," he explained, "that no *exclusive* system of practice can be said to be a good system, for it is impossible that it should suit all the varying states presented by disease."[23]

Thus while Hooker and other regulars viciously attacked unorthodox treatment options, they also conceded the existence of "some good points." Historians briefly mention this fact when they chronicle nine-teenth-century sectarian warfare and its consequences for medical therapeutics and professionalization. The outlines of the story—stressing waves of sectarian challenge and regular co-optation leading to victory—are familiar. What remains unappreciated is the surprising extent to which regulars and their stated enemies, the irregulars, were advocating the same goals.

Hydropathic and Orthodox Parallels

People have used water for therapeutic reasons since ancient times, but not until the nineteenth century did anyone make it the premier therapeutic agent of a medical system. Hydropathy, like Thomson-ianism, was devised during the first third of the century by an unlettered man. Because Silesian peasant Vincent Priessnitz believed that water sus-tained life, he formulated a medical system centered on bathing, wet compresses, steam, massage, exercise, drinking cold water, and eating a plain diet. The peasant's neighbors flocked to him in such numbers that he eventually turned his Graefenberg home into a "water cure" for ad-ministering a wide array of baths, packs, and wet bandages. News of Priessnitz's methods reached the United States in the early 1840s, spark-ing a water-cure craze that lasted until the Civil War. Two regularly edu-cated physicians, Joel Shew and Russell T. Trall, opened the first American water-cure establishments in New York City about 1843. Within a couple of years Mary S. Gove (later Nichols), a veteran health reformer, had opened the city's third water-cure operation. These three pioneers—Shew, Trall, and Nichols—most strenuously promoted the new water system to Americans.[24]

By 1848 at least thirty water-cure institutions existed in Ohio, Mis-sissippi, and seven states along the Atlantic coast. Many more appeared during the 1850s, though some failed quickly, casualties of poor locations and perilous economic times. Between 1843 and 1900, over two hundred water-cure establishments opened, nearly one-third of them in New York state.[25] Weekly fees for treatment plus room and board ranged from five to ten dollars, which meant that most clients were probably drawn from the middle and upper classes. Men comprised a substantial part of the water-cure clientele, but scholars have attributed much of hydropa-thy's popularity to the unique services its establishments provided to women. Characterized by a spirit of female communality, hydropathic settings encouraged bodily freedom and promoted the relief of female reproductive problems.[26]

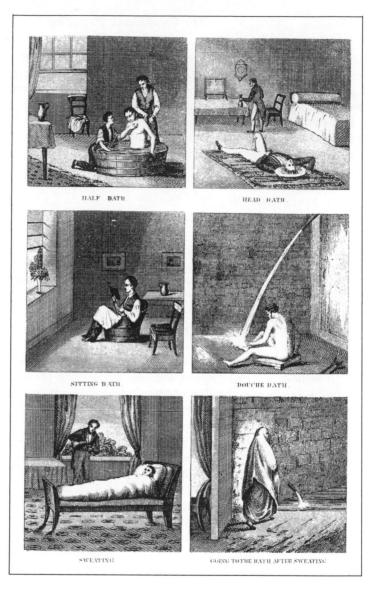

HALF BATH

HEAD BATH

SITTING BATH

DOUCHE BATH

SWEATING

GOING TO THE BATH AFTER SWEATING

This depiction appeared with slight variations in many water-cure publications. Some orthodox writers used it as well, among them James Ewell in *The Medical Companion* (Philadelphia, 1847), facing p. 506.

Hydropathic ideas also appeared in print. Books and pamphlets by native and European authors proliferated, and hydropaths founded several journals to tout the healing powers of water. The most influential periodical was *The Water-Cure Journal,* begun in New York City in the mid-1840s by Joel Shew. Featuring contributions from hydropaths and their patients, the journal also provided advice on domestic treatment, so that people who could not visit a water-cure establishment would be equipped "to prescribe for themselves."[27] Shew also offered to advise by mail, though he required advance payment. *The Water-Cure Journal* floundered until April 1848 when the phrenological publishing house of Fowlers and Wells took it over, adding to its masthead "and Herald of Reforms." At that time, its circulation stood at less than one thousand copies; within four months it had doubled and within four more months had better than doubled again. By July 1849 the magazine's circulation had increased to ten thousand, and after 1850 the editors bragged of a circulation in the vicinity of fifty thousand. No longer struggling, it survived under various names until 1897. There were a number of other hydropathic publications, such as the *Laws of Life,* published at Dansville, New York, by Harriet N. Austin and James Caleb Jackson, prolific writers and hydropathists at Our Home on the Hillside; like this periodical, all were minor in comparison to *The Water-Cure Journal.*[28]

Hydropaths displayed other accoutrements of a profession. The first hydropathic college opened in the autumn of 1851 in New York City, run and staffed by Thomas L. Nichols and his wife, Mary S. Gove Nichols. By May of the following year, however, the couple had moved to a new water-cure establishment in Port Chester, New York, and had founded a School of Integral Education to provide academic and health instruction to young ladies. Two years later Russell T. Trall and a full complement of faculty started a more successful college, the New York Hydropathic School. Within four years Trall had changed the school's name to the New York Hygeio-Therapeutic College and won a charter from the state legislature. There were other, apparently less important hydropathic colleges of which little is known.[29]

Hydropaths also banded together into organizations, beginning with the American Hydropathic Society, formed by water-cure physicians and lay people in 1849. A year later came a new and probably equally short-lived association, the American Hygienic and Hydropathic Association of Physicians and Surgeons. Its constitution listed among mandatory membership requirements both a certificate of a regular medical education and proof of one year's practice of hydropathy. As scholars have demonstrated, hydropaths greeted licensing and educational requirements with such deep ambivalence that they were largely circumvented or ignored. Nonetheless, Harry Weiss and Howard Kemble suspect that two-thirds to three-quarters of the sect's practitioners were doctors of medicine. Even if this estimate is highly exaggerated, a fraction of that number would still be significant testimony to the weight given regular medical education.[30]

Joel Shew, Russell Trall, Mary Gove Nichols, and Thomas Nichols not only took the lead in institutional matters, but they were also the most visible on the popular front. Their writings, as was common with literature for domestic consumption, stressed economy, safety, and self-reliance. Their work displayed other features typical of popular health material, both orthodox and sectarian. They did not advocate that every person be his or her own doctor, but they did want to teach people how to cope with minor medical problems and emergencies, since relatively few had acess to water-cure establishments or physicians. In more serious or complicated cases, they preferred that physicians direct medical treatment, and they emphasized that every individual should assume responsibility for prevention. As was true with other health advisers, hydropaths thus had to walk a fine line between giving enough information to guide domestic action and preserving the treatment authority of the physician. To an even greater extent than was true with orthodox advice, hydropathic literature managed to encourage lay autonomy in medical matters by focusing the nonprofessional's attention on prevention rather than on cure.[31]

Joel Shew has left few traces of his life. Born in Providence, New York, in 1816, he was in the daguerreotype business around 1840, either in New York City or Philadelphia, where he apparently had relatives who were similarly employed. After being "badly impregnated with minerals" as a result of that business, Shew evidently decided to study orthodox medicine, but by 1843 he had embraced hydropathy, which he promoted until his death in 1855.[32]

In 1844 Shew published two books that revealed underlying affinities with orthodox practitioners: *Hand-Book of Hydropathy,* a compendium of treatment options, and *Hydropathy, or Water-Cure,* an anthology of other people's works. Both books reveal that Shew, like the regulars, believed that American society was infested with quacks. Moreover, the reasons he identified for quackery's appeal were reminiscent of the analyses made by his orthodox counterparts. People, wrote Shew, were "easy prey" to the inflated promises of "the villainous quack" because so few knew anything about "the laws of life, health, and disease." To the hydropath, the solution was obvious, and it coincided with orthodox opinion: promote the "general spread of suitable knowledge upon these subjects."[33]

Given the conjunction of their views on quackery, Shew could not understand why the regulars seemed so determined to brand hydropaths as quacks. Quacks, Shew argued, were mercenary and selfish, and rarely ever even saw their suffering patients. Water-cure practitioners, in contrast, were as mentally and physically engaged with the sick as were their regular counterparts. Nor, continued Shew, was hydropathy a medical delusion comparable to the turn-of-the-century tractoration craze or contemporary homeopathy. Shew conceded without hesitation that there were some similarities among these therapies, most notably that each could claim "astounding cures" and that their subjects testified to an "unbounded faith" in the treatments. Though faith was indeed a crucial component of hydropathy, Shew quite logically contended that it was just as central to every other therapeutic relationship. One of the most telling arguments in favor of hydropathy, concluded Shew, was that it had some grounding in "physical truth," which was derived from the effects of water and ancillary therapies.[34]

Nonetheless, many people found it easy to dismiss hydropathy, perhaps because of "the unprofessional manner" in which it had been introduced. Shew, like so many other sectarians, invoked Benjamin Rush to chastise orthodox physicians for condemning therapies that lacked learned pedigrees. Rush, as he reminded his readers, had argued that doctors should be lifelong students, tirelessly gathering information from all possible sources. Such receptivity, Shew hastened to add, would not erode or destroy orthodox medicine. Instead, it would create a stronger system of practice, because it would mandate constant improvement as better therapies, from whatever source, became available. Especially in the area of preventive medicine, hydropathy had much to offer.

Shew reinforced these points by reprinting in his anthology an article by physician John Forbes from the *British and Foreign Medical Review*.[35] Forbes also traced orthodox hostility to hydropathy's "having been originated by a non-medical and uneducated man, and . . . for the most part, adopted and professed by lay practitioners, or by medical men of somewhat equivocal reputation—and yet more, from the system being held out as a *panacea* or cure for all diseases, with an exclusive scorn of medicinal aid." Like Shew and Rush, Forbes argued that all therapies should be objectively judged on their merits, no matter what their source. If the yardstick were efficacy rather than provenance, hydropathy would have much to offer. Whether conducted at "distinct bathing establishments

. . . under the authority and general direction of the ordinary medical attendants" or inside homes by patients themselves, hydropathy had "great power and value."

Forbes tried to soothe the fears of those who thought that accepting hydropathy would spell doom for regular medicine, because it would open the door to all varieties of unorthodox practice, including "stark-naked and rampant quackery itself." Only "the blindest dogmatism or the wildest empiricism could maintain that, because the water treatment is found useful, all other means must be useless." The reverse was also true: just because drugs were sometimes beneficial did not warrant excluding every other type of treatment. "The absolute exclusionist," concluded Forbes, "be he water doctor or drug doctor, is equally unreasonable and equally unjustifiable."

By the time the second edition of *Hydropathy* went to press, Shew had sharpened his attack on orthodox medicine. A large percentage of disease, he now maintained, was tied directly to regular medical practice. This meant that it would be best "if *all* drug medicines were at once wholly abandoned, and people were compelled, with pure clean water, right food, fresh air, and invigorating exercise, to help themselves as they best could."[36] Shew elaborated in *The Water-Cure Manual,* published in 1847. He knew that orthodox physicians contended "that it is not *water*-cure, but more the imagination, the pure air, the exercise, the mental repose, the regularity of habits, and the temperance observed; or that it is not by one circumstance, but by a combination of favorable agencies, that these cures are performed." Shew readily admitted that untangling all these elements would be virtually impossible. But why would it be important to do so? More to the point, he thought, was that "health, like truth and every thing good, must be wrought for." One of the most convincing arguments for the hydropathic system was that cleanliness was next to godliness. "We do not see the cleanly, sober, industrious, temperate and healthy man, committing evil deeds."[37]

Contrary to the accusations of some regulars, Shew neither advocated nor envisioned a world devoid of doctors. In fact, his conception of the doctor-patient relationship resembled that of the regulars. Advising readers to "place confidence in your [hydropathic] physician" and to "follow his directions implicitly," Shew also stressed the extent to which a favorable treatment outcome depended on the patient. While desirable, physicians were not absolutely essential to the success of hydropathy, since hydropathy "[was] admirably calculated for home practice." But if a nonprofessional directed treatment, he or she should proceed cautiously and sensibly, for domestic practice did harbor some pitfalls, not the least of which was the setting itself.

Shew's reservations about home care echoed complaints voiced by regularly educated practitioners. "At home," wrote Shew, "the patient is often annoyed by the fears, importunities, and meddlesomeness of friends. . . . [B]esides all this, he is often thwarted in his efforts, and is unable to carry out his resolutions, however good, amid the temptations and luxuries of home." Most of the problems with home care would disappear, argued Shew, if patients stayed together in one large establishment. In many ways Shew's vision of the advantages of treatment within a water-cure facility paralleled the argument made on behalf of hospitals. In a water-cure establishment, explained Shew, "We have the increased influence of numbers. The strong uphold the weak." Even the faltering patient would be bolstered under the influence of "resolute, industrious, and persevering men and women, who enter right heartily into the work." In addition, residents received incalculable benefits from the establishment's primary physician, the linchpin of the entire enterprise. The example he or she set could be crucial for patients, and his or her influence was often an integral part of the therapeutic regimen. "Better than all, you have the *personal practice* of the presiding genius of the establishment to guide you[,]" enthused Shew. "He lives, and eats and drinks with you, and if he be true to his calling, exhibits in his own life, physical and moral, the precepts you are to follow."[38]

Shew welcomed other unorthodox treatment options, though he examined each with a critical eye. There was no question about Sylvester Graham's teachings, because they were so similar to those of Priessnitz. Each "insist[ed] upon the necessity of simplicity in food, the avoidance of all stimulating substances and drugs, of bathing, exercise, air, and all the natural means of fortifying the general health." He also thought the Thomsonians had been "unmercifully and ignorantly vilified for their use of the vapor bath." Thomsonians, he pointed out, had "often relieved patients in a most remarkable manner, when the 'scientific' practitioner has been compelled to 'give up.'" Unfortunately, the speed with which "a good vapor bath, and a thorough cleansing of the skin" acted often led observers to assume that the relief obtained had been accidental. Even folk remedies could be useful. In sore throats, for example, "whether physicians or others sneer every woman knows that the dirty stocking will benefit the sore throat. The longer the stocking has been worn," he continued, "and the more moist it has become by perspiration, the better does it act."[39]

Many of the same themes resurfaced in Shew's 1854 *Hydropathic Family Physician*. Preventive advice occupied a more subordinate position in this volume, meant to instruct people about coping hydropathically with disease. Shew proselytized that adopting water cure would "not only make the members of communities their own physicians for the most part," but it would also "mitigate, in an unprecedented manner, the extent, the pains, and the perils of disease." Shew's concept of self-treatment did not exclude the physician, nor was it otherwise alien to the orthodox view. The physician's most important responsibility, he thought, was to teach people how to prevent disease, which meant that the public had to learn how to tell the difference between health and disease. What made this difficult was that neither health nor disease was a static concept, but "variable . . . , differing widely in different persons, and in the same person at different times." Since Shew was convinced that disease was an unnatural condition, he believed that "if man were sufficiently intelligent and strong in his moral power to avoid the *causes* of disease, he would live on healthfully from infancy to a good old age." To a large extent, wrote Shew in tones of William A. Alcott, everyone had the choice of whether they would *"manufacture"* disease or preserve health.[40]

As a "family physician," Shew's book was designed to give readers enough information so that they could successfully identify and treat disease. He tried to maximize the volume's utility by using an ample number of illustrations and providing an overview of anatomy, physiology, and hygiene.[41] By doing this, Shew imbedded information about disease treatment within the larger context of achieving and preserving good health. Like his orthodox counterparts, Shew viewed the structure and functioning of the human body within a religious framework. People's behavior should be in line with Divine intentions, but Shew realized that no one was capable of "liv[ing] uniformly in this beautiful and obedient way[.]" As a result, everyone was destined to fall prey to sickness at some point in life. Queried Shew, "Who is there that does not, sometimes at least, do that *knowingly* which he has the best possible evidence must injure his health?" The rare person who never fell sick would still be "liable to accidents . . . , which are . . . to a greater or less extent, unavoidable."[42]

Unfortunately, then, chronic and acute illness prevailed. Shew, like orthodox physicians, placed a premium on the quality of nursing care. Too often, he thought, the physician's best efforts were "wholly thwarted merely for the want of what is termed 'good nursing.'" Shew, however, went one step beyond what an orthodox physician might comfortably have admitted: "So, also, a good and efficient nurse often makes up what is lacking in the medical adviser, and in reality cures the case." Shew echoed his orthodox counterparts, though, when he worried about the number of people usually involved in treating the sick. Visitors, frequently motivated merely by curiosity, added to the problem, since they brought with them "a good deal of advice, too." The danger, of course, was that the interference of visitors, however well-intentioned, would undermine the patient's confidence in his physician and impede his recovery.

Implicit in this scenario was the idea that physicians not only had a role to play as sickroom attendants but were often the only sensible people to direct treatment. For disease to be managed properly, Shew agreed with orthodox healers that every individual should be able to recognize common disease symptoms and understand what each meant. Parents had special obligations to their children, and parental attentiveness could make the difference between life and death in diseases like croup. He accordingly summarized the diagnostic implications of specific changes in pulse, temperature, sleep, respiration, appetite, thirst, appearance, bodily fluids, and so forth. People who did not understand these signs often sent for the doctor at the wrong times, either when no doctor was needed or when the moment had passed for timely medical intervention.[43]

Shew portrayed doctors as necessary but not infallible. In his discussion of fever, he reviewed learned medical opinions on the subject, including the most eminent of the canon: Hippocrates, Galen, Sydenham, Boerhaave, Cullen, Good, Fordyce, Wood, Stahl, Hoffman, Clutterbuck, and Broussais. Despite the individual and collective brilliance of these doctors, wrote Shew, none of their theories had been sanctioned by experience. "Each and all of these theories have led their believers into different and often the most contradictory modes of treatment," which pointed to an obvious conclusion. Even though their intentions were "most benevolent," they had still caused thousands of deaths because their theories led healers to "[treat] a disease the very opposite of what should have been." Not surprisingly, Shew thought "incomparably the safest" route would be to follow the teachings of Hippocrates, which postulated that nature always did "the best in her power to rid the body of the morbid matter which occasions the diseased action." According to this doctrine, any medical treatment "should be practiced with extreme caution, and with a view solely to aid the vital powers in expelling the causes of the disease."[44]

Throughout the *Family Physician* Shew maintained a respectful attitude toward regular doctors. Philadelphia obstetrician Charles D. Meigs, for

instance, he characterized as "a man whose good character and long experience entitle his opinions to much weight." Benjamin Gooch was another "whose opinions are probably equally deserving of respect," and
James Blundell "is certainly very high authority." But "very high authority" did not necessarily correlate with therapeutic success, as the
failure to agree on causal agents and find cures for human ailments so
clearly illustrated.

Shew used learned opinion in another way, plumbing authoritative
works in search of testimonials for water therapy. Croup was one malady
where Shew could insert "a quotation from high authority, showing the
good effects of the cold-water treatment in this disease; a quotation
which shows, by the way, that there are at least some in the profession
who are ready to adopt any measure, so that it promises to be a means of
benefit." Scarlet fever was another disorder in which cold water had been
used to some advantage.[45]

Though receptive to the learned heritage and to some orthodox practice, Shew was discriminating. Orthodox surgical procedures tended to
fall outside the boundaries of his tolerance. Croup again provided a poig-
nant example. "As a desperate resort," wrote Shew "when all other
means fail, and when the child is in danger of strangulation from the
closure of the upper part of the windpipe, it has often been recommended
to cut open the part so low down at the neck as possible, for the purpose
of letting in the air. . . . The doctrine of surgery is always to resort to this
operation, if every thing else fails; and there is no doubt but that all good
and honest surgeons would prefer, by all means, to have it done, rather
than let the child die without it." But, Shew inquired, what was the
utility of the operation? He had never seen a living person with a hole in
the throat. As Shew exclaimed, "What folly . . . or rather what brutality,
to torture a young child . . . just at the point of death!" Because the
surgery never succeeded, it should never be done.[46]

Shew had a similar reaction to using "cutting and scraping" to treat
necrosis. Before resorting to "the knife and saw," he thought "every
other rational means should have a fair trial." He expressed skepticism
about other accepted therapies of the orthodox canon, most notably vaccination for smallpox. Though he conceded that vaccination probably
prevented smallpox and meliorated its worst effects, he thought it inevitably increased the system's vulnerability to other diseases, especially
consumption. Shew had a powerful clincher for this topic. "At any rate,"
he wrote, "I am not willing that any child of my own should be submitted to the process."[47]

Shew recommended a physician's aid without hesitation when he felt it was necessary. Dropsy of the head and ruptures, for example, were serious illnesses, and their treatment would benefit from prompt medical attention. Self-treatment in these cases, he acknowledged, did sometimes seem to work, but he cautioned repeatedly that *"if there should be the least difficulty, lose no time in getting medical advice."* Women, "from motives of false modesty," were especially likely to procrastinate. Those who delayed, he warned, courted death.[48]

The remainder of Shew's *Family Physician* was much like any of the domestic health guides distributed by the regulars. It contained very precise directions for dealing with emergencies, and the first-aid techniques were copiously illustrated. Shew's overall objectives in publishing health-care information were in fact remarkably similar to those of the regulars. Most importantly, he delineated lay and professional duties so that it was the doctor's responsibility to direct treatment and the nonprofessional's responsibility to prevent illness. Other hydropaths published domestic guides equally compatible with the orthodox view of the structure of the doctor-patient relationship.

A Role for Women

Like Thomsonians and regulars, hydropaths emphasized the role of women as providers and consumers of health care. But hydropaths were far more receptive than established physicians to women as *practitioners*. In an age of few female doctors, hydropaths boasted that roughly one-fifth of their number were women. Water-curists of both sexes were also more active participants in the antebellum feminist movement than were their orthodox counterparts.[49] Nonetheless, hydropathic and regular domestic manuals imparted strikingly similar messages to women about how to care for themselves and their families. It was here that female hydropaths, led by Mary Gove Nichols, made their most significant contributions.[50]

Born in 1810 in New Hampshire, Mary Sargeant Neal moved to Vermont with her family when she was about twelve. After that, she attended school only sporadically, but she read so voraciously that by age eighteen she had "commenced reading . . . Medical, Anatomical, Physiological, and Pathological works, as they came [her] way." Subjected to charges of impropriety, the young Quaker woman abandoned her medical studies and taught school until her 1831 marriage to Hiram Gove, a New Hampshire man John Blake has aptly characterized as "an opinionated, greedy dolt."[51]

Unmitigated mental and physical suffering ensued. Mary Gove scrambled to make ends meet as the family breadwinner, and she endured a series of miscarriages and stillbirths. Finding solace once more in medical reading, by 1832 she had begun using cold water therapy occasionally with women patients. Though this was well before Elizabeth Blackwell's pioneering efforts for women in medicine, many physicians supported Gove's quest for knowledge, and she felt tremendously indebted to them. Wrote Gove, "They have loaned me books; they have admitted me to their museums; they have permitted me to see dissections." This unexpected support from the medical profession fed and helped shape Mary Gove's sense of mission.[52]

About 1837 the Goves moved to Lynn, and the young matron resumed teaching. There she discovered Sylvester Graham, whom she thought "one of the greatest benefactors the world ever had." His ideas enhanced her self-taught learning, and Mary Gove became an active crusader for moral and physical salvation through knowledge of physiology and hygiene. She started on a small scale, teaching anatomy and physiology at a Lynn female lyceum and to students in her school. By March 1838, her girls were boarding "on the Graham system."[53]

Mary Gove's reputation grew, particularly after her well-received 1838 address to the women of Boston's newly organized American Physiological Society. The group's unofficial publication, the *Graham Journal,* judged Gove to be a capable and well-informed lecturer. Harvard Medical School professors, they noted, had not only furnished drawings and preparations but had also spoken "very encouragingly of the undertaking." Thanks to their help, Gove had been able to enliven her remarks by demonstrating a skeleton "with the heart, arteries, etc. entire and injected." Each lecture had drawn four to five hundred listeners, and the *Graham Journal* printed synopses of all except "of course" the tenth and eleventh on sexual matters, which had been given separately to unmarried and married women. When Gove offered a free lecture on tight lacing, she attracted an audience of two thousand. In December and January, Gove repeated her course in Boston, Lynn, Harverhill, Providence, and New York, often to standing-room-only crowds.[54]

Not everyone welcomed Mary Gove. Many Quakers criticized her, so much that she eventually left the denomination. Some newspaper editors attacked her. Their moral sense, sputtered the *Lobelian, and Rhode Island Medical Review,* was "so blunted as to be incapable of seeing the difference between gratuitous obscenity and physiological truth." Exhausted from traveling, speaking, and controversy, Gove collapsed in late 1838 from a severe pulmonary hemorrhage. She soon recovered and returned to her crusade to remove "the black pall of ignorance that enveloped" American women. Gove published a lecture on the "solitary vice" in 1839, and several of her articles appeared anonymously in the *Boston Medical and Surgical Journal.* Increasingly estranged from her husband, the health reformer in the early 1840s led a life punctuated by threats, lawsuits, separations, and kidnapping battles over custody of their only child. During this same period, Mary Gove became romantically involved with Henry Gardiner Wright, a British health reformer who introduced her to Priessnitz's work while he was living in the United States.

In June 1845—after Wright's departure for England and a year of illness aggravated by Hiram Gove's abduction of their child—Mary Gove entered Robert Wesselhoeft's new water-cure establishment in Brattleboro, Vermont. After three months of observation and lecturing, Gove became a physician for women at another new water-cure house in Lebanon Springs, New York. Again her health failed, and she moved to Joel Shew's New York water-cure facility. There she soon began to see patients and to give lectures, now illustrated by a "splendid" manikin from Paris. In May 1846 she established her own water-cure operation in New York City.

In mid-1848 Mary Gove, recently divorced, married Thomas Low Nichols, a young writer. Still lecturing, she now illustrated her talks with hundreds of wax and papier-mâché models, which offered an opportunity "for scientific study and practical improvement" such as had "never before been opened to women." She also continued writing and practicing, while Thomas Nichols resumed his medical education at Dartmouth after a fifteen-year absence. When Nichols graduated from New York University in 1850, the couple opened a new and more elaborate water-cure establishment in New York City, and Nichols quickly became a leading contributor to the *Water-Cure Journal.* But after the 1853 publication of Thomas Nichols's *Esoteric Anthropology,* the couple drifted farther and farther away from the main currents of health reform as they focused on more radical prescriptions for sexual relations. Moving to Cincinnati in 1855, they spent five years there before sailing for England, where they resumed more prosaic literary and health reform activities. Mary Gove Nichols died there in 1884.

It was in 1842 that Mary Gove's first book, *Lectures to Ladies on Anatomy and Physiology,* appeared. Preliminary remarks in the *Boston Medical and Surgical Journal* praised the "plainness and strength" of her writing and her "invincible thirst for useful knowledge." They were also pleased that Gove had the support "of many of our most respectable physicians," and that the book was to "be published under the supervision of one of the most accurate scholars and eminent men in the profession."[55] More sustained consideration followed in the journal's next volume. "All liberal-minded medical men," stated the writer, "have given countenance to her efforts, because they saw a need of reformation, and there was nothing objectionable or indelicate for one woman to tell another those important facts which men study with a view to ameliorating their sufferings and promoting their health and longevity." Despite such openness, the reviewer expressed some misgivings about the wisdom of Gove's move from the lecture circuit to print, where she seemed "less forcible, and therefore less interesting." Equally troubling was her reliance on "those who are altogether her inferiors in knowledge," especially Sylvester Graham. Grahamism, in the reviewer's eyes, was "the most grossly absurd . . . of all the great farces of the day," and Graham himself was full of "impudence, officiousness, and offensive self-esteem." Allying herself with Graham, thought the critic, would do Gove's reputation and her work a great deal more harm than good.[56]

Yet Mary Gove's overarching perspective on sickness and health was indistinguishable from that of orthodox physicians. Though she abhorred the standard orthodox remedies, like the regulars she believed that God intended humans to be healthy and that people brought sickness on themselves by disobeying God's laws. "Man," she declared, "came from the hand of his God a noble being, made in the image of his Creator." No longer "that godlike being," she deplored, "now . . . man is depraved, fallen, perverted." She refused to attribute man's condition to "wilful error," because she believed that ignorance was more to blame. Too many Americans assumed "that all diseases are immediate visitations from the Almighty, arising from no cause, but his *immediate* dispensation." Those people did not know "that there are established laws with respect to life and health, and that the transgression of these laws is followed by disease." Her identification of the problem and her strategy for attacking it matched that of regularly educated physicians: educate citizens so that they could make wise decisions. Like orthodox doctors, Gove believed that women should play a central role in this transformation from "the black night of ignorance" to the "dawn of [a new] day."[57] Only later would it be clear that Gove's casting differed significantly from that of the regulars. Orthodox practitioners envisioned women acting as enlightened educators within their own families. While Gove did not repudiate this view, she did increasingly advocate that women follow her own example and operate as physicians.[58]

Four years after the initial appearance of *Lectures to Ladies*, Gove published a revised version, calling it *Lectures to Women on Anatomy and Physiology*. Her goals had not changed; if anything, they were more strident. Announcing herself "fully satisfied of the value and importance to Woman and the Race of hygienic and therapeutic knowledge," she pledged to her readers "to do all in her power to educate women to prevent and cure disease." Prevention remained the key and the framework religious. Wrote Gove, "Let the sick . . . look over the catalogue of their sins; for every violation of the laws of health is sin, and comes back upon us with its penalty of pain."[59] Everyone could attain physical salvation through "WATER[,] . . . the panacea which shall cleanse our land from its disease and defilement." Like everything else, water cure could be abused, and proper use depended primarily on good "sense, knowledge, and experience." But the water cure would not bring miracles, for "there is a point where all diseases become incurable. Water," she said bluntly, "can not raise the dead or cure the incurable." But water cure could accomplish astonishing feats. With rickets, for instance, if the bones were already distorted, little could be done; if less advanced, "the disorder may be cured by any mother who has common sense after reading on water cure, provided that the vital energy of the child is not too far exhausted."[60]

Despite the fact that Mary Gove provided a considerable amount of treatment information to her readers, she did not seek to substitute lay healers for physicians. Instead, though she stressed the superiority of the water cure over heroic medicine, she also emphasized an idea of central importance to the regulars: that the lay person's primary responsibility was preventive living. Thus Gove advocated a Grahamite regimen, including fresh air, exercise, cleanliness, daily cold bathing, whole wheat bread, and abstinence from meat, tea, coffee, and alcohol. She even had cautious praise for homeopathy, believing it had "paved the way for hydropathy, and homoeopathic practitioners unite the two modes of practice." Gove could not convince herself that homeopathy was a "positive good," but she was absolutely "satisfied of [its] negative good[,] . . . [for] any thing that takes man from the horrible dosing and drugging they have so long been guilty of, deserves our thanks."[61]

Attributing her own ill health to tight lacing in her youth, she urged others to "loosen the death grasp of the corset, and send the now imprisoned and poisoned blood rejoicing through the veins of woman." Without changes, the future appeared dismal: "With chest deformed, spine and pelvis distorted, and every organ and tissue of the body imperfectly nourished, can we expect woman to become a mother without indescribable anguish? Or can we expect her offspring to live out half the days allotted to man?" This was a "lamentable, a deplorable picture of society." But it was realistic, she thought, and she urged people to heed her warnings: "If deterioration holds on, at its present rate, especially in our cities, we shall soon be a bed-ridden people."[62]

Though she was the best known and most prolific of the female hydropaths, Mary Gove was not a solitary crusader. In 1844 Marie Louise Shew, wife of Joel Shew, promoted similar ideas in *Water Cure for Ladies.* Physicians, she said, were not the best guardians of health, because they were "employed to *cure,* not to *prevent* disease." Hydropathy, on the other hand, "more than any other [system], implies *the prevention of disease."* Explained Marie Louise Shew: "The pure cool air—the daily appropriate exercise and ablutions—the total abstinence from *all* stimulating and exciting substances—the plain cold food—in short, the *apostolic* temperance which it always implies, tends, in a manner most efficient, to promote health, and to prevent disease. It involves no more nor less than a general removing of the *causes* of disease." Like Mary Gove, Marie Louise Shew emphasized the centrality of woman's role in improving the "the physical condition of our race."[63]

Marie Louise Shew also raised specific questions about the utility of regular medical practice, and effectively buttressed her views by quoting renowned orthodox figures. Benjamin Rush, for instance, had been keenly aware of the extent of human ignorance in medical matters. As he had lamented, *"We have assisted in multiplying disease; we have done more— we have increased their mortality."* A more recent, equally reputable physician had reiterated Rush's sentiments, bemoaning the "trifling good" medicine had conferred on society. Not only was medical practice characterized by *"uncertainty* and *chance,"* charged the French physiologist Magendie, but the typical doctor was too frequently guilty of administering medicines "right or wrong, without for a moment considering the *cause* of the disease, and without a single clear idea of the why and wherefore of what he does."[64]

Marie Louise Shew's object, however, was not to destroy either the medical profession or "trafficking speculators in pills and poisons." Instead, she wanted to teach everyone "the laws of life and health" so that they would be able to live in such a way "that they would seldom need the physician" or the amazing variety "of medicines, cures, and curers." Despite the variety, she warned, "drug medicines cannot be depended on. *Not one* of the whole number." Though the "science of medicine" could do little to relieve suffering, hydropathy offered great promise. Priessnitz, she acknowledged, had been decried as an "illiterate peasant," and she had to concede that "he is, in the common acceptation of the day, *unlearned,"* and his theories have somewhat of rudeness about them." But Priessnitz excelled at *"assisting the inherent energies of the system to throw off its own diseases."* Like other popular medical writers of every affiliation, Marie Louise Shew stressed that the causes of disease and premature

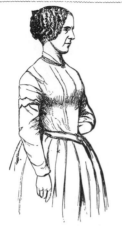

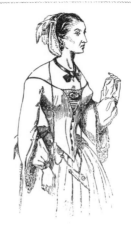

LOOK ON THIS PICTURE:.

A WATER-CURE BLOOMER, WHO BELIEVES IN THE EQUAL RIGHTS OF MEN AND WOMEN TO HELP THEMSELVES AND EACH OTHER, AND WHO THINKS IT RESPECTABLE, IF NOT GENTEEL, TO BE WELL!

AND THEN ON THIS.

AN ALLOPATHIC LADY, OR A PURE COD LIVER OIL FEMALE, WHO PATRON-IZES A FASHIONABLE DOCTOR, AND CONSIDERS IT DECIDEDLY VULGAR TO EN-JOY GOOD HEALTH.

Varieties.

"*Brevity is the soul of wit.*"

A FASHIONABLE YOUNG LADY.—"What is the life of a *would be fashionable* young lady?"

It is to go to a model boarding school, kept by an ex-French milliner; to be put into a room with four promiscuous young ladies, and to learn, in three days, more mischief than her grandmother ever dreamed of. It is to stay there at the tune of thirty dollars per week, for several quarters, and come home "finished," and superficial, with a taste of Latin—a touch of French—a smattering of Italian —German, and Spanish, and a portfolio full of crooked horses, distorted houses, lame sheep, and extraordinary looking abortions of cattle and fowl in general, the types of which were never found in Noah's menagerie. It is to sit in the drawing-room, in a flounced silk dress, with a waist half a yard in circumference, be-curled, be-scented, and be-jeweled; to receive *morning* calls, while mama looks through her spectacles, and tries to mend Mademoiselle's stockings. It is to have Mr. Fitz Humbug, some fine day, get on his knees, and request Mademoiselle to make him, what she has all along been desiring to do, "the happiest of men." It is to wear a white satin dress, an orange wreath, a long, fleecy veil, a diamond pin, and respond Amen to a quantity of things, of which Mad-moiselle does not understand the full import. It is to commence house-keeping where "the old folks" leave off; it is to patronize fast horses, ruinous upholsterers, operas, concerts, theatres, balls and fetes of all kinds. It is to bring a few sickly children into existence, to be tortured into eternity by careless hirelings. It is to find, after a few years probation, that Mr. Fitz Humbug is just what his name imports. It is to have "an execution" in the house; it is for Madame to go into hysterics, and on "coming to," to find herself in the sixth

story of "lodgings," with a tight husband, an air tight stove, a loose wrapper and a crying baby. FANNY FERN.

[Fanny might have added the usual *round* of diseases, drugs, and doctors, slops, pills, and plasters, tea-pots, bottles and death. But the looking glass above is sufficiently large to permit many *poor souls* to see themselves as others see them.]

THE most amusing instance we remember of stilted English is in an apology made by an English Clergyman to his congregation, who had petitioned him to use a simpler style or expression in the pulpit. It was as follows:

"RESPECTED FRIENDS—My oral documents have recently been the subject of your vituperation. I hope it will not be deemed an instance of vain elocution, if I laconically promulgate that, avoiding all syllogical, aristocratic, or peripatetic propositions, whether physiologically, philosophically, politically or polemically considered, all hyperbolical expressions, either in my diurnal peregrinations, in occasional inculpations, I assure you that they shall be categorically assimilated with, considered and rendered congenial to, the caputs, occiputs and cerebrums of you, my most superlatively respected auditors."

It was said at the time the congregation considered the remedy worse than the disease, and concluded to let the minister have his own way.

WHAT an appeal for the Maine Law is thus made by an English writer, who puts the following language in the mouths of those who visit the rumseller's den:

"There's my money—give me drink! There's my clothing and my food—give me drink! There's the clothing, food and fire of my wife and children—give me drink! There is the education of the family, and the peace of the house—give me drink! There's the rent I have robbed from my landlord, fees I have robbed from the schoolmaster, and innumerable articles I have robbed from the shop-keeper—give me drink! Pour me out drink, for more I will yet pay

for it! There's my health of body, and peace of mind! there's my character as a man, and my profession as a christian—I give up my all—give me drink! More yet, I have to give. There is my heavenly inheritance and the eternal friendship of the redeemed—there—there—is all hope of salvation. I give up my Saviour. I give up my God! I resign all! All that is great, good and glorious in the universe, I resign forever, that I may be DRUNK!'"

A popular writer, speaking of the proposed oceanic telegraph, wonders whether the news transmitted through salt water would be fresh!

MORE than half the bar-rooms in the neighborhood of the Crystal have been closed from want of customers.

WANTED, an intended bride who is willing to begin housekeeping in the same style in which her parents began.

THERE is nothing like courage in misfortune; next to faith God, and in His overruling Providence, a man's faith in himself is his salvation.

BYRON says:—"A thousand years scarce serve to form a State." He had never heard of California.

THE "old fogy," who peeped out from "behind the times," has had his head knocked off by a "passing event."

AN old bachelor, having been laughed at by a party of pretty girls, told them, "You are small potatoes!" "We may be small potatoes," said one of them, "but we are *sweet ones!*"

death were well within the control of human beings. As she concluded, "It is therefore unwise, irrational, and unphilosophical to regard such prevailing disease and premature death as the *infliction* of a Divine Providence."[65]

Proselytizers for Preventive Living

Others outside orthodox medicine took up the banner for preventive living, joining a growing chorus within regular ranks.[66] Contrary to orthodox suspicions, they rarely repudiated the physician's role, though, like hydropaths, they hoped that the medical practitioners of the future would be concerned as much or more with prevention than cure. Many of the mid-century crusaders were women who embarked on the lecture circuit; with at least a modicum of training, they delivered a message intended primarily for other women.

Sarah Coates, for instance, was living in Ohio when she wrote physician William Darlington in early 1850 to ask the respected botanist for his endorsement.[67] As had been the case for the past few months, she explained, "I am studying anatomy & physiology, under a physician of this place." It was not her desire "to practice medicine but to teach women—wives, mothers, daughters & sisters, the laws of health, & some of the means of preserving it to themselves & their families." Confident that as a practicing physician he would also have seen the need for this instruction, Coates still felt it necessary to reassure him that she was not trying to usurp the doctor's role: "Don't understand me that I would set anyone to dosing & drugging—Anything but that—Yet I would those who have the care of families & upon whom the health of the whole race may be said to depend, to understand themselves enough to know the importance of pure air, invigorating exercise, wholesome food & that properly administered, comfortable dress, cheerful temper, & most of all cleanliness, that virtue which 'is next to godliness.'" Coates thought she had been fortunate in the training she had been receiving, for she had been studying "with two other ladies, (rare specimens of worth & talent are they & both greatly my seniors)." She had been in the class, "hard at work," for six months, "& having given a good time & attendance to the subject before I came, I hope to be prepared, as early as June, to go and to have classes." In a subsequent letter to Darlington, she reported on her reception, which varied, and her classes, which ranged in size from thirty to forty.

Other mid-nineteenth-century American women, many of them woman's rights advocates, spread anatomical and physiological knowledge among members of their sex. Paulina Kellogg Wright Davis toured the East and Midwest, her lectures to women illustrated with a female manikin imported from Paris. Jane Elizabeth Hitchcock Jones also had a manikin, which she supplemented with engravings in her lectures to Midwestern female audiences. Lydia Folger Fowler, wife of phrenologist Lorenzo Fowler and the second woman to receive a medical degree in America, was an indefatigable writer and lecturer to women on anatomy, physiology, and hygiene.[68]

Another crusader was Harriot K. Hunt, whose personal and professional struggles epitomized those faced by other mid-nineteenth-century women aspiring to be doctors.[69] Writing in 1856 about the first fifty years of her life, she offered medical *Glances and Glimpses* from the perspective of a respectable female practitioner twice barred from formal medical training. Little Harriot had not dreamed from girlhood of becoming a physician; "the great turning-point of my life," she mused, had come in 1830, when her only sister "was prostrated by severe illness."[70] She thought the experience deserved lengthy comment, for it focused her attention on medicine, she wrote, "by leading me, when I had no scientific knowledge of hygeine, to marvel at the dense darkness which surrounds disease, and to wonder at the harsh and severe measures adopted in the treatment of the delicate and sensitive organizations."

The family's "kind allopathic physician" treated her sister, administering the usual battery of blisters, mercurials, and leeches. Nothing worked. "I marvelled—all this agony—all these remedies—and no benefit! The prescriptions seemed wholly experimental, the results entirely unknown," complained Harriot Hunt. Finally the physician called in a colleague for consultation. Pronouncing the malady "a disease of the heart," the doctors insisted that rest and quiet were crucial to recovery. In compliance, the sister retreated to the country, where she made some progress. As soon as she returned, however, she grew rapidly worse, now prey to terrible spasms. Blistering and leeching, judged the doctor, had become "the only hope." The treatment, recorded Hunt, "was certainly 'heroic!'" Seeing no improvement, the doctor next tried a seton, which, Harriot Hunt shuddered, was "truly barbarous."[71]

Though her sister suffered deeply, she did not obey all the doctor's orders without question. In fact, she often argued with her physician, buoyed by her own sense of what the proper course should be. "I well remember," wrote Harriot Hunt, "his ordering her to keep to her room for the winter; but her own *health-instinct* revolted, and she slept in another room where there was no fire;—'on the sly,' as they say." Her course did indeed prove beneficial, and the young women thought it "droll" to witness the doctor taking credit for the favorable outcome.

"After forty-one weeks of sickness, and one hundred and six professional calls," reported Hunt, "my sister was roused to more thought on the subject." They discussed the situation, read some medical books, and concluded that the doctors did not understand her case. But they were perplexed about what to do next. A new symptom attacked, a "severe" and "spasmodic" cough. The doctor simply prescribed "a different train of remedies,—all useless and ineffectual." The situation was nearly insupportable. By this point, Hunt reported, "My sister had lost all confidence in medicine. She reasoned and argued with the doctor: *his* tactics were to arouse her conscience; and then she would tamely submit to a fresh round of torturing prescriptions." Even after fighting successfully to see another respectable physician—this one a member of the Massachusetts Medical Society—the sister's suffering continued.

In June 1833 the two sisters consulted a recently arrived couple named Mott, an act of some controversy because the Motts were suspected to be quacks. The Motts' reputation did not stop the two sisters, "weary and tired out with 'regulars'; and it did not occur to us that to die under regular practice, and with medical etiquette, was better than any other way." They began the new treatment, found themselves impressed beyond anticipation, and eventually became boarders with the couple.[72]

It was here that Harriot Hunt began her quest for medical knowledge, her interest deepening "as physiological, anatomical, pathological laws were unfolded." Very quickly she lost all remaining patience with regular medicine. Concluded Hunt, "Medical science, full of unnecessary details, lacked, to my mind, a soul; it was a huge, unwieldy body—distorted, deformed, inconsistent, and complicated." She wanted to learn more about general and specific anatomy, but Harvard refused to admit her to "dissections in connection with close study and able lectures[.]" Physiology, however, she found more accessible, "with all its thousand ramifications . . . —use, abuse—cause, effect—beginning, and end—all were significant in the light of a science undarkened by technicalities, doubtful assumptions, tedious dissertations, controversies, and contradictions." Eschewing medication, "we endeavored to trace diseases to violated laws, and learn the science of prevention. That word—preventive—seemed a great word . . . ; curative, was small beside it."

The sisters thought their exclusion from orthodox medicine put them at a disadvantage compared to the novice who had been accredited by a regular medical faculty. No matter how inexperienced or uncertain, the orthodox beginner "had older heads to sustain him—a code of laws to obey—a mistake would not be fatal to him, though it might be to the patient!—and if he reverently looked to the centre, the centre would kindly regard him." But as the patients trickled in, the two women quickly realized their advantages. Though it was true that they had no one to turn to for guidance or support, the adjunct to that was that they were not bound by "formal rules." Neither disciples nor proselytes of any medical sect, they were wide-ranging in their choice of therapies, eclectic without being indiscriminate.[73] Thus the two sisters found Thomsonianism, homeopathy, and hydropathy to be beneficial in some cases, and they welcomed the ideas of contemporary lecturers on health. In 1838 Mary Gove impressed Harriot Hunt with "her deep interest in anatomy and physiology." Since that time, Gove had been successful as a physician and lecturer on physiology, "fluent and correct in expression," speaking "with enthusiasm and power." The only blemish Hunt could find from this period of Gove's life was her adherence to Grahamism; her later years were another matter, and Hunt lamented "the peculiar doctrines" the health reformer espoused toward the end of her life.

A much more important influence was George Combe, who filled a vacuum created by the sisters' "being entirely shut out from the medical world, having no minds with which to interchange views, compare thoughts, and examine experiences, and whose sympathy would have cheered and encouraged [them]." When the acclaimed phrenologist began a course of lectures in Boston in the autumn of 1838, the two women rejoiced at having finally found "a clear, exploring light." Harriot Hunt's enthusiasm was nearly boundless. Combe's lectures, she said, instilled in her "a more earnest consciousness of laws" and the realization "that they govern every department of life." These lectures "gave the bones, joints, sinews, arteries, nerves, and veins of the human body a deeper language. They snapped the fetters that had manacled thought." Hunt altered her perception of all kinds of relationships, for Combe's lectures "brought to light hidden affinities, . . . revealed indirect influences; and thus robbed metaphysical subtleties of their mysticism, effecting a reconciliation in the mind between sin and its consequences."[74]

Not surprisingly, Hunt also praised Spurzheim, but Combe occupied a special niche, partly because he was "a philisophical physician" and a phrenologist. Combe's "dietetics of the mind" reinforced her own ideas about the physician's role and the doctor-patient relationship. Like Combe, Hunt believed that diseases frequently resulted from "departures from duty, or law." Medicines alone, then, would not cure. Rather, the physician's "first and most powerful means of cure" was "to win the patient back to normality—to duty— . . . Obedience to spiritual and physical laws—hygeine of the body, and hygeine of the spirit—is the surest warrant for health and happiness." Once the healing relationship was conceived in this way, it was obvious that "the medicine, and the diagnosis, are both above the region of physics, in the domain of metaphysics." A doctor, no matter how skilled, could not cure disease on his own. Instead, Hunt wrote, there had to be a "oneness between the doctor and the patient," for only "*together* [could they] cure or mitigate the disease. They must be coworkers. In order to be so, there must be the fullest—the most cordial sympathy and frankness between them."[75]

This relationship had clear consequences for proper medical etiquette. The doctor had to recognize that the patient lived within a nexus of personal relationships that had enormous significance for him or her. In many cases, relatives gave "months of untiring care" and faithfully executed the doctor's instructions. Under these circumstances, it was "an outrage on common sense and propriety" to exclude these people from consultation. It was only logical to "suppose that the anxious mother, sister, or friend, who had watched the case day and night, would have some valuable facts—some observations about symptoms—some suggestions to offer." The doctor also owed "a frankness, a candor, and a confidence . . . to . . . patients, and their families and friends." If the patient's relatives wanted to be present during the doctor's visits, they should be, and the doctor should keep them fully informed. This would help everyone concerned: the doctor, the patient, and the caregivers. Giving relatives the opportunity to advise the doctor should not undermine professional authority, argued Hunt, but should instead increase the likelihood that professionally directed treatment would be successful.[76]

Hunt warned the profession to listen to her views. Times were changing, she said, and the profession could not afford to be complacent. "The public are getting enlightened," she wrote, "and you must recognize it. Families are reading works on hygiene, and preparing themselves to meet you in sickness. The day of blind obedience, or foolish deference, to you, is entirely gone; you now stand on your merits." The physician had an awesome responsibility, "as high a mission as God has permitted to his beings on earth. To you [has been] committed the care of bodies, and through them of souls, suffering with pain and anguish." But the physician's sphere of action should be influenced by other considerations: "You have your mission; they have theirs. Your patients have their duties. They must rely on you with faith; but their judgment must be taken whenever practicable. They have a health-instinct; and it must be consulted. They have reason; and it must be respected. They, in suffering moments, often *catch glimpses* of their real maladies, by chance gleams of intuition, which may help you, and may prove hints guiding you to more accurate knowledge. Stand fearlessly on your own merits; they are eminence enough for you. You have got wisdom; now get understanding. Must you drape yourselves in mystery and secrecy, and demand privacy as a condition whereby you are to work your cures?" There should, Harriot Hunt reiterated, be a "oneness" and "perfect frankness" between the physician and patient.[77]

Female practitioners did achieve such oneness with their female patients, proclaimed Hunt, because women spoke more freely to other women. In addition, she believed that female practitioners were more likely to educate women about anatomy and physiology. Teaching people, especially women, about physical laws, became increasingly important to Hunt, and she welcomed the 1843 formation of a Ladies' Physiological Society in Charlestown because she anticipated that "it would enable them to dispense in great measure with physicians, put them on their own responsibilities, and be a blessing to themselves and their children." Hunt acted on her convictions in her own practice, and she bragged about the fact that "many people I attended can bear testimony to their being their own physicians after my visits, except in cases of emergency."[78]

Despite the emphasis she placed on the female role in health care, Hunt saw preventive living as a duty to be borne by Americans of both sexes and all ages. She upbraided those who "disregard the laws of the body until sickness ensues, and then tax the skill and ingenuity of the physician to renew the lease of life for them, or their children;—parents, who when emergencies are passed, and self-reproach forgotten, relapse into carelessness and thus bring upon themselves severer lessons, which indeed they need." Parents, especially mothers, "should pay the strictest attention to the diet, air, exercise, sleep, and bathing of [themselves] and [their] children." The child himself could be of great assistance to achieving good health, because, like adults, each child had "a health-instinct" that indicated what actions were "appropriate" and "necessary." This "the true mother" recognized and heeded, treating each child according to his or her own unique temperament.[79]

Though it was important that women be informed about physiological laws, that knowledge should be diffused throughout the entire society. Americans would "then know when to apply for medical aid." Physicians should meet this lay reformation with changes of their own. Though Hunt wanted to see improvements in the doctor-patient relationship and in medical therapeutics, she thought that it was equally important for the medical profession to alter its fundamental orientation. As

Hunt envisioned it, "The true way [to practice medicine] would be to have a physician examine well people, advise them how *to keep well,* tell them what their hereditary and acquired tendencies are," and explain to them the impact of all factors on health.[80]

Homeopathic Domestic Medicine

Homeopathy proved to be nineteenth-century orthodox medicine's greatest threat as well as its greatest lesson. Invented by a regularly educated German physician, Samuel Hahnemann, during the last decade of the eighteenth century, homeopathy was based in large part upon the healing power of nature and two fundamental principles, the law of similars and the law of infinitesimals. According to the first law, diseases were cured by medicines capable of producing in healthy persons symptoms similar to those of the disease. A feverish patient, for example, would be treated with a drug known to increase the pulse or temperature of a healthy person. Hahnemann's second law held that medicines worked better in smaller doses, even in dilutions up to one-millionth of a gram.[81]

The first American homeopath of any importance was physician Hans Burch Gram, who returned to the United States in 1825 after nearly twenty years in his ancestral Denmark. Gram settled in New York, but the more significant hub of homeopathic fervor was in Pennsylvania. There the influx of German-speaking physicians included Henry Detweiler, William Wesselhoeft, and Constantin Hering. In 1835 they won incorporation for the Allentown Academy, which paved the way for the 1848 establishment of the Homoeopathic College of Pennsylvania, the most important of the sect's colleges prior to 1860.

Not until the early 1840s did homeopathy spread beyond the narrow following it had attracted in New York and Pennsylvania. Translations of homeopathic works appeared, and Allentown graduates joined a steady infusion of European homeopaths in preaching the doctrine. By midcentury there were homeopathic medical societies in many states. In 1844 the American Institute of Homeopathy became the first national medical society, antedating by three years the orthodox American Medical Association. By 1849 one thousand doctors and lay people had organized a homeopathic society in Cincinnati, and the following year a homeopathic college was founded in Cleveland. Three years later, homeopathy claimed more than three hundred practitioners in New York state, twenty in greater Boston, and fifty-three in Philadelphia. When the Civil War began, there were nearly two thousand five hundred homeopathic

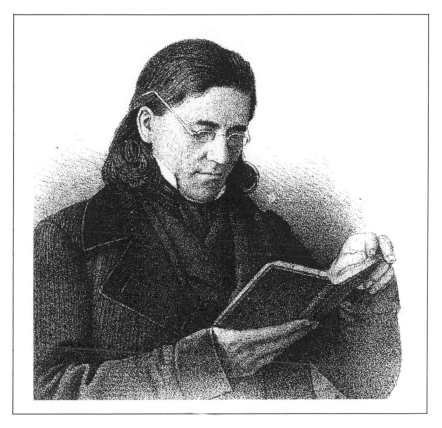

Portrait of prominent homeopathic doctor Constantin Hering from the frontispiece of his *Domestic Physician* (Philadelphia, 1845).

physicians, concentrated largely in New England, New York, Pennsylvania, and the Midwest. Before 1860, however, most homeopathic practitioners were still orthodox doctors who had abandoned their system in favor of a safer and seemingly more effective one.[82]

Part of homeopathy's attraction was its mildness. Instead of the "heroic" remedies of the regulars or the equally rigorous therapies of the Thomsonians, homeopaths prescribed pleasant-tasting pills ("infinitesimals") that rarely produced side effects. Many people thought homeopathic medicines were especially suitable for babies and small children. As Oliver Wendell Holmes, its most devastating critic, observed, homeopathy "does not offend the palate, and so spares the nursery those scenes of single combat in which infants were wont to yield at length to the pres-

sure of the spoon and the imminence of asphyxia." Scholars have specu-
lated that homeopathy's suitability for children won the support of large
numbers of American women, who constituted approximately two-
thirds of its patrons and were among its most active propagators. "Many
a woman, armed with her little stock of remedies, has converted an entire
community," announced the American Institute of Homeopathy with
delight.[83]

Central to the home practice of homeopathy was the "domestic kit,"
which typically contained a case of infinitesimal medicines and a guide.
Available in a variety of combinations, they ranged from small pocket
cases with tiny guides to large family chests with thick volumes. Often
the books appeared in foreign languages as well as in English, and sometimes they covered homeopathic treatments for domestic animals.
Leipzig-educated Constantin Hering, one of the most important and active of the American homeopaths, produced and distributed the first domestic kit. It accompanied his two-part *The Homoeopathist, or Domestic
Physician,* which appeared in 1835 and 1838 respectively. The mahogany
box contained small, numbered vials filled with infinitesimal pills, the
numbers of the vials corresponding to the numbered remedies in the
books. After making a diagnosis, the individual had a simple task: to
select the proper number of pills from the vial recommended in the
manual.[84]

Like Hahnemann and Hering, most homeopaths were trained physicians, and many had recently arrived from Germany. They envisioned an
important but circumscribed role for domestic practitioners. Hering, for
example, wrote his book not to replace the physician but to assist families
in treating minor complaints and to provide medical advice for students,
travellers, mariners, and "those living in remote parts of the country."
Like virtually all of his homeopathic colleagues, he urged his readers to
seek qualified medical assistance in serious cases, such as dropsy or ty-
phoid fever. This, Hering explained, was because his book alone could
"make no one a homoeopathic physician. . . . No one could be a successful disciple of *Hahnemann,* who is not well versed, as *Hahnemann*
himself was, in the learning of the medical schools; and it would be . . .
impossible for him to act judiciously without a knowledge of anatomy,
physiology, pathology, surgery and materia medica, together with chemistry and botany."[85]

Hering did urge Americans to abandon the "irrational and pernicious
practice" of orthodox medicine in favor of the "judicious and rational"
practice of homeopathy. But Hering had much in common with his
orthodox counterparts. He sought to reduce popular reliance on "the so-

called domestic remedies, . . . and . . . nostrums or patent medicines, some of which are to be found in almost every nursery, and the habitual use of which is such a prolific cause of innumerable drug-diseases." Despite his antagonism to common domestic remedies, Hering wanted to *guide* domestic treatment, not jettison it. Domestic practice could be improved, Hering believed, only if nonprofessionals honed their diagnostic and treatment skills. To help his audience, Hering provided lengthy "directions for prescribing." There, Hering instructed his readers to scan the table of contents until they found the chapter pertinent to the complaint needing treatment. To make the search easier, Hering arranged diseases according to their principal symptoms, not according to their proper medical nomenclature. As a further aid to nonprofessionals, Hering divided his book into two sections. In the first part, he treated "the most common causes of diseases," including such things as "consequences of overeating, immoderate exertion and great exhaustion" and "consequences of spirituous liquors, coffee, tea, tobacco, acids, etc." Part 2 covered diseases that manifested themselves in specific parts of the body. This section began "with *head, neck, chest,* and so on downward, enumerating under each head the disease to which that part is principally subject." In order to diagnose and prescribe properly, Hering also expected his readers to imitate the physician's habit of making an exhaustive initial investigation. It was, he acknowledged, "troublesome, but you can have no success without it; if you succeed without this troublesome examination, it is by chance, not by skill." Hering's list of questions to ask, conditions to ascertain, and symptoms to monitor was indeed comprehensive, covering a full seven pages.[86]

Other homeopathic domestic guides utilized a similar organization, but some pointedly discouraged self-treatment. Egbert Guernsey wrote that his 1855 *Gentleman's Handbook of Homoeopathy* was not intended to make every person his own doctor but was to be used in emergency situations and minor illnesses. His aim had been the same in his lengthier *Homoeopathic Domestic Practice* of 1853.[87] He wanted, he said in the earlier volume, "to prepare as clear and practical a guide as possible for the sickroom and domestic practice," but had "no wish . . . to supersede . . . the physician." No one could hope to fulfill "the high and holy duties of the physician" without devoting "years to the investigation of the human system, the causes of sickness, [and] the power of remedial agents." Only after such training would a person be "able to look beneath the surface and trace from apparent unimportant symptoms the true seat and cause of the difficulty." What each individual could—and should—do, Guernsey pointed out, was to take responsibility for preventing disease.

A TABLE OF A NUMBER OF THE AFFECTIONS OF THE EYES, WITH THEIR PROPER REMEDIES.

	Aconit.	Ant. crud.	Arnica.	Arsenic.	Bryonia.	Culcarea.	Cham.	China.	Cina.	Drosera.	Euphr.	Hepar.	Hyos.	Ignat.	Mercur.	Nux vom	Puls.	Rhus.	Spigel.	Staph.	Stram.	Sulph.	Veratrum.	Bell.
1. THE EYES AND EYEBALLS.																								
Pain	*		*		*	*			*		*						*	*	*	*		*		*
Bloodshot eyes	*														*				*		*			*
Itching				*	*	*		*		*	*				*	*		*		*	*		*	*
Stinging	*			*	*	*					*				*	*	*		*		*		*	*
Burning	*		*	*	*	*	*				*				*	*	*	*		*		*		*
Pressure outward	*												*		*					*				
do inward															*					*				
Inflammation	*		*	*	*		*	*			*		*		*	*	*	*	*		*	*	*	*
Discharge of tears			*	*		*	*		*			*	*		*	*	*	*	*		*	*	*	*
2. THE EYLIDS.																								
Burning					*	*									*		*		*			*		
Inflammation	*				*	*	*			*		*			*	*	*		*	*	*	*	*	*
Sty																*	*		*					
Swelling	*				*	*	*			*		*			*	*	*		*		*	*		*
Itching					*			*	*					*	*	*		*			*	*		
Difficulty of opening	*				*		*					*		*	*	*	*		*			*	*	
Redness		*			*	*	*							*	*	*				*		*		
Stitches			*																*	*		*		
Closing					*	*	*				*		*	*	*	*	*		*	*	*	*	*	*
Aggravated in the																								
Morning	*	*			*		*	*	*					*		*	*	*	*	*				
Forenoon		*			*			*						*		*								
Afternoon					*				*						*				*	*				
Evening					*			*	*		*		*		*	*	*	*		*		*		
At Night	*				*	*					*	*	*	*	*	*	*	*		*				
SYMPTOMS WORSE.																								
By moving the eyes	*						*	*										*	*					
After wakening					*										*		*			*				
In the open air					*						*			*	*	*	*		*		*			
By reading						*			*	*	*	*				*		*				*		
By look'g at the light	*	*							*			*	*			*	*			*		*		*
By closing the eyes		*												*					*			*		
By rubbing																*		*						
SYMPTOMS RELIEVED																								
After rising																*		*						
By closing the eyes																*		*						
By external pressure					*											*							*	
In the open air													*			*	*							
By rubbing							*									*		*		*				

Only those who were knowledgeable about how their bodies worked could sensibly exercise this responsibility. Thus both of Guernsey's books provided some coverage of anatomy, physiology, and hygiene.[88]

George E. Shipman argued in a similar vein. "No *very* sensible person," said Shipman in his *Homoeopathic Family Guide,* "will ever attempt to treat himself or his family, who can obtain the advice of a well-qualified physician. If those fail too often, who make the study of diseases and their remedies the sole business of their lives, what success can they expect, who know little or nothing of either?" Shipman advised readers to consult doctors when they had to cope with colic, consumption, scald head, scarlet fever, croup, or another serious illness.[89]

Despite their qualms about home treatment, homeopaths had no doubt that domestic guides and kits were valuable "messengers of mercy and usefulness" which "traveled with, and often ahead of, the regular practitioners of Homoeopathy." As such, continued Joseph Hippolyt Pulte in *Homoeopathic Domestic Physician,* domestic guides were "the silent, but efficient missionaries of truth, declaring it everywhere by facts and conquests over disease, won by the people themselves." Thus most homeopaths viewed domestic manuals not as competitors but "as necessary allies in the great work of reforming the medical state of the world." For this reason, Pulte wrote, "the profession . . . bestows a great deal of care on their constantly increasing perfection, by making them more practical and definite, progressing in their improvement as the science itself progresses."[90] Even orthodox physicians did not dispute their effectiveness. Many an "impecunious practitioner" had failed to get a case, complained one regular, because of "Dr. Humphrey's book and box that preceded him in the domestic corner."[91]

Homeopaths did not worry much about domestic excesses and errors because they realized their system was relatively harmless, particularly when compared to the heroic remedies of the regularly educated doctors. Even if the patient took the wrong medicine, there was no need for alarm, wrote Hering, "for Homoeopathic medicine is so prepared that it will help, when it is the right one, but it will not injure should a mistake occur." The very worst possibility would be a slight delay in the healing process. Readers of British reformer John Epps's manual, for example, were assured that "no life was ever lost by homoeopathic medicine used carelessly, or otherwise," a point conceded by sarcastic regulars. Homeopathy, sneered Oliver Wendell Holmes, "gives the ignorant, who have such an inveterate itch for dabbling in physic, a book and a doll's medicine chest, and lets them play doctors and doctresses without fear of having to call in the coroner."[92]

Many lay practitioners shared the belief that homeopathy was safe even when misused. In 1854 South Carolina politician and plantation owner James Henry Hammond embraced homeopathy after rejecting orthodox medicine and then Thomsonianism. In an 1861 letter to William Gilmore Simms, Hammond first expressed his condolences on the death of the novelist's little boy and then chastised him for "allow[ing] too much use of medicine in your family." Vehemently opposed to heroic medicine, Hammond advised: "Throw, as I did seven years ago, all medicine into the River. Get Pulte's Family Physician, Hull, Jahr, and a box of Homoeopathic pellets not tinctures, nor powders. Treat every case symptomatically ignoring the name of the disease. When you hit right you make a speedy cure. If you miss, you do no harm."[93]

The confidence of other nonprofessionals was more shaky. For days Calvin Fletcher confided in his diary about his uncle's precarious health, noting on 9 April 1857 further deterioration after a local doctor predicted that homeopathy would kill rather than cure him. Nine more days passed before his uncle seemed beyond danger, and only then did Fletcher write the details about that incident and its aftermath: "While sick here & at the worst moment an allopathy Doctor sent a messenger to him to say that if he did not take calomel he would die that his liver did not perform its office & consequently the fluids stagnated & became poisonous & were being diffused thro his whole system & that he might as well take arsenic & die by that as to die as he was dying." Convinced that "this word was sent for a malicious purpose," Fletcher angrily recalled that it had indeed "had a very bad effect on him & took some days to get over it." Aided by good nursing and rest, however, "his Homopa'mest Doctor . . . at last quietted his nerves & the last 4 or 5 days has recovered very fast."[94]

As the century advanced and homeopathy waned, homeopaths wrote less to the general public and more to their own profession.[95] The domestic guides that appeared during the latter part of the century were less comprehensive and focused more on emergency care and minor illnesses. However, at mid-century, homeopaths—like hydropaths and female practitioners—stressed the necessity of preventive living and helped spread knowledge of anatomy, physiology, and hygiene. Despite the hostility shown by the regulars to sectarian therapeutic challenges, most grudgingly agreed with Dan King. Homeopathy, asserted King in his 1858 *Quackery Unmasked,* was clearly "absurd," but he had to acknowledge one benefit. "Through the use of [Hahnemann's] empty and inert means, we have been enabled to see what the innate powers of the animal organization can accomplish without medical interference." Thus mankind had been benefited by the "ineffable delusion."[96] Worthington Hooker reached the same conclusion with equal reluctance. Homeopathy, Hooker wrote in 1849, "is doing a good work in helping to destroy . . . undue reliance upon positive medication." The legacy, he thought, would endure, "unwittingly" bringing "more good than harm to the permanent interests of medical science."[97]

The Transformation of Domestic Medicine

Homeopathy enjoyed great popularity in the two decades after the Civil War. Especially strong in urban areas of the Northeast and Midwest, it continued to have the backing of many prominent Americans. Despite the growth of homeopathy and other sects, regular physicians still greatly outnumbered their challengers. Joseph Kett has estimated that sectarians comprised roughly ten percent of the total number of physicians between 1835 and 1860. By 1871, according to J. M. Toner's count published that year, they represented about thirteen percent, or nearly six thousand sectarians compared to thirty-nine thousand regulars. Yet there were four thousand eight hundred doctors Toner could not classify, and his figures also failed to include another ten thousand to fourteen thousand practitioners. Paul Starr suggests that twenty percent of all physicians were sectarians during the last decades of the century.[98]

But statistics do not tell the whole story. The existence and success of rival sects called into question orthodox preemption of professional legitimacy and scientific reputability. The regulars' hostility to medical alternatives endured beyond the Civil War and indeed continues to the present.[99]

Beleaguered and fragmented, orthodox physicians used institutional and organizational means to strengthen their profession. They formed associations, lobbied for licensing laws, and tried to reform medical schools. They had a dual aim: improving the quality of regular medical practice and excluding practitioners who were not properly qualified. One important consequence would be a public better equipped to distinguish among legitimate and illegitimate healers.

Yet to stress the battle lines obscures and misleads as much as it enlightens. It fails to take into account the degree to which regulars and their rivals shared the same goals. For a hundred years prior to the Civil War, orthodox doctors and reform-minded writers had been articulating new ideas about the proper roles for the professional and nonprofessional in meeting disease. The doctor, they increasingly argued, should be given primary responsibility for directing medical treatment. Though this conception ousted the lay person from the supervisory position to which he or she had been accustomed, writers gave the lay person a new assignment: prevention, which they deemed equally or more important to the nation's survival. Scholars have neglected the campaign for preventive living, which was an integral part of the regulars' professionalizing efforts and was also central to the work of unorthodox healers.

Medical science and practice changed radically in the half-century following the Civil War, sparked by the dramatic bacteriological breakthroughs of Pasteur and Koch in the 1860s and 1870s. Until the last decade of the century, however, the most obvious applications of these discoveries were in public hygiene. To use Erwin Ackerknecht's classification, this was preeminently "an era of public health." Said one physician in 1893, bacteriology had "rendered great service to the art by adding to the power of preventive medicine. It has not done much for the drug treatment of disease."[100] Yet by the end of the first quarter of the twentieth century, bacteriology had begun to revolutionize the way Americans lived. "Our work in the past ten years has changed tremendously," stated a Minnesota physician in 1923. "Ten years ago no parent brought a child to the physician for examination to make sure that nothing was wrong. Today, I venture to say that the greatest part of the work a pediatrician has is in preventive medicine."[101]

In this century, Americans have reaped astounding rewards from changes in medical knowledge and health care. Many should be attributed to the multitude of great scientific and technological achievements, but the widespread adoption of prevention-oriented ways of living has also played a significant role.[102] On the eve of the twenty-first century, however, it is ironic that health publicists—both professionals and nonprofessionals—are articulating many of the same fundamental themes that their predecessors of the past two centuries voiced in very different social, cultural, and medical contexts.

Contemporary crusaders still stress prevention as the lay person's primary duty, but a growing chorus is calling for every person to assume a newly proactive role in his or her own health care. This is essential, say the analysts, because both lay people and doctors have placed far too much faith in the power of medicine and technology to work miracles. For a host of different reasons and from a variety of different perspectives, health advocates are calling on each person to "accept a certain measure of responsibility for his or her own recovery from disease or disability."[103]

What would this entail? There are probably as many answers to this question as there are respondents, but it is striking to note how many of the solutions would have been familiar to our ancestors who lived between 1760 and 1860. One recurring idea, for instance, is that each person knows his or her own constitution and history best, and therefore has a duty to communicate that knowledge to medical personnel. Another is the refurbished concept of *vis medicatrix naturae,* the belief that many diseases are self-limiting and therefore do not require much medical intervention—and certainly not the amount or the sort to which contemporary Americans are accustomed. Most significantly, today's analysts are calling on professionals and nonprofessionals to build and nurture a health-care partnership very much like that envisioned by nineteenth-century health publicists: a partnership based on mutual respect, clear understanding, and faithful execution. In that scenario, both as it originally evolved and in its updated version, it is the doctor who directs treatment, but crucial to a successful outcome are the informed and responsible actions of the patient, other caregivers, and the patient's family and friends.

Journalist Norman Cousins in many ways epitomizes this stance. In 1964 Cousins was diagnosed with a crippling condition that experts believed was irreversible. Instead of submitting to the prognosis and its attendant therapies, Cousins critically evaluated the care he was being given and then rejected it in favor of one he conceived himself. Of course, as Cousins wrote in his acclaimed *Anatomy of an Illness,* he was fortunate to have had a good, long-standing relationship with an open-minded doctor. Cousins's doctor encouraged his patient to learn as much as he could about his disease and its treatment, and then to apply that knowledge to his own case. As a result, explained Cousins, he felt like a valuable part of his own medical team: "I would say that the principal contribution made by my doctor to the taming, and possibly the conquest, of my illness was that he encouraged me to believe that I was a respected partner with him in the total undertaking."[104]

Though Cousins's story is inspirational, there are probably few contemporary observers who would adopt the Cousins model as a depiction of the ideal doctor-patient relationship. Nor would they endorse the idea that lay people abdicate all treatment responsibility to the doctor. Most would probably agree with Cousins that the ideal doctor-patient relationship is one in which both parties acknowledge that they form a partnership characterized by mutual respect, informed judgment, and responsible execution.

This concept exhibits obvious parallels to the ideas promoted between the American Revolution and the Civil War. Today, however, the situation is reversed. Instead of living in a world where lay healers are perceived as having too much authority, we are confronted with exactly the opposite problem. Health publicists between 1760 and 1860 left a legacy that still has great relevance as we work to improve health-care delivery in the United States.[105]

Notes

Abbreviations Used

AHR	*American Historical Review*
AQ	*American Quarterly*
BHM	*Bulletin of the History of Medicine*
BMSJ	*Boston Medical and Surgical Journal*
DAB	*Dictionary of American Biography*
DNB	*Dictionary of National Biography*
enl.	enlarged [edition]
JAH	*Journal of American History*
JHMAS	*Journal of the History of Medicine and Allied Sciences*
JIH	*Journal of Interdisciplinary History*
J. Soc. Hist.	*Journal of Social History*
J. Southern Hist.	*Journal of Southern History*
JUH	*Journal of Urban History*
MVHR	*Mississippi Valley Historical Review*
NUC	*National Union Catalogue, Pre-1956 Imprints*
rev.	revised [edition]
t.p.	title page
WMQ	*William and Mary Quarterly*

Unless otherwise indicated, all emphases appeared in the original texts. Spelling and punctuation have also been retained from the original texts, and the term *sic* is used only when it appeared in the original texts.

Preface

1. Leo Hershkowitz and Isidore S. Meyer, eds., *The Lee Max Friedman Collection of American Jewish Colonial Correspondence: Letters of the Franks Family (1733–1748)*. *Studies in American Jewish History*, no. 5 (Waltham, Mass.: American Jewish Historical Society, 1968), pp. 86–87. Brackets in original.

2. Carol F. Karlsen and Laurie Crumpacker, eds., *The Journal of Esther Edwards Burr, 1754–1757* (New Haven and London: Yale University Press, 1984), p. 279.

3. Ibid., pp. 285–87. Bracketed ellipsis points in original.

4. Raymond C. Werner, "Diary of Grace Growden Galloway," *Pennsylvania Magazine of History and Biography* 55(1931): 32–94; 58(1934): 152–89, at p. 66.

5. Three historiographical essays discuss this point from different perspectives: Gerald Grob, "The Social History of Medicine and Disease in America: Problems and Possibilities," *J. Soc. Hist.* 10(1977): 391–409; Charles E. Rosenberg, "The Medical Profession, Medical Practice, and the History of Medicine," in Edwin Clarke, ed., *Modern Methods in the History of Medicine* (London: Althone Press, 1971), pp. 22–35; and Ronald L. Numbers, "The History of the American Medicine: A Field in Ferment," *Reviews in American History* 10(1982): 245–63.

6. Particularly during the past five years the focus on doctors has begun to shift to other participants. See, for example, Judith Walzer Leavitt, *Brought to Bed: Childbearing in America, 1750 to 1950* (New York: Oxford University Press, 1986). Roy Porter and Dorothy Porter have recently published several path-breaking volumes: Dorothy Porter, *Patient's Progress: Doctors and Doctoring in Eighteenth-Century England* (Cambridge: Polity Press, 1989); Roy Porter, ed., *Patients and Practitioners: Lay Perceptions of Medicine in Pre-Industrial Society* (Cambridge: Cambridge University Press, 1985); and Roy Porter and Dorothy Porter, *In Sickness and In Health: The British Experience, 1650–1850* (New York: Basil Blackwell, 1989 [1988]). In an earlier study, Jean Strouse did justice to the nuances of the invalid-doctor relationship and its larger familial and social contexts: *Alice James: A Biography* (Boston: Houghton Mifflin, 1980).

7. For an extended historigraphical discussion, see my dissertation: Mary Lamar Riley, "The 'Family Physician': Health Advice and Domestic Medicine from the American Revolution to the Civil War" (unpublished Ph.D. dissertation, University of Chicago, 1985), pp. 4–23.

8. I do not view those who have social and cultural authority as necessarily coercive or conspiratorial, though they may be either or both. To describe people and objects invested by their societies and cultures with authority, I prefer the German historian Momsen's terse definition: "more than advice and less than a command, an advice which one may not safely ignore." Quoted in Paul Starr, *The Social Transformation of American Medicine* (New York: Basic Books, 1982), p. 14.

9. There are no systematic discussions of the genres within popular health literature, but two works provided extremely helpful orientation: Guenter B. Risse, Ronald L. Numbers, and Judith Walzer Leavitt, eds. *Medicine Without Doctors: Home Health Care in American History* (New York: Science History

Publications, 1977), especially John B. Blake, "From Buchan to Fishbein: The Literature of Domestic Medicine," pp. 11–30; and Madge E. Pickard and R. Carlyle Buley, *The Midwest Pioneer: His Ills, Cures, and Doctors* (Crawfordsville, Ind.: R. E. Banta, 1945). In a provocative book, Jeffrey Brooks has examined the origins of a very different type of popular writing and placed it within the context of larger social, cultural, and economic changes: *When Russia Learned to Read: Literacy and Popular Literature, 1861–1917* (Princeton: Princeton University Press, 1985).

10. As many scholars have shown, it is very difficult to pinpoint the extent to which advice literature reflects or prescribes actual social and cultural practices and then to tie those conclusions to particular groups of people. See, for example, Carl Degler, "What Ought To Be and What Was: Women's Sexuality in the Nineteenth Century," *AHR* 79(1974): 1479–90. John Haller and Robin Haller inadequately heed this warning in arguing that Victorian sexual ideology, largely promulgated and perpetuated by physicians, was a means whereby white, middle-class men were able to exercise control over women: *The Physician and Sexuality in Victorian America* (Urbana: University of Illinois Press, 1974). Ann Douglas Wood's strident feminism greatly weakens a similar argument in " 'The Fashionable Diseases': Women's Complaints and Their Treatment in Nineteenth Century America," *JIH* 4(1973–74): 25–52. Regina Markell Morantz has sensibly observed that Wood's portrait of the Victorian doctor borders on caricature: "The Perils of Feminist History," *JIH* 4(1973–74): 649–60; and "The Lady and Her Physician," in Mary Hartmann and Lois Banner, eds., *Clio's Consciousness Raised: New Perspectives on the History of Women* (New York: Harper and Row, 1974), pp. 38–53.

11. The pioneer in broadening the study of medical history was Richard H. Shryock. In addition to numerous articles and monographs, two of his books in particular have remained standard, if now somewhat outdated, references: *The Development of Modern Medicine: An Interpretation of the Social and Scientific Factors Involved* (New York: Alfred A. Knopf, 1947); and *Medicine and Society in America: 1660–1860* (New York: New York University Press, 1960). Several of Shryock's medically trained contemporaries stressed similar themes, but Charles E. Rosenberg has been more influential in redirecting research energies, beginning with *The Cholera Years: The United States in 1832, 1849, and 1866*, Phoenix paperback ed. (Chicago: University of Chicago Press, 1962). For a good overview of current scholarship, see Judith Walzer Leavitt and Ronald L. Numbers, eds., *Sickness and Health in America: Readings in the History of Medicine and Public Health* (Madison: University of Wisconsin Press, 1978); a revised, second edition appeared in 1985.

12. As is customary in discussing American medical history, I use interchangeably the adjectives *orthodox, established,* and *regular* to refer to allopathic doctors. Their nineteenth-century competitors—irregular or unorthodox practitioners—were sectarians, including Thomsonians, hydropaths, homeopaths, and many others.

13. My argument bears superficial resemblance to that presented in Anita Clair Fellman and Michael Fellman, *Making Sense of Self: Medical Advice Literature in Late Nineteenth Century America* (Philadelphia: University of Pennsylvania Press, 1981). More a speculative series of essays than a definitive study, the book does not characterize in any systematic way the late-nineteenth-century

health writers under review, though it assumes—probably correctly—that they were important supporters of established medicine. In addition, their claims to have used a wide range of sources is misleading. Most significantly, however, the Fellmans focus on the late nineteenth century and only allude to the foundation laid in the preceding hundred years.

14. The most comprehensive study of the popularization of health is John C. Burnham's *How Superstition Won and Science Lost: Popularizing Science and Health in the United States* (New Brunswick and London: Rutgers University Press, 1987). Burnham identifies and characterizes successive phases of popularization, beginning with the antebellum period. Late-nineteenth- and twentieth-century evidence leads Burnham to the conclusion encapsulated in the title. Changing concepts of health are discussed in James C. Whorton, *Crusaders for Fitness: The History of American Health Reformers* (Princeton: Princeton University Press, 1982); and Martha H. Verbrugge, *Able-Bodied Womanhood: Personal Health and Social Change in Nineteenth-Century Boston* (New York: Oxford University Press, 1988).

15. Richard W. Wertz and Dorothy C. Wertz make the argument that the campaign was not at first predicated on excluding women in *Lying-In: A History of Childbirth in America* (New York: Free Press, 1977), pp. 29–76. Dorothy Porter agrees in *Patient's Progress,* pp. 173–85. Regina Markell Morantz-Sanchez, however, finds exclusionary motives among most doctors from the beginning, as she explains in *Sympathy and Science: Women Physicians in American Medicine* (New York: Oxford University Press, 1987 [1985]), pp. 8–27.

1. The Family Physician

1. Quoted in Keith Thomas, *Religion and the Decline of Magic* (London: Weidenfeld and Nicolson, 1971), p. 12. Earlier versions of this chapter were presented as follows: "Domestic Practice in the New Republic," to the Midwest Society of Medical Historians (North of Forty Group), 22 October 1983; and "The 'Family Physician': Professional Advice and Domestic Medicine in the New American Republic," to the University of Chicago Workshop in the Social Sciences, 31 January 1984.

2. Roy Porter, "The Language of Quackery in England, 1660–1800," in Peter Burke and Roy Porter, eds., *The Social History of Language* (Cambridge: Cambridge University Press, 1987), pp. 73–103, quote on p. 77; Lucinda McCray Beier, "In Sickness and in Health: A Seventeenth Century Family's Experience," in Roy Porter, ed., *Patients and Practitioners: Lay Perceptions of Medicine in Pre-Industrial Society* (Cambridge: Cambridge University Press, 1985), pp. 101–28. Also very useful is Matthew Ramsey, *Professional and Popular Medicine in France, 1770–1830: The Social World of Medical Practice* (Cambridge and New York: Cambridge University Press, 1988).

3. Joseph F Kett provides a cogent overview of the British background in *The Formation of the American Medical Profession: The Role of Institutions, 1780–1860* (New Haven: Yale University Press, 1968), pp. 1–13. A more detailed treatment is Lester S. King, *The Medical World of the Eighteenth Century* (Chicago: University of Chicago Press, 1958), pp. 1–58. See also Eric H. Christianson, "Medicine in New England," in Ronald L. Numbers, ed., *Medicine in the New World: New Spain, New France, and New England* (Knoxville: Univer-

sity of Tennessee Press, 1987), pp. 101–53; and Beier, "In Sickness and in Health."

4. King, *Medical World of the Eighteenth Century*, pp. 1–29.

5. Kett, *American Medical Profession*, pp. 1–13; Roy Porter, "Language of Quackery"; and Ramsey, *Professional and Popular Medicine in France*, pp. 129–276.

6. Kett, *American Medical Profession*, pp. 1–13, quote on p. 4; and Beier, "In Sickness and in Health."

7. Quoted in Thomas, *Religion and the Decline of Magic*, p. 14.

8. Kett, *American Medical Profession*, p. 5 (quote); Beier, "In Sickness and in Health."

9. The discussion in this paragraph and the two following is based on the following sources: Charles E. Rosenberg, "The Therapeutic Revolution: Medicine, Meaning, and Social Change in Nineteenth-Century America," in Morris J. Vogel and Charles E. Rosenberg, eds., *The Therapeutic Revolution: Essays in the Social History of American Medicine* (Philadelphia: University of Pennsylvania Press, 1979), pp. 3–25, quote on p. 8; J. Worth Estes and David M. Goodman, *The Changing Humors of Portsmouth: The Medical Biography of an American Town, 1623–1983* (Boston: Francis A. Countway Library of Medicine, 1986), pp. 1–12; Christianson, "Medicine in New England," pp. 110–12, 137–42; and Edward C. Atwater, "Touching the Patient: The Teaching of Internal Medicine in America," in Judith Walzer Leavitt and Ronald L. Numbers, eds., *Sickness and Health in America: Readings in the History of Medicine and Public Health*, 2nd ed., rev. (Madison: University of Wisconsin Press, 1985), pp. 129–47.

10. Two pioneering books give us valuable insights into how a person living centuries ago viewed illness and health: Roy Porter and Dorothy Porter, *In Sickness and In Health: The British Experience, 1650–1850* (New York: Basil Blackwell, 1989 [1988]); and Dorothy Porter, *Patient's Progress: Doctors and Doctoring in Eighteenth-Century England* (Cambridge: Polity Press, 1989).

11. Laurel Thatcher Ulrich, "Housewife and Gadder: Themes of Self-Sufficiency in Eighteenth-Century New England," in Carol Groneman and Mary Beth Norton, eds., *"To Toil the Livelong Day": America's Women at Work, 1780–1980* (Ithaca: Cornell University Press, 1987), pp. 21–34; Annegret S. Ogden, *The Great American Housewife: From Helpmate to Wage Earner, 1776–1986* (Westport, Conn.: Greenwood Press, 1986), pp. 13–15; Beier, "In Sickness and in Health," pp. 111–26. The social nature of medical care persisted until at least the late nineteenth century, as described in Lida L. Greene, ed., "Diary of a Young Girl," *Annals of Iowa*, 3rd ser., 36(1962): 437–57.

12. Plantation families, slaves, and Southern practitioners operated in an even more complex healing environment, as documented by Todd L. Savitt in "Black Health on the Plantation: Masters, Slaves, and Physicians," in Leavitt and Numbers, eds., *Sickness and Health* (1985), pp. 313–30. A more extended discussion is Savitt's *Medicine and Slavery: The Health Care and Diseases of Blacks in Antebellum Virginia* (Urbana: University of Illinois Press, 1978).

13. William G. Rothstein, *American Physicians in the Nineteenth Century: From Sects to Science* (Baltimore: Johns Hopkins University Press, 1972), pp. 26–38; Christianson, "Medicine in New England," pp. 117–42; Estes and Goodman, *Changing Humors*, pp. 1–41.

14. Paul Starr, *The Social Transformation of American Medicine* (New York: Basic Books, 1982), pp. 30–59.
15. Richard D. Brown briefly treats the interpenetration of popular and professional medicine in "The Healing Arts in Colonial and Revolutionary Massachusetts: The Context for Scientific Medicine," in Philip Cash, Eric H. Christianson, and J. Worth Estes, eds., *Medicine in Colonial Massachusetts, 1620–1820,* vol. 57 of the *Publications* of The Colonial Society of Massachusetts (Boston: Colonial Society of Massachusetts, 1980), pp. 35–47. Charles E. Rosenberg stresses the overlap between vernacular and academic medical practice during a slightly later period in his "Introduction to the New Edition," *Gunn's Domestic Medicine, or, Poor Man's Friend* (Knoxville, Tenn.: Printed under the immediate superintendance of the author, a physician of Knoxville, 1830; facsimile ed., Tennesseana Editions, Knoxville: University of Tennessee Press, 1986), pp. [v]–xxi. For other perspectives on the same point, see Judith Walzer Leavitt, *Brought to Bed: Childbearing in America, 1750 to 1950* (New York: Oxford University Press, 1986), pp. 4–12; and Louis K. Wechsler, *The Common People of Colonial America: As Glimpsed Chiefly Through the Dusty Windows of the Old Almanacks, Chiefly of New-York* (New York: Vantage Press, 1978), pp. 86–96.
16. The best overview is Whitfield J. Bell, Jr., "A Portrait of the Colonial Physician," in Whitfield J. Bell, Jr., *The Colonial Physician & Other Essays* (New York: Science History Publications, 1975), pp. 5–25. Bell treats Franklin in another article in the same volume, "Benjamin Franklin and the Practice of Medicine," pp. 119–30. Private libraries with extensive medical collections included those of Cotton Mather, William Byrd, and Quakers James Logan and Isaac Norris. For the latter two and interesting comments on Quakers and medicine, consult Frederick B. Tolles, *Meeting House and Counting House: The Quaker Merchants of Colonial Philadelphia, 1682–1763* (New York: W. W. Norton and Co., 1963 [1948]), pp. 161–204.
17. Guenter B. Risse, "Introduction," in Guenter B. Risse, Ronald L. Numbers, and Judith Walzer Leavitt, eds., *Medicine Without Doctors: Home Health Care in American History* (New York: Science History Publications, 1977), pp. 1–8. William Coleman provides more extended discussion in two excellent articles: "Health and Hygiene in the *Encyclopédie*: A Medical Doctrine for the Bourgeoisie," *JHMAS* 29(1974): 399–421; and "The People's Health: Medical Themes in 18th-Century French Popular Literature," *BHM* 51(1977): 55–74. See also John B. Blake, *"The Compleat Housewife,"* *BHM* 49(1975): 30–42. There are several pertinent articles in Roy Porter, ed., *Patients and Practitioners*: Joan Lane, "'The Doctor Scolds Me': The Diaries and Correspondence of Patients in Eighteenth Century England," pp. 205–48; Ginnie Smith, "Prescribing the Rules of Health: Self-help and Advice in the Late Eighteenth Century," pp. 249–82; and Roy Porter, "Laymen, Doctors and Medical Knowledge in the Eighteenth Century: The Evidence of the *Gentleman's Magazine*," pp. 283–314.
18. Historians usually emphasize the undeniable degree to which intrafaculty acrimoniousness weakened the profession by splintering it into factions. Fighting was notorious, and some feuds—like those between Benjamin Rush and Adam Kuhn or between John Morgan and William Shippen, Jr.—had far-reaching consequences. However, it should also be remembered that these

squabbles simultaneously kept the public informed about a wide range of medical matters. Carl Bridenbaugh and Jessica Bridenbaugh discuss this briefly in *Rebels and Gentlemen: Philadelphia in the Age of Franklin* (New York: Reynal and Hitchcock, 1942), pp. 295–99. The 1793 yellow fever epidemic in Philadelphia is an excellent example of the duality of this process, as John H. Powell demonstrates in *Bring Out Your Dead: The Great Plague of Yellow Fever in Philadelphia in 1793* (Philadelphia: University of Pennsylvania Press, 1949). See also Laurel Thatcher Ulrich, " 'The Living Mother of a Living Child': Midwifery and Mortality in Post-Revolutionary New England," *WMQ*, 3rd ser., 46(1989): 27–48, esp. pp. 40–41.

19. On Cornaro, see William B. Walker, "Luigi Cornaro, A Renaissance Writer on Personal Hygiene," *BHM* 28(1954): 525–34. Weems's letters are collected in E[mily] E. F. Skeel, ed., *Mason Locke Weems: His Works and Ways*, 3 vols. (New York: Richmond Mayo-Smith, 1929), vol. 2, pp. 38–45; quote at p. 45.

20. Henry R. Viets, "George Cheyne, 1673–1743," *BHM* 23(1949): 435–52; and Lester S. King, "George Cheyne, Mirror of Eighteenth-Century Medicine," *BHM* 48(1974): 517–39.

21. George E. Gifford, Jr., "Botanic Remedies in Colonial Massachusetts, 1620–1820," in Cash, Christianson, and Estes, eds., *Medicine in Colonial Massachusetts*, pp. 263–88. See also David L. Cowen, "The Boston Editions of Nicholas Culpeper," *JHMAS* 11(1956): 156–65; *DNB* 5: 286–87 (Culpeper); and *DNB* 20: 1214–25 (Wesley).

22. William Buchan, *Domestic Medicine; Or, The Family Physician: Being an Attempt to Render the Medical Art More Generally Useful, by Shewing People What Is in Their Own Power Both with Respect to the Prevention and Cure of Diseases. Chiefly Calculated to Recommend a Proper Attention to Regimen and Simple Medicines* (Edinburgh: Balfour, Auld, and Smellie, 1769), pp. ix–xiv. For biographical details see *DNB* 3: 180–81.

23. Ibid., pp. 1–154 and passim; Coleman, "Health and Hygiene," pp. 399–400.

24. Charles E. Rosenberg, "Medical Text and Social Context: Explaining William Buchan's *Domestic Medicine*," *BHM* 57(1983): 22–42. See also C. J. Lawrence, "William Buchan: Medicine Laid Open," *Medical History* 19(1975): 20–33; and *NUC* 81: 610–16.

25. Lyman H. Butterfield, ed., *Diary and Autobiography of John Adams*, 4 vols. (Cambridge: Belknap Press of Harvard University Press, 1961), at vol. 3, p. 158 (28 June 1784).

26. Vicesimus Knox, "On the Rashness of Young and Adventurous Writers in Medicine," in his *Winter Evenings: Or, Lucubrations on Life and Letters*, 3 vols., 3rd ed. (London: Printed for Charles Dilly, 1795; facsimile ed., New York: Garland Publishing Co., 1972), vol. 1, pp. 106–10; quotes are from pp. 109–10. Biographical information is in *DNB* 11: 334–36.

27. Benjamin Rush, "Observations on the Duties of a Physician, and the Methods of Improving Medicine. Accommodated to the Present State of Society and Manners in the United States," in his *Medical Inquiries and Observations*, 4th ed., 4 vols. in 2 (Philadelphia: Printed for E. Kimber and S. W. Conrad by Griggs and Dickinsons, Printers, 1815), vol. 1, pp. [251]–264; all quotes in this paragraph are from pp. 261–62. Rush reiterated these sentiments in his personal correspondence. See, for example, advice given to John Foulke on

25 April 1780 about how best to spend his time abroad: Lyman H. Butterfield, ed., *Letters of Benjamin Rush,* 2 vols. (Princeton: Published for the American Philosophical Society by Princeton University Press, 1951), at vol. 1, pp. 250–51. A copy of this list was sent the following year to Samuel Powel Griffitts prior to his departure for European study, and John Adams received a letter in 1790 with similar remarks; see vol. 1, p. 545.

28. Benjamin Rush, "Upon the Causes Which Have Retarded the Progress of Medicine, and the Means of Promoting Its Certainty and Greater Usefulness," in his *Six Introductory Lectures, To Courses of Lectures Upon the Institutes and Practice of Medicine, Delivered in the University of Pennsylvania* (Philadelphia: John Conrad and Co., etc., 1801), pp. [143]–168, at pp. 148, 151. The same lecture was reprinted for Rush's *Sixteen Introductory Lectures, To Courses of Lectures Upon the Institutes and Practice of Medicine, with a Syllabus of the Latter. To Which Are Added, Two Lectures Upon the Pleasures of the Senses and of the Mind; with an Inquiry into Their Proximate Cause. Delivered in the University of Pennsylvania* (Philadelphia: Bradford and Innskeep, 1811), pp. [141]–165, at pp. 146, 148.

29. Cecil K. Drinker, *Not So Long Ago: A Chronicle of Medicine and Doctors in Colonial Philadelphia* (New York: Oxford University Press, 1937), p. 41. Biographical details are from Anne Firor Scott, "Self Portraits: Three Women," in Richard L. Bushman et al., eds., *Uprooted Americans: Essays to Honor Oscar Handlin* (Boston: Little, Brown and Co., 1979), pp. 43–76.

30. Drinker, *Not So Long Ago,* p. 126. This excerpt is particularly interesting in light of the vitriolic feud between Rush and Kuhn.

31. [Devereux Jarratt], *The Life of the Reverend Devereux Jarratt, Rector of Bath Parish, Dinwiddie County, Virginia. Written by Himself, in a Series of Letters Addressed to the Rev. John Coleman, One of the Ministers of the Protestant Episcopal Church, in Maryland* (Baltimore: Printed by Warner and Hanna, 1806), pp. 140–69.

32. Seth Ames, ed., *Works of Fisher Ames. With a Selection from His Speeches and Correspondence,* vol. 1 (Boston: Little Brown and Co., 1854), pp. 175–76.

33. Jack P. Greene, ed., *The Diary of Colonel Landon Carter of Sabine Hall, 1752–1778,* 2 vols. (Charlottesville: Published for the Virginia Historical Society by the University Press of Virginia, 1965), at vol. 2, p. 627 (11 September 1771). Daniel Blake Smith puts Carter in a larger context in *Inside the Great House: Planter Family Life in Eighteenth-Century Chesapeake Society* (Ithaca: Cornell University Press, 1980), pp. 249–80. Weymouth T. Jordan has compiled a sample of typical plantation remedies from the papers of Alabama's Martin Marshall in *Herbs, Hoecakes, and Husbandry: The Daybook of a Planter of the Old South* (Tallahassee: Florida State University Press, 1960). Planters' wives also handled medical care, as summarized by Catherine Clinton in *The Plantation Mistress: Woman's World in the Old South* (New York: Pantheon Books, 1982), pp. 143–50.

34. Jack Greene, ed., *Diary,* vol. 2, pp. 692–93 (26 May 1772); and vol. 2, p. 783 (30 September 1773). Carter's knowledge of medical writings is apparent throughout the diary.

35. Ibid. All quotes in this paragraph are from vol. 2, pp. 840–42 (27 June 1774), 854 (25 August 1774). Costiveness is constipation.

36. Ibid. This paragraph is based on vol. 1, pp. 315–17 (7–9 July 1776). The

lochial discharge is secreted from the vagina and uterus after delivery and normally lasts two to four weeks. Carter's participation in delivery and its aftermath was unusual for the period, though the idea of male attendance during childbirth was gaining acceptance. See, for example, Judith Walzer Leavitt, "'Science' Enters the Birthing Room: Obstetrics in America since the Eighteenth Century," *JAH* 70(1983): 281–304. Other citations on this subject may be found in the next chapter.

37. Jack Greene, ed., *Diary*; all quotes in this paragraph and the next two are from vol. 1, pp. 320–27 (24 July–20 August 1766). Despite Carter's comment, I find no record in the diary of the first "indecent and abusive" letter sent to him by the doctor.

38. Ibid. Carter was obsessive in his attention to the state of his own health. See, for instance, vol. 1, pp. 318–19 (21 July 1766), and vol. 2, pp. 850–90 (14 August–27 November 1774).

39. Ibid., vol. 2, pp. 1129–30 (14 September 1777).

40. The quote is from the title page of an identical edition: William Buchan, *Domestic Medicine: Or, A Treatise on the Prevention and Cure of Diseases, by Regimen and Simple Medicines. With an Appendix, Containing a Dispensatory for the Use of Private Practitioners. Revised and Adapted to the Diseases of the United States of America, by Samuel Powel Griffitts, M.D.,* 2nd ed. (Philadelphia: Thomas Dobson, 1797). For biographical information on Griffitts, see James Thacher, *American Medical Biography: Or Memoirs of Eminent Physicians Who Have Flourished in America. To Which Is Prefixed a Succinct History of Medical Science in the United States, from the First Settlement of the Country* (Boston: Richardson and Lord and Cottons and Barnard, 1828), pp. 275–85; Whitfield J. Bell, Jr., "Philadelphia Medical Students in Europe, 1750–1800," in his *Colonial Physician*, pp. 41–69; and Joseph Carson, *A History of the Medical Department of the University of Pennsylvania, From Its Foundation in 1765. With Sketches of the Lives of Deceased Professors* (Philadelphia: Lindsay and Blakiston, 1869), pp. 93, 102–103.

41. Buchan, *Domestic Medicine* (Griffitts, 1797), pp. [iii] (quote), 241–51 (inoculation), and 218–24 (yellow fever).

42. Isaac Cathrall used roughly the same title: William Buchan, *Domestic Medicine: Or, A Treatise on the Prevention and Cure of Diseases, by Regimen and Simple Medicines: With an Appendix, Containing a Dispensatory for the Use of Private Practitioners. Adapted to the Climate and Diseases of America, by Isaac Cathrall* (Philadelphia: Printed by Richard Folwell, for Robert Campbell and Co., 1797). As Charles Rosenberg points out, in 1797 Folwell produced nine different issues for booksellers in Philadelphia, Baltimore, and New York (Rosenberg, "Medical Text and Social Context," p. 41n).

43. Biographical details are from Thacher, *American Medical Biography*, pp. 214–17. Cathrall's article on yellow fever, different from that of Griffitts, is in Buchan, *Domestic Medicine* (Cathrall, 1797), pp. 152–67.

44. Robert Wallace Johnson, *Friendly Cautions to the Heads of Families and Others, Very Necessary to Be Observed in Order to Preserve Health and Long Life: With Ample Directions to Nurses Who Attend the Sick, Women in Child-Bed, etc.,* 3rd ed., with additions; 1st American ed., with notes and additions (Philadelphia: Printed and sold by James Humphreys, 1804). Reviewed in *Phila-*

delphia Medical Museum 1(1805): 239–40, quote on p. 239. For publishing information, see *NUC* 282: 364.

45. *Medical Repository*, second hexade, 2(1805): 424.

46. [James Parkinson], *The Town and Country Friend and Physician; Or an Affectionate Address on the Preservation of Health, and the Removal of Disease on Its First Appearance: Supposed To Be Delivered by a Country Physician to the Circle of His Friends and Patients on His Retiring from Business. With Some Cursory Observations on the Treatment of Children, etc.* (Philadelphia: J. Humpreys, 1803). Biographical details are in "James Parkinson," *Medical Classics* 2(1938): 957–61; and *DNB* 15: 314–15. For publishing information, see *NUC* 442: 569–71.

47. *Medical Repository*, second hexade, 1(1804): 64–76; all quotes in this paragraph are from p. 65.

48. Shadrach Ricketson, *Means of Preserving Health, and Preventing Diseases: Founded Principally on an Attention to AIR AND CLIMATE, DRINK, FOOD, SLEEP, EXERCISE, CLOTHING, PASSIONS OF THE MIND, AND RETENTIONS AND EXCRETIONS. With an Appendix, Containing Observations on Bathing, Cleanliness, Ventilation, and Medical Electricity; and on the Abuse of Medicine. Enriched with Apposite Extracts from the Best Authors. Designed not Merely for Physicians, but for the Information of Others. To Which Is Annexed, a Glossary of the Technical Terms Contained in the Work* (New York: Collins, Perkins, and Co., 1806). I know very little about Ricketson except that he published frequently in the *Medical Repository* in its early years, and his articles were written from Duchess County, New York.

49. *Medical Repository*, second hexade, 4 (1807): 194–96; quote on p. 195.

50. Ricketson, *Means of Preserving Health*, t.p.; *NUC* 494: 135.

51. Henry Wilkins, *The Family Adviser; Or, a Plain and Modern Practice of Physic; Calculated for the Use of Private Families, and Accommodated to the Diseases of America. To Which Is Annexed, Mr. Wesley's Primitive Physic, Revised* (Philadelphia: Parry Hall, 1793). For facts about Wilkins's life, see John R. Quinan, *Medical Annals of Baltimore. From 1608 to 1880, Including Events, Men and Literature* (Baltimore: Press of Isaac Friedenwald, 1884), pp. 178–79; and Eugene F Cordell, *The Medical Annals of Maryland, 1799–1899* (Baltimore: Press of Williams and Wilkins Co., 1903), pp. 668–700.

52. Bibliographical information has been compiled from the following: *NUC* 664: 24–25; Robert Austin, *Early American Medical Imprints: A Guide to Works Printed in the United States, 1668–1820* (Washington, D.C.: U.S. Department of Health, Education, and Welfare, 1961); and Charles Evans and Clifton K. Shipton, eds., *American Bibliography: A Chronological Dictionary of All Books, Pamphlets, and Periodical Publications Printed in the United States of America from the Genesis of Printing in 1639 down to and Including the Year 1820. With Bibliographical and Biographical Notes*, 14 vols. (New York: P. Smith, 1941–59).

53. By the 1816 edition, which I have used, the title had changed slightly: James Ewell, *The Medical Companion. Treating, According to the Most Successful Practice: I. The Diseases Common to Warm Climates on Ship Board. II. Common Cases in Surgery, as Fractures, Dislocations, etc. III. The Complaints Peculiar to Women and Children. With A Dispensatory and Glossary. To Which Are Added, A Brief Anatomy of the Human Body; An Essay on Hygiene, Or the Art of Preserving Health and Prolonging Life; An American Materia Medica, Instructing Country*

Gentlemen in the Very Important Knowledge of the Virtues and Doses of Our Medicinal Plants; Also, A Concise and Impartial History of the Capture of Washington, and the Diseases Which Sprung from that most Deplorable Disaster, 3rd ed., greatly improved (Philadelphia: Printed for the Author by Anderson and Meehan, 1816). For publishing information, see *NUC* 164: 379–80.

54. James Ewell, *Medical Companion,* pp. [iii]–vi. For biographical information, see *DAB* 6: 229; Wyndham Blanton, *Medicine in Virginia in the Nineteenth Century* (Richmond: Garrett and Massie, 1933), pp. 344–46; and Stuart Galishoff's entry in Martin Kaufman, Stuart Galishoff, and Todd L. Savitt, eds., *Dictionary of American Medical Biography* (Westport, Conn.: Greenwood Press, 1984), vol. 1, p. 236.

55. *Philadelphia Medical Museum* 5(1808): [190]–[196], at pp. [190]–[193]; *Medical Repository,* second hexade, 5(1808): 387–96, at p. 388. Brackets are part of the pagination in the original for the first citation.

56. James Parkinson, *Medical Admonitions to Families, Respecting the Preservation of Health, and the Treatment of the Sick. Also, A Table of Symptoms, Serving to Point Out the Degree of Danger, and, To Distinguish One Disease from Another: With Observations on the Improper Indulgence of Children, etc.,* 1st Am., from the 4th Eng. ed. (Portsmouth, N.H.: Printed for Charles Peirce, by N. S. and W. Peirce, 1803). Parkinson discusses the dangers of domestic quackery throughout; see, for example, pp. 111–28, esp. p. 113 (inflammation); 302–306, esp. p. 305 (hemorrhage from the lungs); and [45]–51 ("prefatory observations").

57. Thomas Cooper, *A Treatise of Domestic Medicine, Intended for Families, in Which the Treatment of Common Disorders Are Alphabetically Enumerated. To Which Is Added, A Practical System of Domestic Cookery, Describing the Best, Most Economical, and Most Wholesome Methods of Dressing Victuals; Intended for the Use of Families Who Do Not Affect Magnificence in Their Style of Living. Also, the Art of Preserving all Kinds of Animal and Vegetable Substances for Many Years, by M. Appert* (Reading: George Getz, 1824), pp. 6–22. For a capsule biography of this prominent and controversial scientist, lawyer, educator, and physician, see *DAB* 4: 414–16. The best guide to Cooper's scientific and educational interests in the decade prior to the manual's publication is Whitfield J. Bell, Jr., "Thomas Cooper as Professor of Chemistry at Dickinson College, 1811–1815," *JHMAS* 8(1953): 70–87. For publishing information, see *NUC* 122: 22–27.

58. Thomas Ewell, *American Family Physician; Detailing Important Means of Preserving Health, from Infancy to Old Age: The Offices Women Should Perform to Each Other at Births, and the Diseases Peculiar to the Sex: With Those of Children and of Adults. With an Appendix, Containing Hints Respecting the Treatment of Domestic Animals, and the Best Means of Preserving Fish and Meat* (Georgetown, D.C.: James Thomas, 1824), pp. xi–xii. Biographical details may be found in: *DAB* 6: 230–31; Blanton, *Medicine in Virginia in the Nineteenth Century,* pp. 335, 344; and Howard A. Kelly and Walter L. Burrage, eds., *American Medical Biographies* (Baltimore: Norman Remington Co., 1920), pp. 373–74. For bibliographical information, see *NUC* 164: 382.

59. See, for example: [Anthony A. Benezet], *The Family Physician; Comprising Rules for the Prevention and Cure of Diseases; Calculated Particularly for the Inhabitants of the Western Country, and for Those Who Navigate Its Waters. With a*

Dispensatory and Appendix. This Work Affords, in Simple Language, a Concentration of all the Practical Matter Which Can Be Derived from the Best Authorities. With Original Remarks. By a Graduate of the Pennsylvania University, and Honorary Member of the Medical Society of Philadelphia Who Has for Years Been Acquainted with the Modes of Living, and with the Diseases of the West (Cincinnati: W. Hill Woodward, [1826], pp. 463–85 (surgery and accidents); and Horatio Gates Jameson, *The American Domestick Medicine; or, Medical Admonisher: Containing, Some Account of Anatomy, the Senses, Diseases, Casualties; a Dispensatory, and Glossary. In Which The Observations, and Remedies, Are Adapted to the Diseases, etc. of the United States. Designed for the Use of Families* (Baltimore: F Lucas, Jun[ior], 1817), pp. 100–14 (taking a pulse), 422–76 (casualties), [134]–166 (treatment of yellow fever).

60. James Ewell, *Medical Companion*, pp. xiii, 461–596. Ewell was Parson Weems's brother-in-law. Information about the medicine chests that Ewell sold is in Skeel, ed., *Mason Locke Weems*, vol. 2, pp. 294–95n; see also Savitt, "Black Health," p. 325. A more general discussion of medicine chests may be found in Estes and Goodman, *Changing Humors*, pp. 69–76. For other examples of handbooks that included dispensaries, see Benezet, *Family Physician*, pp. [497]–539, and Jameson, *American Domestick Medicine*, pp. [585]–[657].

61. See, for example, Jameson's section on anatomy, *American Domestick Medicine*, pp. [16]–49. Biographical details about Jameson may be found in Quinan, *Medical Annals of Baltimore*, pp. 115–17; Cordell, *Medical Annals of Maryland*, pp. 85–100, 685–704, 779–95; and Genevieve Miller, "A Nineteenth Century Medical School: Washington University of Baltimore," *BHM* 14(1943): 14–29. For bibliographical information, see *NUC* 277: 46.

62. A good example of James Ewell's style is his discussion of the passions: *Medical Companion*, pp. 110–244.

63. Respectful modifiers are sprinkled throughout these texts. See, for example, Jameson, *American Domestick Medicine*, pp. 364–65 (Sydenham) and pp. 263–65 (Mead).

64. Ibid., pp. 215, 380–85, 465–71.

65. Benezet, *American Family Physician*, pp. [iii]–iv, [5]–13, 67 (quote), 189. Much of Benezet's section on scrofula (pp. 343–46) is reproduced exactly from William Buchan, *Domestic Medicine: Or, a Treatise on the Prevention and Cure of Diseases, by Regimen and Simple Medicines. With an Appendix, Containing a Dispensatory for the Use of Private Practitioners. To Which Are Added, Observations on Diet; Recommending a Method of Living Less Expensive, and More Conducive to Health, than the Present. Also, Advice to Mothers, On the Subject of Their own Health; and of the Means of Promoting the Health, Strength, and Beauty of Their Offspring*, new, correct ed., enl. from the author's last revisal (Boston: Joseph Bumstead, 1811) pp. 274–76. Benezet's opening essay on fevers (pp. 99–100) is almost entirely rewritten as compared to the 1811 Bumstead text (pp. 117–21). Though Benezet's book was published anonymously, the title page identified the author as "a graduate of the Pennsylvania University, and honorary member of the Medical Society of Philadelphia." Since I have not been able to locate biographical material about Benezet, I cannot confirm the truth of his claims, though John B. Blake verifies his status in "From Buchan to Fishbein: The Literature of Domestic Medicine," in Risse, Numbers, and Leavitt, eds., *Medicine Without Doctors*, pp. 11–30, at

p. 15. There is no evidence to suggest that he was the same Anthony Benezet who was an eminent humanitarian of the period. For bibliographical information, see *NUC* 21: 126. Scrofula is defined in n. 103 of this chapter.

66. See several articles in Cash, Christianson, and Estes, eds., *Medicine in Colonial Massachusetts*: Eric H. Christianson, "The Medical Practitioners of Massachusetts, 1630–1800: Patterns of Change and Continuity," pp. 49–67; Philip Cash, "The Professionalization of Boston Medicine, 1760–1803," pp. 69–100; C. Helen Brock, "The Influence of Europe on Colonial Massachusetts Medicine," pp. 101–43; and Whitfield J. Bell, Jr., "Medicine in Boston and Philadelphia: Comparisons and Contrasts, 1750–1820," pp. 159–83.

67. Biographies of practitioners of the time often contain much information. Among the most useful have been Betsy Copping Corner, *William Shippen, Jr., Pioneer in American Medical Education* (Philadelphia: American Philosophical Society, 1951), which reprints Shippen's London diary; Richard L. Blanco, *Physician of the American Revolution, Jonathan Potts* (New York: Garland STPM Press, 1979); Whitfield J. Bell, Jr., *John Morgan, Continental Doctor* (Philadelphia: University of Pennsylvania Press, 1965); Frederick B. Tolles, *George Logan of Philadelphia* (New York: Oxford University Press, 1953; reprint ed., New York: Arno Press, 1972); Nathan G. Goodman, *Benjamin Rush: Physician and Citizen, 1746–1813* (Philadelphia: University of Pennsylvania Press, 1934). Also indispensable for Rush (in addition to his *Letters*, cited above) are Donald J. D'Elia, "The Republican Theology of Benjamin Rush," *Pennsylvania History* 33(1966): 187–203; and George W. Corner, ed., *The Autobiography of Benjamin Rush* (Princeton: Princeton University Press, 1948).

68. Quoted in Bell, "Philadelphia Medical Students," p. 55.

69. Bell, *John Morgan*, p. 58.

70. Douglas Sloan, *The Scottish Enlightenment and the American College Ideal* (New York: Teachers College Press, 1971), quote from pp. 5–6n.

71. Quoted in Blanco, *Potts*, p. 27.

72. Butterfield, ed., *Rush Letters*, vol. 1, p. 41.

73. Letter of 8 March 1784 from Griffitts to Rush quoted in J. Rendall, "The Influence of the Edinburgh Medical School on America in the Eighteenth Century," in R. G. W. Anderson and A. D. C. Simpson, eds., *The Early Years of the Edinburgh Medical School* (Edinburgh: Royal Scottish Museum, 1976), pp. 95–124, at p. 97.

74. Quoted in Whitfield J. Bell, Jr., "Some American Students of 'That Shining Oracle of Physic,' Dr. William Cullen of Edinburgh, 1755–1766," American Philosophical Society, *Proceedings*, 94(1950): 275–81, at p. 275. See also Guenter B. Risse's excellent survey, *Hospital Life in Enlightenment Scotland: Care and Teaching at the Royal Infirmary of Edinburgh* (Cambridge and New York: Cambridge University Press, 1986).

75. Fothergill is quoted in Betsy Corner, *Shippen*, p. 93. On George Logan, see Bell, "Philadelphia Medical Students," pp. 51–52; and Rendall, "Influence of the Edinburgh Medical School," p. 103.

76. Butterfield, ed., *Rush Letters*, vol. 1, p. 61 (27 July 1768).

77. Ibid., vol. 1, p. 66 (21 October 1768).

78. William Frederick Norwood, *Medical Education in the United States Before the*

Civil War (Philadelphia: University of Pennsylvania Press, 1944); and George W. Corner, *Two Centuries of Medicine: A History of the School of Medicine, University of Pennsylvania* (Philadelphia: J. B. Lippincott Co., 1965). Charles Caldwell's caustic evaluations of this instruction are well known; see Harriot W. Warner, ed., *Autobiography of Charles Caldwell, M.D.* (Philadelphia: Lippincott, Grambo, and Co., 1855), p. 124 on Adam Kuhn.

79. Bell, *John Morgan*, pp. 144–46. See also Richard H. Shryock, "Empiricism Versus Rationalism in American Medicine, 1650–1950," American Antiquarian Society, *Proceedings*, 79(1969): 99–150.

80. Quoted in Christianson, "Medical Practitioners," p. 63. There were some earlier licensing and regulatory efforts, but they were not very successful; see Christianson, "Medicine in New England," pp. 129–37.

81. John Morgan, *A Discourse Upon the Institution of Medical Schools in America; Delivered at a Public Anniversary Commencement, Held in the College of Philadelphia May 30 and 31, 1765. With a Preface Containing, Amongst Other Things, The Author's Apology for Attempting to Introduce the Regular Mode of Practicing Physic in Philadelphia* (Philadelphia: Printed and Sold by William Bradford, 1765). Quotes in the next paragraph are from pp. 15–24.

82. Richard W. Wertz and Dorothy C. Wertz argue that this campaign was not originally predicated on excluding women from medical practice in *Lying-In: A History of Childbirth in America* (New York: Free Press, 1977), pp. 29–76. Dorothy Porter agrees in *Patient's Progress*, pp. 173–85. Regina Markell Morantz-Sanchez gives the opposite interpretation in *Sympathy and Science: Women Physicians in American Medicine* (New York: Oxford University Press, 1987 [1985]), pp. 8–27.

83. Robert E. Shalhope, "Republicanism and Early American Historiography," *WMQ*, 3rd ser., 39(1982): 334–56; Linda K. Kerber, *Women of the Republic: Intellect and Ideology in Revolutionary America* (Chapel Hill: Published for the Institute of Early American History and Culture by the University of North Carolina Press, 1980); Gordon S. Wood, *The Creation of the American Republic, 1776–1787* (New York: W. W. Norton and Co., 1972); Garry Wills, *Inventing America: Jefferson's Declaration of Independence* (Garden City, N.Y.: Doubleday and Co., 1978); and Rhys Isaac, *The Transformation of Virginia, 1740–1790* (Chapel Hill: Published for the Institute of Early American History and Culture by the University of North Carolina Press, 1982).

84. Linda K. Kerber, *Federalists in Dissent: Imagery and Ideology in Jeffersonian America* (Ithaca: Cornell University Press, 1970).

85. Benjamin Rush, "A Plan for the Establishment of Public Schools and the Diffusion of Knowledge in Pennsylvania; To Which Are Added, Thoughts Upon the Mode of Education, Proper in a Republic. Addressed to the Legislature and Citizens of the State," in Frederick Rudolph, ed., *Essays on Education in the Early Republic* (Cambridge: Belknap Press of Harvard University Press, 1965), pp. 1–23, at p. 17.

86. Wills, *Inventing America*, pp. 175–91. Also useful are Daniel J. Boorstin, *The Lost World of Thomas Jefferson* (New York: Henry Holt and Co., 1948); Henry May, *The Enlightenment in America* (New York: Oxford University Press, 1976); and Charles Camic, *Experience and Enlightenment: Socialization for Cultural Change in Eighteenth-Century Scotland* (Chicago: University of Chicago Press, 1983).

87. Benjamin Rush, "An Eulogium upon Dr. William Cullen, Professor of the Practice of Physic in the University of Edinburgh; Delivered Before the College of Physicians of Philadelphia, on the 9th of July, Agreeably to Their Vote of the 4th of May, 1790, and Afterwards Published at Their Request," in his *Essays, Literary, Moral and Philosophical* (Philadelphia: Printed by Thomas and Samuel Bradford, 1798), pp. 321–43, at pp. 340–41.

88. Benjamin Rush, "Thoughts on Common Sense," in his *Essays,* pp. 249–56, at p. 251.

89. The E. H. Smith quote is from James E. Cronin, ed., *The Diary of Elihu Hubbard Smith (1771–1798)* (Philadelphia: American Philosophical Society, 1973), p. 150 (30 March 1796). Sloan quoted Samuel Stanhope Smith in *Scottish Enlightenment and American College Ideal,* p. 210.

90. Quoted by Lawrence A. Cremin in *American Education: The National Experience, 1783–1876* (New York: Harper and Row, 1980), p. 103.

91. Benjamin Rush, "An Address to the People of the United States," *American Museum* 1(January 1787): 8–11, at p. 8. As Jan Goldstein points out, Philippe Pinel's "creation" of the moral treatment of insanity demonstrates a parallel connection between republican political values and medical thought. See her *Console and Classify: The French Psychiatric Profession in the Nineteenth Century* (Cambridge: Cambridge University Press, 1987), pp. 64–119.

92. Benjamin Rush, "Upon the Causes Which Have Retarded the Progress of Medicine," in his *Six Introductory Lectures* (1801), pp. 156–57; same lecture, in his *Sixteen Introductory Lectures* (1811), pp. 154–56. In *Medical Admonitions,* James Parkinson agreed, despite his "philippics against domestic quackery." Indeed, he expressed confidence that "the most effectual mode of checking the career of empiricism would be, by more frequently admitting the study of anatomy, physiology, pathology, and chemistry, as part of a liberal education." For this passage, see p. 468.

93. *The Diary of William Bentley, D.D., Pastor of the East Church, Salem, Massachusetts. Volume 1, April 1784–December 1792* (Salem: Essex Institute, 1905), pp. 163 (28 April 1790), 232 (30 January 1791).

94. Carl Bridenbaugh, ed., *Gentleman's Progress: The Itinerarium of Dr. Alexander Hamilton, 1774* (Chapel Hill: Published for the Institute of Early American History and Culture by the University of North Carolina Press, 1948), pp. 148, 116–17.

95. Jameson, *American Domestick Medicine,* p. 115.

96. Parkinson, *Medical Admonitions,* pp. [45]–47.

97. Ibid., pp. [7]–43 (table of symptoms), 70–78 (slow nervous fever), 145–49 (putrid or malignant ulcerated sore throat). He gave treatment information on pp. 205–10 (inflammation of the stomach) and pp. 216–21 (inflammation of the liver).

98. Johnson, *Friendly Cautions,* pp. 137–38.

99. Parkinson, *Medical Admonitions,* pp. 392–93. Johnson complains about the same behavior in *Friendly Cautions,* p. 153.

100. Benezet, *Family Physician,* pp. 88, 89n.

101. Johnson, *Friendly Cautions,* p. 46.

102. James Ewell, *Medical Companion,* pp. [13]–55, esp. p. 14; Benezet, *Family Physician,* p. 36. See also Jameson, *American Domestick Medicine,* pp. [16]–49.

103. Jameson, *American Domestick Medicine*, p. 247. The modern word for consumption is tuberculosis; scrofula was the term used for the tubercular condition which manifested itself especially in a chronic enlargement and cheesy degeneration of the lymph glands, particularly those of the neck. Both also bore the connotation of moral contamination.
104. *The Manual for Invalids*, 3rd ed. (London: Edward Bull, 1829), p. iv. For bibliographical information, see *NUC* 360: 48.
105. Benjamin Rush, "An Inquiry into the Comparative State of Medicine, in Philadelphia, Between the Years 1760 and 1766, and the Year 1809," in his *Medical Inquiries and Observations* (1815), vol. 4, pp. [225]–249, at p. 247.

2. The Maternal Physician

1. Judith Walzer Leavitt, *Brought to Bed: Childbearing in America, 1750–1950* (New York: Oxford University Press, 1986), pp. 36–53, 87–115; quote on p. 39. An earlier version does not make this point as forcefully: Judith Walzer Leavitt, "'Science' Enters the Birthing Room: Obstetrics in America since the Eighteenth Century," *JAH* 70(1983): 281–304; the same quote is on p. 283. See also the work by Catherine M. Scholten: "'On the Importance of the Obstetrick Art'; Changing Customs of Childbirth in America, 1760 to 1825," *WMQ*, 3rd ser., 34(1977): 426–45; and *Childbearing in American Society, 1650–1850* (New York: New York University Press, 1985).
2. The most extreme examples are the polemical works of Barbara Ehrenreich and Deirdre English: *Complaints and Disorders: The Sexual Politics of Sickness* (Old Westbury, N.Y.: Feminist Press, 1973); *Witches, Midwives and Nurses: A History of Women Healers* (Old Westbury, N.Y.: Feminist Press, 1973); and *For Her Own Good: 150 Years of the Experts' Advice to Women* (New York: Anchor Press/Doubleday, 1978).
3. Jane B. Donegan, *Women and Men Midwives: Medicine, Morality and Misogyny in Early America* (Westport, Conn.: Greenwood Press, 1978); Richard W. Wertz and Dorothy C. Wertz, *Lying-In: A History of Childbirth in America* (New York: Free Press, 1977); Regina Markell Morantz-Sanchez, *Sympathy and Science: Women Physicians in American Medicine* (New York: Oxford University Press, 1987 [1985]), pp. 15–27; and Gerda Lerner, "The Lady and the Mill Girl," *American Studies (Midcontinent American Studies Journal)* 10(1969): 5–15.
4. The long-term consequences obviously did not fulfill this early vision. From different perspectives two other books make a similar point about the disjunction between original goals and eventual outcome: Wertz and Wertz, *Lying-In*, pp. 29–76; and Dorothy Porter, *Patient's Progress: Doctors and Doctoring in Eighteenth-Century England* (Cambridge: Polity Press, 1989), pp. 173–85. Morantz-Sanchez, on the other hand, believes a stronger case can be made that the doctors began their crusade with exclusionary aims; see *Sympathy and Science*, pp. 8–27.
5. In addition to the sources cited above, see Laurel Thatcher Ulrich's chapter on "Travail" in her *Good Wives: Image and Reality in the Lives of Women in Northern New England, 1650–1750* (New York: Alfred A. Knopf, 1982), pp. 126–45; Daniel Blake Smith, "Autonomy and Affection: Parents and Children in Chesapeake Families," in Michael Gordon, ed., *The American*

Family in Social-Historical Perspective, 3rd ed. (New York: St. Martin's Press, 1983), pp. 209–28; and Adrian Wilson, "Participant or Patient? Seventeenth Century Childbirth from the Mother's Point of View," in Roy Porter, ed., *Patients and Practitioners: Lay Perceptions of Medicine in Pre-Industrial Society* (Cambridge: Cambridge University Press, 1985), pp. 129–44. Carroll Smith-Rosenberg has argued that this powerful all-female experience was one of the fundamental bonds of women's domestic culture: "The Female World of Love and Ritual: Relations Between Women in Nineteenth-Century America," *Signs* 1(1975): 1–29.

6. Midwives were often important figures in their communities, and some earned as much as merchants, lawyers, and government officials. See Mary Beth Norton, *Liberty's Daughters: The Revolutionary Experience of American Women, 1750–1800* (Boston: Little, Brown and Co., 1980), pp. 139–41; and Morantz-Sanchez, *Sympathy and Science,* pp. 11–15.

7. Charles Eventon Nash, *The History of Augusta: First Settlements and Early Days as a Town, Including the Diary of Mrs. Martha Moore Ballard (1785 to 1812)* (Augusta, Me.: Charles E. Nash and Son, 1904), quote on p. 327. For occasions on which Ballard summoned a doctor, see pp. 243, 338; on p. 314 is a record of a time the doctor was too late. Ballard even served as a midwife to at least one of the doctors' wives: see pp. 273, 283, 336. Laurel Thatcher Ulrich draws on the manuscript version of Ballard's diary in "'The Living Mother of a Living Child': Midwifery and Mortality in Post Revolutionary New England," *WMQ,* 3rd ser., 46(1989): 27–48.

8. Information about Ballard's making and dispensing medicines is sprinkled through Nash, *History of Augusta.* See, for example, pp. 240, 242, 243, 428, and passim. A case Ballard nursed for Cony is described on p. 379. Quotes are on pp. 377, 290.

9. Ibid., pp. 299 (swollen thigh), 378 (grandson's illness). Ballard suffered very frequently from bone displacements, which she typically brought to the attention of a physician; see pp. 363, 364, 383 for a few examples.

10. Ibid., pp. 390, 386.

11. Margaret Morris's diary and correspondence appear in John Jay Smith, ed., *Letters of Doctor Richard Hill and His Children: Or, The History of a Family, as Told by Themselves* (Philadelphia: Privately Printed, 1854), pp. 333–466. Quotes in this paragraph and the next are from pp. 424–25.

12. *Letters from John Pintard to his Daughter Eliza Noel Pintard Davidson, 1816–1833,* 4 vols. (New York: New-York Historical Society Collections, 1937–40), vol. 1, p. 200 (21 June 1819).

13. Ibid., vol. 1, p. 179 (8 April 1819); vol. 2, p. 91 (1 October 1821). Brackets in original.

14. Ibid., vol. 1, p. 229 (28 September 1819); vol. 3, pp. 243–44 (21 April 1831). Brackets in original.

15. Ibid., vol. 2, pp. 94–95 (12 October 1821); vol. 3, pp. 94 (6 September 1829), 300–301 (29 November 1831).

16. Eliza Cope Harrison, ed., *Philadelphia Merchant: The Diary of Thomas P. Cope, 1800–1851* (South Bend, Ind.: Gateway Editions, 1978); all quotes in this paragraph are from p. 172 (20 January 1805).

17. Ibid., p. 398 (14 August 1843).

18. As many scholars have demonstrated, it is hard to pinpoint the extent to

which advice literature reflects or influences social and cultural practices and then to tie those conclusions to a particular group of people. See: Jay Mechling, "Advice to Historians on Advice to Mothers," *J. Soc. Hist.* 9(Fall 1975): 44–63; and Carl Degler, "What Ought To Be and What Was: Women's Sexuality in the Nineteenth Century," *AHR* 79(1974): 1479–90. As I hope to show throughout this book by juxtaposing personal accounts with advice literature, there *were* connections between "what ought to be" and "what was," though the relationships were not always what the advisers would have wished. One study that uses diaries to document these connections is Nancy Schrom Dye and Daniel Blake Smith, "Mother Love and Infant Death, 1750–1920," *JAH* 73(1986): 329–53.

19. Jacqueline S. Reiner, "Rearing the Republican Child: Attitudes and Practices in Post-Revolutionary Philadelphia," *WMQ*, 3rd ser., 39(1982): 150–63. See also Ruth H. Bloch, "American Feminine Ideals in Transition: The Rise of the Moral Mother, 1785–1815," *Feminist Studies* 4(1978): 101–26; Elizabeth Andrews Wilson, "Hygienic Care and Management of the Child in the American Family Prior to 1860" (unpublished M.A. thesis, Duke University, 1940); Robert Sunley, "Early Nineteenth-Century American Literature on Child Rearing," in Margaret Mead and Martha Wolfenstein, eds., *Childhood in Contemporary Cultures* (Chicago: University of Chicago Press, 1963 [1955]), pp. 150–67; Anne L. Kuhn, *The Mother's Role in Childhood Education: New England Concepts, 1830–1860* (New Haven: Yale University Press, 1947); David Lundberg and Henry F. May, "The Enlightened Reader in America: 1700 to 1813," *AQ* 28(1976): 262–71 and appendix; Robert H. Bremner et al., eds., *Children and Youth in America: A Documentary History. Volume 1: 1600–1865* (Cambridge: Harvard University Press, 1970), pp. 282–306; and Abigail J. Stewart et al., "Coding Categories for the Study of Child-Rearing from Historical Sources," *JIH* 4(1975): 687–701.

20. Reiner, "Rearing the Republican Child," p. 151.

21. William Buchan, *Domestic Medicine; Or, The Family Physician: Being an Attempt to Render the Medical Art More Generally Useful, by Shewing People What Is in Their Own Power Both with Respect to the Prevention and Cure of Diseases. Chiefly Calculated to Recommend a Proper Attention to Regimen and Simple Medicines* (Edinburgh: Balfour, Auld, and Smellie, 1769), pp. 1–51 and passim. For biographical and bibliographical information, consult sources listed in chapter 1.

22. F. B. Smith, *The People's Health, 1830–1910* (New York: Holmes and Meier Publishers, 1979), pp. 65–69; P. J. Corfield, *The Impact of English Towns, 1700–1800* (Oxford and New York: Oxford University Press, 1982), pp. 106–23; George Rosen, "Disease, Debility, and Death," in H. J. Dyos and Michael Wolff, eds., *The Victorian City: Images and Realities* (London and Boston: Routledge and Kegan Paul, 1973), vol. 2, pp. 625–77.

23. Quotes in this paragraph and the next two are from Buchan, *Domestic Medicine*, pp. 1–8. During this period many people debated the utility and morality of using wet nurses, as described by Valerie A. Fildes in two books: *Breasts, Bottles and Babies: A History of Infant Feeding* (Edinburgh: Edinburgh University Press, 1986), pp. 121, 162–204; and *Wet Nursing: A History from Antiquity to the Present* (Oxford: Basil Blackwell, 1988), pp. 79–241.

24. Buchan, *Domestic Medicine*, pp. 9–51 (preventing diseases in children), 557–78 (women's diseases), 578–94 (children's diseases), 593–94 (quote).
25. [Anthony A. Benezet], *The Family Physician; Comprising Rules for the Prevention and Cure of Diseases; Calculated Particularly for the Inhabitants of the Western Country, and for Those Who Navigate Its Waters. With a Dispensatory and Appendix. This Work Affords, in Simple Language, a Concentration of all the Practical Matter Which Can Be Derived from the Best Authorities. With Original Remarks. By a Graduate of the Pennsylvania University, and Honorary Member of the Medical Society of Philadelphia Who has for Years Been Acquainted with the Modes of Living, and with the Diseases of the West* (Cincinnati: W. Hill Woodward, [1826]), pp. 415–32 (women's diseases), 432–62 (children's diseases); and James Ewell, *The Medical Companion. Treating, According to the Most Successful Practice: I. The Diseases Common to Warm Climates on Ship Board. II. Common Cases in Surgery, as Fractures, Dislocations, etc. III. The Complaints Peculiar to Women and Children. With a Dispensatory and Glossary. To Which Are Added, A Brief Anatomy of the Human Body; An Essay on Hygiene, Or the Art of Preserving Health and Prolonging Life; An American Materia Medica, Instructing Country Gentlemen in the Very Important Knowledge of the Virtues and Doses of Our Medicinal Plants; Also, A Concise and Impartial History of the Capture of Washington, and the Diseases Which Sprung from that most Deplorable Disaster*, 3rd ed., greatly improved (Philadelphia: Printed for the Author by Anderson and Meehan, 1816), pp. 418–45 (women's diseases), 445–60 (infants' complaints). For biographical and bibliographical details, consult sources listed in chapter 1.
26. James Parkinson, *Medical Admonitions to Families, Respecting the Preservation of Health, and the Treatment of the Sick. Also, A Table of Symptoms, Serving to Point Out the Degree of Danger, and, To Distinguish One Disease from Another: With Observations on the Improper Indulgence of Children, etc.*, 1st Am., from the 4th Eng. ed. (Portsmouth, N.H.: Printed for Charles Peirce, by N. S. and W. Peirce, 1803), pp. 312–16 (menses), 435–38 (inflammation of the breast), 149–61 (croup), 167–74 (teething), and passim; and Josiah Burlingame, *The Poor Man's Physician, The Sick Man's Friend; or, Nature's Botanic Garden Exhibited to View: Its Medical Qualities Unfolded, Symptoms of Diseases Described, and Cures Made Easy. Designed Wholly for the Use and Benefit of Families* (Norwich, N.Y.: Printed by William G. Hyer, for the Author, 1826). For biographical and bibliographical information about Parkinson, consult sources listed in chapter 1. For publishing information about Burlingame, see *NUC* 85: 462.
27. Horatio Gates Jameson, *The American Domestick Medicine; or, Medical Admonisher: Containing, Some Account of Anatomy, the Senses, Diseases, Casualties; a Dispensatory, and Glossary. In Which The Observations, and Remedies, Are Adapted to the Diseases, etc. of the United States. Designed for the Use of Families* (Baltimore: F. Lucas, Jun[ior], 1817), pp. 504–57 (women's medical problems), 564–84 (children's ailments), 564 (explanatory remark). For biographical and bibliographical information, consult sources listed in chapter 1.
28. William Buchan, *Domestic Medicine: Or, a Treatise on the Prevention and Cure of Diseases, by Regimen and Simple Medicines. With an Appendix, Containing a Dispensatory for the Use of Private Practitioners. To Which Are Added, Observa-*

tions on Diet; Recommending a Method of Living Less Expensive, and More Condu-cive to Health, than the Present. Also, Advice to Mothers, On the Subject of Their own Health; and of the Means of Promoting the Health, Strength, and Beauty of Their Offspring, new, correct ed., enl. from the author's last revisal (Boston: Joseph Bumstead, 1809), pp. 507, 509, 566.

29. Ibid. Quotes in this paragraph and the next are from pp. 558–60.
30. J. G. Coffin, "On the Management of Infants," New-England Journal of Medi-cine 6(1817): 130–34; quotes on p. 133.
31. William Cadogan, An Essay Upon Nursing, and the Management of Children, From Their Birth to Three Years of Age. By a Physician. In a Letter to One of the Governors of the Foundling Hospital. Published by the Order of the General Com-mittee for Transacting the Affairs of the said Hospital (London: J. Roberts, 1748); quotes in this paragraph are from pp. [3]–4, 28. Biographical information may be found in Arthur F. Abt, ed., Abt-Garrison History of Pediatrics (Phila-delphia: W. B. Saunders Co., 1965), pp. 76–77; and DNB 3: 639. Excerpts from the Essay are printed in John Ruhrah, Pediatrics of the Past (New York: Paul B. Hoeber, 1925), pp. 382–99. For publishing information, see NUC 88: 651–53.
32. Fildes, Breasts, Bottles and Babies, pp. 114–21, 162–204, 398–400, 446–49; Roy Porter, "Laymen, Doctors and Medical Knowledge in the Eighteenth Century: The Evidence of the Gentleman's Magazine," in Roy Porter, ed., Patients and Practitioners, pp. 283–314.
33. George Armstrong, An Account of the Diseases Most Incident to Children, From Their Birth till the Age of Puberty; With a Successful Method of Treating Them. To Which Is Added, an Essay on Nursing. Also A General Account of the Dispensary for the Infant Poor, from Its First Institution in 1769 to the Present Time (London: T. Cadell, 1777), pp. [v]–vii. Biographical and bibliographical information is from Leslie T. Morton, A Medical Bibliography (Garrison and Morton). An An-notated Check-List of Texts Illustrating the History of Medicine, 3rd ed. (Phila-delphia: J. B. Lippincott Co., 1970), p. 729. See also Fildes, Breasts, Bottles and Babies, pp. 343–45, 446–47; Abt, ed., History of Pediatrics, p. 77; Ruhrah, Pediatrics of the Past, pp. 440–46; DNB 1: 564; and NUC 21: 436–37.
34. William Moss, An Essay on the Management and Nursing of Children in the Ear-lier Periods of Infancy: and on the Treatment and Rule of Conduct Requisite for the Mother During Pregnancy, and in Lying-In. Including the Diseases to Which the Mother and Child are Liable; with the Methods of Curing, and Particularly of Pre-venting Many of, Those Diseases. The Whole addressed, as well, to the Medical Faculty, as to the Public at Large; and Purposely Adapted to a Female Comprehen-sion, in a Manner Perfectly Consistent with the Delicacy of the Sex (London: J. Johnson, 1751), t.p. See also Fildes, Breasts, Bottles and Babies, p. 448; and NUC 397: 491–92.
35. Quotes in this paragraph and the next are from Moss, Essay, pp. [vii]–xxxi.
36. Ibid. For examples of areas where Moss omitted information, see pp. 217, 255.
37. Michael Underwood, A Treatise on the Diseases of Children, With General Di-rections for the Management of Infants from the Birth, 2 vols. in 1, new ed., rev. and enl. (Philadelphia: Printed by T. Dobson, 1793), pp. 48, 2. For bio-graphical and bibliographical background, see Abt, ed., History of Pediatrics, p. 78; Morton, Medical Bibliography, p. 729; Robert B. Austin, Early American

Medical Imprints: A Guide to Works Printed in the United States, 1668–1820 (Washington, D.C.: U.S. Department of Health, Education, and Welfare, 1961), p. 206; Ruhrah, *Pediatrics of the Past,* pp. 447–53; Fildes, *Breasts, Bottles and Babies,* p. 449; *DNB* 20: 31–32; and *NUC* 607: 589–91.

38. Underwood, *Treatise,* pp. vi–vii, 3–4, 6–7.

39. The quotes in this paragraph are paraphrases of the 1793 text from Michael Underwood, *A Treatise on the Disorders of Childhood, and Management of Infants from the Birth; Adapted to Domestic Use,* 3 vols., 2nd ed., with additions (London: Printed for J. Mathews, by J. Smeeton, Printer, 1801), vol. 1, pp. 2, 261 (compare with 1793 text, pp. 2, 184–85); vol. 2, p. iii (1793 text, passim). John Syer had a similar approach in his *Treatise on the Management of Infants: Containing the General Principles of Their Domestic Treatment. With the History and Method of Cure of Some of Their Most Prevalent and Formidable Diseases* (London: Printed for John Murray, etc., 1812), pp. 6–9, 46, 64–65, 105–107. Syer's volume was favorably reviewed in *The Eclectic Repertory and Analytical Review, Medical and Philosophical* 4(October 1813–July 1814): 481–88. For publishing information, see *NUC* 579: 672.

40. Alexander Hamilton, *A Treatise on the Management of Female Complaints, and of Children in Early Infancy,* new ed., with large improvements (New York: Printed and sold by Samuel Campbell, 1792), pp. 6 (quote), [346]–375 (cures), 376–78 (consulting doctors by letter), 378–79 (choosing a nurse), [13]–79 (anatomy and physiology). Publishing history may be traced in Austin, *Medical Imprints,* pp. 95–96; and *NUC* 228: 387–89. See also Fildes, *Breasts, Bottles and Babies,* pp. 447–48; and *DNB* 8: 1017–18. "Prescribing by post" was quite common, as described by Dorothy Porter and Roy Porter, *Patient's Progress: Doctors and Doctoring in Eighteenth-Century England* (Cambridge: Polity Press, 1989), pp. 76–78.

41. Alexander Hamilton, *The Family Female Physician: or, A Treatise on the Management of Female Complaints, and of Children in Early Infancy,* 1st Worcester ed. (Worcester, Mass.: Isaiah Thomas, 1793).

42. I have used Hugh Smith, *Letters to Married Women, on Nursing and the Management of Children,* 1st Am. ed. from 6th London ed. (Philadelphia: Mathew Carey, 1792), pp. 117–18, vii. Publishing information may be garnered from Austin, *Medical Imprints,* pp. 185–86; and *NUC* 551: 314–15. Limited biographical details are available in *DNB* 18: 463 and Fildes, *Breasts, Bottles and Babies,* p. 449.

43. Smith, *Letters to Married Women,* pp. 101–102, 117–18, 149.

44. Parkinson, *Medical Admonitions,* pp. [471], 474, 481–87.

45. Ibid., p. 495. Other examples of serious diseases that could not be weathered without docility were whooping cough (p. 496) and inflammation of the stomach and bowels (pp. 492–93).

46. John Herdman, *Discourses on the Management of Infants and the Treatment of their Diseases. Written in a Plain Familiar Style, To Render Them Intelligible and Useful to All Mothers* (London: Printed by Ruffy and Evans, for Jordan and Maxwell, etc., 1807), pp. [1]–5, 27. For bibliographical and biographical information, see *NUC* 242: 10; and *DNB* 9: 688–89.

47. Ibid., pp. 5–13.

48. Ibid., p. 127 and passim.

49. Sir Arthur Clarke, *The Mother's Medical Assistant, Containing Instructions for*

the Prevention and Treatment of the Diseases of Infants and Children (London: Printed for Henry Colburn and Co., 1820), pp. [v]–x, 146, 78. For publishing information, see *NUC* 83: 622.

50. Ibid., pp. [v]–x, 2, 77. Emphasis added.

51. Thomas Bull, *The Maternal Management of Children, in Health and Disease* (London: Longman, Orme, Brown, Green, and Longmans, 1840), t.p., pp. 184, 299, 185.

52. Sydney A. Halpern, *American Pediatrics: The Social Dynamics of Professionalism, 1880–1980* (Berkeley and Los Angeles: University of California Press, 1988), pp. 37–47.

53. The seminal statement about the historical importance of this period for children is Bernard Wishy, *The Child and the Republic: The Dawn of Modern American Child Nurture* (Philadelphia: University of Pennsylvania Press, 1968). A more concise and precise argument is Reiner, "Rearing the Republican Child." On the mother's role, see Kuhn, *The Mother's Role;* Linda K. Kerber, "The Republican Mother: Women and the Enlightenment—An American Perspective," *AQ* 28(1976): 187–205; and Barbara Welter, "The Cult of True Womanhood," *AQ* 18(1966): 151–74.

54. Bloch, "American Feminine Ideals in Transition."

55. Linda K. Kerber, "Daughters of Columbia: Educating Women for the Republic, 1787–1805," in Stanley Elkins and Eric McKitrick, eds., *The Hofstadter Aegis: A Memorial* (New York: Alfred A. Knopf, 1974), pp. 36–59. A more extended discussion can be found in Kerber's *Women of the Republic: Intellect and Ideology in Revolutionary America* (Chapel Hill: Published for the Institute of Early American History and Culture by the University of North Carolina Press, 1980).

56. Carroll Smith-Rosenberg and Charles E. Rosenberg, "Pietism and the Origins of the American Public Health Movement: A Note on John H. Griscom and Robert M. Hartley," *JHMAS* 23(1968): 16–35; Charles E. Rosenberg, "Social Class and Medical Care in 19th-Century America: The Rise and Fall of the Dispensary," *JHMAS* 29(1974): 32–54; Virginia A. Metaxas Quiroga, "Female Lay Managers and Scientific Pediatrics at Nursery and Child's Hospital, 1854–1910," *BHM* 60(1986): 194–208.

57. Samuel K. Jennings, *The Married Lady's Companion, or Poor Man's Friend. In Four Parts. I. An Address to the Married Lady, Who is the Mother of Daughters. II. An Address to the Newly Married Lady. III. Some Important Hints to the Midwife. IV. An Essay on the Management and Common Diseases of Children. To Which Will Be Added a Short Note on Fever,* 2nd ed., rev., corrected and enl. by the author (New York: Lorenzo Dow, 1808; reprint ed., New York: Arno Press, 1972). Biographical information has been compiled from Wyndham B. Blanton, *Medicine in Virginia in the Nineteenth Century* (Richmond: Garrett and Massie, 1931), p. 346; John R. Quinan, *Medical Annals of Baltimore. From 1608 to 1880, Including Events, Men and Literature* (Baltimore: Press of Isaac Friedenwald, 1884), pp. 117–18; and Eugene F. Cordell, *The Medical Annals of Maryland, 1799–1899* (Baltimore: Press of Williams and Wilkins Co., 1903), pp. 76–90, 126, 704 and passim. For discussion of Jennings's vapor bath, see *American Medical Recorder* 4(April 1821): 383–91, 594–95. Jennings worked with Horatio Gates Jameson and others to found the Washington Medical

College; see Cordell, *Medical Annals of Maryland,* pp. 779–95. For publishing information, see *NUC* 279: 409–10.

58. Jennings, *Married Lady's Companion,* pp. [98]–162 (hints for midwives), 5–8, [98]–99.

59. Ibid. This paragraph and the next are based on pp. 198–204.

60. Joseph Brevitt, *The Female Medical Repository. To Which Is Added A Treatise on the Primary Diseases of Infants: Adapted to the Use of the Female Practitioners and Intelligent Mothers; The Technical Terms Are Explained, and an Attempt Hath Been Made to Reduce These Branches of "The Healing Art," to Conciseness and Perspicuity* (Baltimore: Hunter and Robinson, 1810), t.p., p. [121]. Quotes in the next three paragraphs from pp. 7, 192, 206, 56. Biographical details are from Quinan, *Medical Annals of Baltimore,* p. 67; bibliographical details are in *NUC* 74: 663.

61. Leavitt summarizes some of the far-reaching consequences of ideals about female modesty in *Brought to Bed,* pp. 40–43. For biographical and bibliographical details on Ewell, see sources listed in chapter 1.

62. Most of Ewell's *American Family Physician* was based on his 1808 *Letters to Ladies,* of which Ewell boasted approximately three thousand copies sold. In the *Family Physician,* he omitted some "exceptionable" information from the earlier volume, but he explained that he had retained enough so that women could minister to each other during normal deliveries, without interference from male midwives. Thomas Ewell, *American Family Physician; Detailing Important Means of Preserving Health, from Infancy to Old Age: The Offices Women Should Perform to Each Other at Births, and the Diseases Peculiar to the Sex: With Those of Children and of Adults. With an Appendix, Containing Hints Respecting the Treatment of Domestic Animals, and the Best Means of Preserving Fish and Meat* (Georgetown, D.C.: James Thomas, 1824), p. xv.

63. Ibid., pp. xvi–xviii, 140.

64. Ibid., p. xii.

65. Thomas Ewell, *The Ladies Medical Companion: Containing, In a Series of Letters, An Account of the Latest Improvements and Most Successful Means of Preserving Their Beauty and Health; Of Relieving the Diseases Peculiar to the Sex, and an Explanation of the Offices They Should Perform to Each Other at Births. With Engraved Figures Explanatory. Also, The Best Means of Nursing, Preventing and Curing the Diseases of Children* (Philadelphia: William Brown, 1818), p. x. The review was a letter to the editor, signed by Philo, in the *Philadelphia Medical Museum* 4(1808): clix–clx. Philo's subject was Ewell's chemistry book.

66. Thomas Ewell, *Ladies Medical Companion,* p. 57. Both statements are also found in Ewell's *Am. Fam. Physician* (1824), p. xviii.

67. Thomas Ewell, *Am. Fam. Physician* (1824), pp. 140–43; quote on p. 143.

68. Thomas Ewell, *Ladies Medical Companion,* p. 261; *Am. Fam. Physician* (1824), p. 245; and Thomas Ewell, *American Family Physician; Detailing Important Means of Preserving Health, from Infancy to Old Age: The Offices Women Should Perform to Each Other at Births, and the Diseases Peculiar to the Sex: With Those of Children and of Adults. With an Appendix, Containing Hints Respecting the Treatment of Domestic Animals, and the Best Means of Preserving Fish and Meat,* 2nd ed., improved (Georgetown, D.C.: James Thomas, 1826), p. 264.

69. Thomas Ewell, *Am. Fam. Physician* (1824), pp. 140–43.

70. Ibid., pp. 110–11; Thomas Ewell, *Am. Fam. Physician* (1826), pp. 121–23.
71. Hugh Smith, *Letters to Married Ladies, To Which Is Added, a Letter on Corsets, and Copious Notes, By an American Physician* (New York: E. Bliss and E. White, etc., 1827), p. iii; see also Fildes, *Breasts, Bottles and Babies*, p. 449.
72. Smith, *Letters to Married Ladies*, pp. iii–v.
73. Ibid., pp. vi–ix.
74. Dr. G. Ackerley, *On the Management of Children in Sickness and in Health*, 2nd ed., enl. (New York: Bancroft and Holley, 1836), p. [4]. Publishing information is from *NUC* 3: 4.
75. Ackerley, *On the Management of Children*, pp. [7]–10, 38–41. According to Barbara Rosenkrantz, Massachusetts children under five accounted for over 43 percent of all deaths in that state during the 1830s (Barbara Gutmann Rosenkrantz, *Public Health and the State: Changing Views in Massachusetts, 1842–1936* [Cambridge: Harvard University Press, 1972], p. 18).
76. Ackerley, *On the Management of Children*, pp. 35–38.
77. Ibid., pp. 13–17.
78. "Prospectus," *Journal of Health* 1(September 1829): 1–2. Editors of the Philadelphia periodical were John Bell and D. Francis Condie, both orthodox physicians.
79. Untitled filler, *Journal of Health* 1(September 1829): 26.
80. Untitled introductory material, *Journal of Health* 1(November 1829): 65–69, at p. 66. See also from the same journal: "Domestic Doctoring of Children," 1(December 1829): 100–102; and untitled introductory material, 1(February 1830): 161–64.
81. Anthony Todd Thomson, *The Domestic Management of the Sick-Room, Necessary, in Aid of Medical Treatment, for the Cure of Diseases*, 1st Am., from the 2nd London ed. Revised, with additions, by R. E. Griffith, M.D. (Philadelphia: Lea and Blanchard, 1845); quotes in this paragraph are from pp. [iii], 69. For publishing information, see *NUC* 592: 131–34.
82. An American Matron, *The Maternal Physician; A Treatise on the Nurture and Management of Infants, From the Birth Until Two Years Old. Being the Result of Sixteen Years' Experience in the Nursery. Illustrated by Extracts from the Most Approved Medical Authors* (New York: Isaac Riley, 1811), t.p., pp. 59, 52–53. For publishing information, see *NUC* 13: 287.
83. American Matron, *Maternal Physician*, pp. [5], 7, 73.
84. Ibid., pp. 16, 73, 171–72, 226. Emphasis in first quote added. Quinsy is a severe inflammation of the throat or adjacent parts accompanied by swelling and fever.
85. Ibid., pp. 172, 248–75.
86. Ibid., pp. 175, 202. See chapter 1 for the Ewell brothers' feelings on the subject.
87. [Margaret Jane King Moore, Countess of Mount Cashell], *Advice to Young Mothers on the Physical Education of Children. By a Grandmother*, 1st Am. ed., with additions (New York: Hilliard, Gray and Co.), t.p., pp. [v]–vi. For publishing information, see *NUC* 398: 243.
88. Moore, *Advice to Young Mothers*, pp. v, viii, 334–35.
89. [Lydia Maria] Child, *The Family Nurse; or Companion of the Frugal Housewife. Revised by a Member of the Massachusetts Medical Society* (Boston: Charles J. Hendee, 1837), t.p. Bibliographical details are in *NUC* 106: 639–48. The

most convenient summary of her life is Louis Filler's entry in Edward T. James et al., eds., *Notable American Women: A Biographical Dictionary* (Cambridge: Belknap Press of Harvard University Press, 1971), vol. 1, pp. 330–33.
90. The remainder of this paragraph and the following one are based on Child, *Family Nurse*, pp. [3]–4, 6–9.
91. Ibid., pp. 8–13.
92. James et al., eds., *Notable American Women*, vol. 1, pp. 330–33.
93. [Louisa Mary Bacon] Barwell, *Infant Treatment: With Directions to Mothers for Self-Management Before, During, and After Pregnancy. Addressed to Mothers and Nurses. Revised, Enlarged, and Adapted to Habits and Climate in the United States, By a Physician of New York, Under the Approval and Recommendation of Valentine Mott, M.D.* 1st Am. ed. (New York: James Mowatt and Co., 1844), t.p., p. [viii]. Biographical information may be found in *DNB* 1: 1269–70. For publishing details, see *NUC* 38: 169–70.
94. Barwell, *Infant Treatment*, pp. 15–16, 57.
95. Ibid., pp. 25, 57–58.
96. Ibid., pp. 120–37 (supplementary chapter), 125 (quote).

3. 'Every Man His Own Doctor'

1. Joseph F. Kett, *The Formation of the American Medical Profession: The Role of Institutions, 1780–1860* (New Haven: Yale University Press, 1968), pp. 97–131; William G. Rothstein, *American Physicians in the Nineteenth Century: From Sects to Science* (Baltimore: Johns Hopkins University Press, 1972), pp. 125–51.
2. George E. Gifford, "Botanic Remedies in Colonial Massachusetts, 1620–1820," in Philip Cash, Eric H. Christianson, and J. Worth Estes, eds., *Medicine in Colonial Massachusetts, 1620–1820*, vol. 57 of the *Publications* of The Colonial Society of Massachusetts (Boston: The Colonial Society of Massachusetts, 1980), pp. 263–88; and William G. Rothstein, "The Botanical Movement and Orthodox Medicine," in Norman Gevitz, ed., *Other Healers: Unorthodox Medicine in America* (Baltimore: Johns Hopkins University Press, 1988) pp. 29–51.
3. Gifford, "Botanic Remedies," pp. 270–79, where the books I mention and others are discussed. For Culpeper, see David L. Cowen, "The Boston Editions of Nicholas Culpeper," *JHMAS* 11(1956): 156–65; and *NUC* 129: 202 et seq.
4. Bibliographical information may be found in Charles Evans and Clifton K. Shipton, eds., *American Bibliography: A Chronological Dictionary of All Books, Pamphlets, and Periodical Publications Printed in the United States of America from the Genesis of Printing in 1639 down to and Including the Year 1820. With Bibliographical and Biographical Notes*, 14 vols. (New York: P. Smith, 1941–1959). The Theobald edition I used was published earlier: John Theobald, *Every Man His Own Physician. Being a Complete Collection of Efficacious and Approved Remedies for Every Disease Incident to the Human Body. With Plain Instructions for Their Common Use. Compiled at the Command of His Royal Highness the Duke of Cumberland*, 10th ed., improved (London: Printed for W. Griffin; Boston: Printed for Cox and Berry, 1767).

5. [John Tennent], *Every Man His Own Doctor, or, The Poor Planter's Physician. Prescribing Plain and Easy Means for Persons to Cure Themselves of All, or Most of the Distempers, Incident to this Climate, and with very Little Charge, the Medicines Being Chiefly of the Growth and Production of this Country,* 4th ed., with additions (Williamsburg: Printed and sold by William Hunter, 1751). For bibliographical details, see Evans and Shipton, eds., *American Bibliography*; and *NUC* 586: 363–64. For biographical information, see Wyndham B. Blanton, *Medicine in Virginia in the Eighteenth Century* (Richmond: Garrett and Massie, 1931), pp. 119–29; Richard M. Jellison, "Dr. John Tennent and the Universal Specific," *BHM* 37(1963): 336–46; Norman Gevitz, "Three Perspectives on Unorthodox Medicine," in Gevitz, ed., *Other Healers,* pp. 1–28; and the entry by P. Addis in Martin Kaufman, Stuart Galishoff, and Todd L. Savitt, eds., *Dictionary of American Medical Biography,* 2 vols. (Westport, Conn.: Greenwood Press, 1984), at vol. 2, pp. 734–35. Tennent's book in turn was often bound with other volumes. One such pairing was with the ninth edition of George Fisher's *American Instructor* (Philadelphia: Benjamin Franklin, 1748).
6. Though not entirely satisfactory, the most extended treatment of Stearns is John C. L. Clark, "The Famous Doctor Stearns," American Antiquarian Society, *Proceedings* 45, part I(1935): 317–24.
7. Gifford, "Botanic Remedies," pp. 280–83.
8. Ibid., pp. 282–85; Rothstein, "Botanical Movement," p. 33.
9. A good discussion is David L. Cowen, "Materia Medica and Pharmacology," in Ronald L. Numbers, ed., *The Education of American Physicians: Historical Essays* (Berkeley and Los Angeles: University of California Press, 1980), pp. 95–121. Martin Kaufman, however, does not mention botanical study in his synthesis, *American Medical Education: The Formative Years* (Westport, Conn.: Greenwood Press, 1976). William F. Norwood gives only slight attention to the subject in his *Medical Education in the United States Before the Civil War* (Philadelphia: University of Pennsylvania Press, 1944).
10. Madge E. Pickard and R. Carlyle Buley, *The Midwest Pioneer: His Ills, Cures, and Doctors* (Crawfordsville, Ind.: R. E. Banta, 1945), pp. 35–89. See also Gerald Carson, *One for a Man, Two for a Horse: A Pictorial History, Grave and Comic, of Patent Medicines* (Garden City, N.Y.: Doubleday and Co., 1961), pp. 23–29.
11. Peter Smith, *The Indian Doctor's Dispensatory, Being Father Smith's Advice Respecting Diseases and Their Cure; Consisting of Prescriptions for Many Complaints: And a Description of Medicines, Simple and Compound, Showing Their Virtues and How To Apply Them. Designed for the Benefit of his Children, his Friends and the Public, but More Especially the Citizens of the Western Parts of the United States of America* (Cincinnati: Printed by Browne and Looker, for the Author, 1813). D. L. Cowen has summarized biographical information about Smith in Kaufman, Galishoff, and Savitt, eds., *Dictionary of American Medical Biography,* vol. 2, pp. 697–98. For publishing details, see *NUC* 552: 9.
12. Jonas Rishel, *The Indian Physician, Containing a New System of Practice, Founded on Medical Plants, Together with a Description of Their Properties, Localities and Method of Using, and Preparing Them. A Treatise on the Causes and Symptoms of Diseases, Which Are Incident to Human Nature, With a Safe and Sovereign Cure for Them, and the Mode of Treatment, In any Stage of Disease. For*

the Use of Families and Practitioners of Medicine (New Berlin, Pa.: Printed for the Author and Proprietor, by Joseph Miller, 1828). Though Samuel North did not label himself an Indian doctor, his text draws on Rishel: *The Family Physician and Guide to Health, Together with some Remarks on Surgery: Containing a Familiar and Accurate Description of the Symptoms of Most Diseases Incident to Mankind; Together with their Gradual Progress and Method of Cure; and Tables of Preparation, with a Medical Herbal. The Whole Selected and Compiled from the Writings of Various Authors in Europe and America* (Waterloo, N.Y.: William Child, printer, 1830). North also recommended Thomsonian remedies. See, for example, pp. 217–30 (Rishel's table of preparations), 173–76, 239–40 (Thomsonian advice). For publishing information, see *NUC* 496: 205 (Rishel), 422: 45 (North).

13. Ammon Monroe Aurand, ed., *John George Hohman's Pow-Wows; or, Long Lost Friend. A Collection of Mysterious and Invaluable Arts and Remedies for Man as well as Animals. With Many Proofs of Their Virtue and Efficacy in Healing Diseases, etc., the Greater Part of which Never Published until They Appeared in Print for the First Time in the U.S. in the Year 1820* (Harrisburg, [Pa.]: n.p., 1930 [1820]).

14. Samuel Curtis, *A Valuable Collection of Recipes, Medical and Miscellaneous. Useful in Families, and Valuable to Every Description of Persons* (Amherst, N.H.: Printed by Elijah Mansur, 1819); Samuel Henry, *A New and Complete American Medical Family Herbal, Wherein, Is Displayed the True Properties and Medical Virtues of the Plants, Indigenous to the United States of America: Together with Lewis' Secret Remedy, Newly Discovered, Which Has Been Found Infallible in the Cure of that Dreadful Disease Hydrophobia; Produced by the Bite of a Mad Dog. Being the Result of More than Thirty Years Experienced Practice of the Author, While a Prisoner, Towards the Close of the Last War, among the Creek Indians; and his Travels through the Southern States, Whilst Making Botanic Discoveries on the Real Medical Virtues of our Indigenous Plants, Wherein he has Made Known All his New Discoveries, with the Method How to Use Them, in the Cure of Most Diseases Incident to the Human Body. Adapted for the Benefit of Masters and Mistresses of Families, and for the Country at Large, of our United, Free and Independent States of America. With an Appendix, of Many Choice Medical Secrets, Never Made Known to the World Before* (New York: Samuel Henry, 1814). For publishing information, see *NUC* 130: 115 (Curtis), and 241: 157 (Henry).

15. Since sectarian literature has typically been used by scholars studying particular sects, there are few discussions of it as a genre, and there are no extended, systematic analyses of its authors and contents. One source of useful information, especially for little-known books and writers, is Pickard and Buley, *Midwest Pioneer.* A more recent scholarly overview is John B. Blake, "From Buchan to Fishbein: The Literature of Domestic Medicine," in Guenter B. Risse, Ronald L. Numbers, and Judith Walzer Leavitt, eds., *Medicine Without Doctors: Home Health Care in American History* (New York: Science History Publications, 1977), pp. 11–30.

16. Josiah Burlingame, *The Poor Man's Physician, The Sick Man's Friend; or, Nature's Botanic Garden Exhibited to View: Its Medical Qualities Unfolded, Symptoms of Diseases Described, and Cures Made Easy. Designed Wholly for the Use and Benefit of Families* (Norwich, N.Y.: Printed by William G. Hyer, for the Au-

thor, 1826), pp. 10–11, [7]. For biographical and bibliographical information, see sources listed in chapter 2.

17. A. G. Goodlett, *The Family Physician, or Every Man's Companion, Being a
Compilation from the Most Approved Medical Authors, Adapted to the Southern
and Western Climates. To Which Is Added an Account of Herbs, Roots and Plants,
Used for Medical Purposes, with Directions How They Are To Be Prepared, So
That Every Man Can Be His Own Physician, Together with a Glossary of Medical
Terms. With an Appendix, Containing a New and Successful Mode of Treating
Asiatic Cholera, By the Compiler* (Nashville, Tenn.: Printed at Smith and
Nesbit's Steam Press, 1838), t.p., p. 628. For publishing information, see
NUC 206: 320.

18. Burlingame, *Poor Man's Physician*, pp. [iii]–v.

19. For biographical and bibliographical information on John Gunn, see Ben H.
McClary, "Introducing a Classic: *Gunn's Domestic Medicine*," *Tennessee Histor-
ical Quarterly* 45(Fall 1986): 210–16; S. R. Bruesch's entry in Kaufman,
Galishoff, and Savitt, eds., *Dictionary of American Medical Biography*, vol. 1,
pp. 311–12; and especially Charles E. Rosenberg, "Introduction to the New
Edition," *Gunn's Domestic Medicine, or, Poor Man's Friend* (Knoxville, Tenn.:
Printed under the immediate superintendance of the author, a physician of
Knoxville, 1830; facsimile ed., Tennesseana Editions, Knoxville: University
of Tennessee Press, 1986), pp. [v]–xxi. For publishing information, see *NUC*
223: 333–37.

20. Michael H. Harris, "Books on the Frontier: The Extent and Nature of Book
Ownership in Southern Indiana, 1800–1850," *Library Quarterly* 42(1972):
416–30. See also Edward Stevens, Jr., "Books and Wealth on the Frontier:
Athens County and Washington County, Ohio, 1790–1859," *Social Science
History* 5(1981): 417–43; and Howard H. Peckham, "Books and Reading on
the Ohio Valley Frontier," *MVHR* 44(1957–58): 649–63, esp. pp. 660–61.

21. John Gunn, *Gunn's Domestic Medicine, or Poor Man's Friend, Describing in Plain
Language, the Diseases of Men, Women, and Children, and the Latest and Most
Approved Means Used in Their Cure; Designed Especially for the Use of Families.
It Also Contains Descriptions of the Medical Roots and Herbs of the United States,
and How They Are to be Used in the Cure of Diseases. Arranged on a New and
Simple Plan, by which the Practice of Medicine Is Reduced to Principles of Common
Sense*, 13th ed. (Pittsburgh: J. Edwards and J. J. Newman, 1839), pp. 9–17,
520–23; quotes on pp. [9], 10, 520. These were commonplace ideas in nine-
teenth-century America, as Charles E. Rosenberg explains in *The Cholera
Years: The United States in 1832, 1849, and 1866*, Phoenix paperback ed. (Chicago: University of Chicago Press, 1962), pp. 40–54, 121–50, and passim.

22. Kett, *American Medical Profession*, pp. 123–31. A larger historical context is
provided by Hans Huth, *Nature and the American: Three Centuries of Changing
Attitudes* ([Lincoln]: University of Nebraska Press, 1972 [1957]).

23. See, for example, Richard Carter, *Valuable Vegetable Medical Prescriptions, For
the Cure of All Nervous and Putrid Disorders* (Frankfort, Ky.: Gerard and Berry,
1815), p. 38. For publishing information, see *NUC* 97: 209.

24. Richard Carter, *A Short Sketch of the Author's Life, And Adventures from his
Youth Until 1818, in the First Part. In Part the Second, A Valuable, Vegetable,
Medical Prescription, with a Table of Detergent and Corroborant Medicines to Suit*

the Treatment of the Different Certificates (Versailles, Ky.: Printed by John H. Wilkins, Commonwealth Office, 1825), pp. [16]–58.

25. Richard Carter, *Valuable, Vegetable, Medical Prescriptions*, p. 38; Richard Carter, *Short Sketch*, p. 308.

26. Richard Carter, *Short Sketch*, p. 362.

27. Gunn, *Domestic Medicine* (1839), t.p.; Goodlett, *Family Physician*, t.p.

28. Pickard and Buley, *Midwest Pioneer*, pp. 47–71, at p. 47.

29. Richard Carter, *Short Sketch*, p. 5. Carter, of course, recommended the ubiquitous Benjamin Rush; he also praised Cullen, Sydenham, Boerhaave, and other European and American colleagues of equal celebrity. For example, Carter suggested that those afflicted with sore legs read works by physicians Townsend, Cooper, and Benjamin Bell (p. 92).

30. Richard Carter, *Valuable, Vegetable, Medical Prescriptions*, p. [120]; Richard Carter, *Short Sketch*, pp. 309–10.

31. Richard Carter, *Short Sketch*, pp. 228–29, 308–12, 379–80 (attacks on regulars); 152–53 (Indian lexicon); 93, 118–19 (folk cures); 224, 231 (God's aid).

32. Gunn, *Domestic Medicine* (1839), pp. 657, 130–33. Despite the nationalism implied in his title, another who was eclectic in his choice of remedies was Thomas W. Ruble, *The American Medical Guide for the Use of Families, In Two Parts, Part 1st. A MATERIA MEDICA. Being a Treaties on All the Most Usefull Articles Used as Medicine, Including the Which Are the Produce of our own Country. Part 2nd. THERAPEUTICS, or, The Art of Curing the Various Diseases of the HUMAN BODY* (Richmond, [Ky.]: Printed by E. Harris, for the Author, 1810). Like Gunn, Ruble saw no harm in using calomel and other heroic remedies in the right circumstances. See, for example, pp. iii–viii, 1–54. For publishing information on Ruble, see *NUC* 508: 540.

33. Gunn, *Domestic Medicine* (1839), p. 130. Paul Starr gives a good synopsis of these democratic and antielitist impulses in *The Social Transformation of American Medicine* (New York: Basic Books, 1982), pp. 54–59.

34. Gunn, *Domestic Medicine* (1839), pp. 595–99 (bleeding); 272, 290, 702–705 (catheters); 295, 417, 427–28, 599–607 (enemas). Charles Rosenberg has argued that Gunn's provision of this kind of medical information demonstrates his lack of concern with the need "to define careful boundaries between lay and professional spheres and to place certain areas of practice off-limits . . . [to] the nonprofessional." In Rosenberg's view, Gunn went further than previous authors of household health guides in "erasing boundaries between the nonspecialist and the physician" (Rosenberg, "Introduction," pp. x, xvi). But when Gunn's manual is placed in the context of the guides discussed in the first two chapters of this book, it is clear that the type of information that Gunn provided was more typical than not. In addition, despite his fervent democratic rhetoric, Gunn shared his predecessors' concerns about defining appropriate professional and nonprofessional responsibilities. As they had, Gunn assumed that domestic and professional medicine coexisted. Like theirs, Gunn's ability to demarcate precise boundaries was both limited and undermined by his determination to educate people, especially those in sparsely populated areas remote from medical aid, about proper medical care. Gunn *did* intimate broad boundaries, but they were by necessity extremely fluid and fuzzy. I would agree with Rosenberg, however, that Gunn's

later manuals did diverge more and more from the increasingly prevention-oriented volumes countenanced by orthodox physicians.

35. Gunn, *Domestic Medicine* (1839), pp. [378]–383 (lockjaw), 491–93 (convulsions in children).

36. Ibid., pp. 657, 384. Examples of Gunn's support for orthodox practitioners and remedies may be found on pp. 369, 382–88.

37. In his *Family Physician*, Goodlett's discussion of catheters (pp. 627–28) comes directly from Gunn's section (pp. 702–705). Goodlett's introduction (pp. xv–xvi) is very similar to William Buchan's *Domestic Medicine: Or, a Treatise on the Prevention and Cure of Diseases, by Regimen and Simple Medicines. With an Appendix, Containing a Dispensatory for the Use of Private Practitioners. To Which Are Added, Observations on Diet; Recommending a Method of Living Less Expensive, and More Conducive to Health, than the Present. Also, Advice to Mothers, On the Subject of Their Own Health; and of the Means of Promoting the Health, Strength, and Beauty of Their Offspring*, new, correct ed., enl. from the author's last revisal (Boston: Joseph Bumstead, 1811), pp. 17–47. Most of the remainder of the text follows James Ewell's *Medical Companion. Treating, According to the Most Successful Practice: I. The Diseases Common to Warm Climates on Ship Board. II. Common Cases in Surgery, as Fractures, Dislocations, etc. III. The Complaints Peculiar to Women and Children. With A Dispensatory and Glossary. To Which Are Added, A Brief Anatomy of the Human Body; An Essay on Hygiene, Or the Art of Preserving Health and Prolonging Life; An American Materia Medica, Instructing Country Gentlemen in the Very Important Knowledge of the Virtues and Doses of Our Medicinal Plants; Also, A Concise and Impartial History of the Capture of Washington, and the Diseases Which Sprung from that most Deplorable Disaster*, 3rd ed., greatly improved (Philadelphia: Printed for the Author by Anderson and Meehan, 1816). Sections that are apparently Goodlett's own appear on pp. 621–81.

38. Goodlett, *Family Physician*, pp. 642, 682.

39. John L. Thomas, "Romantic Reform in America, 1815–1865," *AQ* 17(1965): 656–81; Ronald G. Walters, *American Reformers, 1815–1860* (New York: Hill and Wang, 1978); and Alice Felt Tyler, *Freedom's Ferment: Phases of American Social History from the Colonial Period to the Outbreak of the Civil War*, Harper Torchbook ed. (New York: Harper and Row, 1962 [1944]).

40. Alex Berman's still-unpublished dissertation and derivative articles were until very recently the most substantive treatments of the Thomsonian movement: "The Impact of the Nineteenth Century Botanico-Medical Movement on American Pharmacy and Medicine" (unpublished Ph.D. dissertation, University of Wisconsin, 1954); "The Thomsonian Movement and Its Relation to American Pharmacy and Medicine," *BHM* 25(1951): 405–28, 519–38; and "Neo-Thomsonianism in the United States," *JHMAS* 11(1956): 133–55. Ronald L. Numbers offers a brief history of the movement in his "Do-It-Yourself the Sectarian Way," in Risse, Numbers, and Leavitt, eds., *Medicine Without Doctors*, pp. 49–72, on pp. 49–57. Kett's discussion of Thomsonianism as political and cultural expression is very good: *American Medical Profession*, pp. 97–131. A valuable synthesis of the secondary literature is Rothstein, *American Physicians*, pp. 123–51. Pickard and Buley, *Midwest Pioneer*, also discuss the Thomsonians, pp. 167–68. A more narrowly focused examination is James O. Breeden, "Thomsonianism in Virginia," *Virginia*

Magazine of History and Biography 82(1974): 150–80. Thomson's own account, of course, is indispensable: Samuel Thomson, *A Narrative of the Life and Medical Discoveries of Samuel Thomson; Containing an Account of his System of Practice, and the Manner of Curing Disease with Vegetable Medicine, upon a Plan Entirely New; To Which Is Added an Introduction to his New Guide to Health, or Botanic Family Physician, Containing the Principles upon Which the System Is Founded, with Remarks on Fevers, Steaming, Poison, etc.* (Boston: Printed for the Author, by E. G. House, 1822). Frequently reissued, the text changed remarkably little over time, except for the additions of bitter attacks on Thomsonian agents and of radical "supplements." Editions printed in Ohio in the late 1820s and early 1830s were especially vocal on democratic themes.

41. Thomson, *Narrative* (1822), pp. 16, 27. The same text appears in Samuel Thomson, *New Guide to Health: Or Botanic Family Physician. Containing A Complete System of Practice, On a Plan Entirely New: with a Description of the Vegetables Made Use of, and Directions for Preparing and Administering Them, to Cure Disease. To Which Is Prefixed, A Narrative of the Life and Medical Discoveries of the Author* (Boston: Printed for the Author, and Sold by his General Agent, at the Office of the Boston Investigator; J. Q. Adams, Printer, 1835), pp. 16, 27. Both the *Narrative* and *New Guide* were frequently reprinted by Thomson and his agents. Despite the marked resemblance of each edition to the others, none of the dozen and a half versions I consulted were exactly alike. Among other things, Thomson and his agents used these books to air grievances against one another. For an orientation to the publishing history, see *NUC* 592: 313–16.

42. Samuel Thomson, *New Guide to Health; Or, Botanic Family Physician. Containing A Complete System of Practice, on a Plan Entirely New; with a Description of the Vegetables Made Use of, and Directions for Preparing and Administering Them, to Cure Disease. To Which Is Prefixed, A Narrative of the Life and Medical Discoveries of the Author*, 3rd ed. (Boston: Printed for the Author, by J. Howe, 1832), pp. 39–42. The same text appears in Thomson, *New Guide* (1835), pp. 39–42.

43. Except for the final one, these quotes are from Thomson, *Narrative* (1822), pp. 43–44; the same language appeared in Thomson, *New Guide* (1835), p. 43. The concluding quote is from Thomson's *New Guide to Health; or, Botanic Family Physician. Containing A Complete System of Practice, Upon a Plan Entirely New; with a Description of the Vegetables Made Use of, and Directions for Preparing and Administering Them to Cure Disease. To Which Is Prefixed a Narrative of the Life and Medical Discoveries of the Author* (Boston: Printed for the Author, by E. G. House, 1822), pp. 185–86. For summaries of the derivative nature of Thomson's theory, see Kett, *American Medical Profession*, p. 107; and Rothstein, *American Physicians*, pp. 136–37.

44. Samuel Thomson, *A Narrative of the Life and Medical Discoveries of Samuel Thomson: Containing an Account of his System of Practice, and the Manner of Curining Diseases with Vegetable Medicine, upon a Plan Entirely New; To Which Is Added an Introduction to his New Guide to Health, or Botanic Family Physician; Containing the Principles upon Which the System Is Founded, with Remarks on Fevers, Steaming, Poison, etc.*, 6th ed. (Columbus, Ohio: Pike, Platt, and Company, 1832), pp. 20, 44; Thomson, *New Guide* (1832), pp. 20–78.

45. Thomson, *New Guide* (1832), pp. 44–45, 59.

46. Samuel Thomson, *New Guide to Health; Or Botanic Family Physician. Containing A Complete System of Practice, Upon a Plan Entirely New; with a Description of the Vegetables Made Use of, and Directions for Preparing and Administering Them to Cure Disease. To Which Is Added a Description of Several Cases of Disease Attended by the Author, with the Mode of Treatment and Cure* (Montpelier, [Vt.]: Printed for the Publisher, 1851), pp. 34–35. Though the words were slightly different in earlier editions, the meaning was the same.

47. Thomson, *New Guide* (1832), pp. 46–47. Very similar language appears in Thomson, *New Guide* (1835), pp. 46–47.

48. John Tebbel discusses the American Tract Society in *A History of Book Publishing in the United States,* 4 vols. (New York: R. R. Bowker, 1972–1975), at vol. 1, pp. 513–16. Michael Hackenberg's article is "Hawking Subscription Books in 1870: A Salesman's Prospectus from Western Pennsylvania," *Papers of the Bibliographical Society of America* 78(1984): 137–53. I am indebted to Michael Hackenberg for orienting me to sources about nineteenth-century book publishers and publishing. The Howard volume used by Hackenberg is fascinating: [Horton Howard], *Howard's Domestic Medicine: Being a Revised Edition of Horton Howard's Anatomy and Physiology, and Midwifery, Diseases of Women and Children. Practice of Medicine and Materia Medica, Founded Upon Correct Physiological Principles, and Especially Adapted to Family Use; Containing All the Important Discoveries and Improvements Down to the Present Time. Forming a Complete Family Medical Guide,* new enl. ed., embellished with over one hundred useful engravings, 3 vols. in one; publisher's prospectus (Philadelphia: Quaker City Publishing House, etc., 1869). For publishing information on Howard, see *NUC* 256: 603–604.

49. These are common estimates of Thomsonian popularity. See, for instance, Rothstein, *American Physicians,* p. 141, and Berman, "Thomsonian Movement," p. 407.

50. *NUC* 592: 313.

51. Daniel Drake, "The People's Doctors: A Review by 'The People's Friend,'" *Western Journal of the Medical and Physical Sciences* 3(1829): 407; quoted in Numbers, "Do-It-Yourself," p. 50. Excerpts from Drake's essay are included in Henry D. Shapiro and Zane L. Miller, eds., *Physicians to the West: Selected Writings of Daniel Drake on Science and Society* (Lexington: University Press of Kentucky, 1970), pp. 195–202.

52. Thomson, *Narrative* (1822), p. 25; Thomson, *New Guide* (1832), p. 25.

53. J. H. Smith, *A Guide to Health; Being a Compendium of Medical Instruction, Upon Botanic Principles: Designed for the Use of Families, and Private Individuals* (Ann Arbor, Mich.: N. Sullivan, Printer, 1842), pp. 105–107. For publishing information, see *NUC* 551: 338.

54. Frank G. Halstead, "A First-Hand Account of a Treatment by Thomsonian Medicine in the 1830's," *BHM* 10(1941): 680–87, at pp. 681–83.

55. Thomson, *New Guide* (1822), pp. [183]–184. See also Samuel Thomson, *A Narrative of the Life and Medical Discoveries of Samuel Thomson; Containing an Account of his System of Practice, and the Manner of Curing Disease with Vegetable Medicine, upon a Plan Entirely New; To Which Is Added an Introduction to his New Guide to Health, or Botanic Family Physician; Containing the Principles upon Which the System Is Founded, with Remarks on Fevers, Steaming, Poison, etc.,* 5th

ed. (St. Clairsville, [Ohio]: Published by Horton Howard; Howard and Little, Printers, 1829), p. 29.

56. Thomson, *Narrative* (1822), pp. 188–90; New York senator quoted by Kett, *American Medical Profession,* p. 123.

57. This is a common theme in Thomson's writings. See, for example, Thomson, *Narrative* (1822), p. 27.

58. Thomson, *Narrative* (1832), pp. 243–44, 254; Thomson, *New Guide* (1835), pp. 203, 213.

59. Thomson, *Narrative* (1832), pp. 245–46; Thomson, *New Guide* (1835), pp. 204–205.

60. Sumner Stebbins, *An Address in Refutation of the Thomsonian System of Medical Practice. Delivered in the Lecture Room of the Chester Co. Cabinet of Natural Science, West Chester, Pa., on December 31, 1836* (West Chester, Pa.: n.p., 1837), pp. 37–39.

61. Quoted in Cecil K. Drinker, *Not So Long Ago: A Chronicle of Medicine and Doctors in Colonial Philadelphia* (New York: Oxford University Press, 1937), pp. 150–51.

62. See, for instance, Norwood, *Medical Education;* and Kaufman, *American Medical Education.*

63. Unless otherwise noted, the following account is based on J. Marion Sims, *The Story of My Life* (New York: Appleton, 1884), pp. 138–46.

64. John Harley Warner argues that during this period knowledge (education) was essential but subordinate to practice (experience): essential because it defined practice, but subordinate because practice was what distinguished the regulars from their sectarian rivals. As Warner points out, morality was the third critical element in making up the professional medical identity. Based on the evidence I have used, experience and education seem to have had roughly equal weight. See Warner's excellent *The Therapeutic Perspective: Medical Practice, Knowledge, and Identity in America, 1820–1885* (Cambridge: Harvard University Press, 1986), pp. 11–36.

65. "Medical Reflection—No. III. On Medical Experience," *BMSJ* 12(February–August 1835): 12–13.

66. Sir Henry Halford, "On the Education and Conduct of a Physician," *BMSJ* 10(February–August 1834): 149–54, at p. 153.

67. Worthington Hooker, *Physician and Patient; or, A Practical View of the Mutual Duties, Relations and Interests of the Medical Profession and the Community* (New York: Baker and Scribner, 1849), p. 58.

68. "Medical Improvement—No. VIII," *BMSJ* 9(August 1833–February 1834): 202–205, at p. 203.

69. "Steam Doctoring," *BMSJ* 4(February–August 1831): 135.

70. For biographical details, consult Lois Wood Burkhalter, *Gideon Lincecum, 1793–1874: A Biography* (Austin: University of Texas Press, 1965). My discussion is based more closely on "Autobiography of Gideon Lincecum," *Publications of the Mississippi Historical Society* 8(1904): 443–519, esp. pp. 493–503.

71. "Medical Improvement—No. XI," *BMSJ* 9(August 1833–February 1834): 286–88, at p. 286.

72. Physicians faced a great deal of criticism from the public about the fees they

charged, and the economics of medical practice were at the center of debates about professionalizing; see George Rosen, *Fees and Fee Bills: Economic Aspects of Medical Practice in Nineteenth Century America* (Baltimore: Johns Hopkins University Press, 1946).

73. Samuel Robinson, *A Course of Fifteen Lectures, on Medical Botany, Denominated Thomson's New Theory of Medical Practice; In Which the Various Theories That Have Preceded It, Are Reviewed and Compared; Delivered in Cincinnati, Ohio* (Columbus, Ohio: Printed and Published by Horton Howard, 1829), p. 9. Robinson's book was reprinted using the same title in Boston by J. Q. Adams in 1835; these quotes are on p. 10. For publishing information, see *NUC* 498: 663.

74. Simon B. Abbott, *The Southern Botanic Physician: Being a Treatise on the Character, Causes, Symptoms and Treatment of the Diseases of Men, Women and Children of all Climates, on Vegetable or Botanical Principles, as Taught at the Reformed Medical Colleges in the U.S. Containing Also Many Valuable Recipes for Preparing Medicines. The Whole Preceded by Practical Rules for the Prevention of Disease and the Preservation of Health. Compiled from the Best Works Now Published on the Reformed Practice* (Charleston: Published for the Author, 1844), pp. xii, vii. For publishing information, see *NUC* 1: 469.

75. One follower was so enthusiastic about Thomson that his volume consisted primarily of strings of passages from Thomson's own work: [L. Meeker Day], *The Improved American Family Physician; Or, Sick Man's Guide to Health: Containing a Complete Theory of the Botanic Practice of Medicine, on the Thomsonian and Hygiean System, with Alterations and Improvements. To Which Is Appended, a Concise Formula for Compounding Medicines for the Cure of Every Complaint Incident to Human Nature. Also, a Complete Digest of Midwifery, So That 'Every Man May Be His Own Physician'* (New York: n.p., 1833). As suggested in the title, even Meeker did not believe that Thomson's remedies were the best in every case. Bound with his *Improved American Family Physician* was *The Botanic Family Physician; or the Secret of Curing All Diseases, on Improved Hygiean Principles, Fully Disclosed; Containing Also, Formulas, or Recipes, for the Cure of Every Disease Incidental to Human Nature: Together with a Valuable Digest on Midwifery, From the Best and Most Approved Botanical Publications, with Improvements, by Which 'Every One May Truly Now Be Their Own Physician, and Enjoy a Sound Mind in a Sound Body, at a Cheap Rate'* (New York: n.p., 1833).

76. Benjamin Colby, *A New Guide to Health; Being an Exposition of the Principles of the Thomsonian System of Practice, and Their Mode of Application in the Cure of Every Form of Disease; Embracing a Concise View of the Various Theories of Ancient and Modern Practice* (Nashua, N.H.: Charles T. Gill, 1844), pp. vii–ix. For publishing information, see *NUC* 114: 494. Charles Fourier's version of socialism enjoyed only brief success in America after the failure of several communities modeled on his utopian ideas.

77. Similar points will be made in chapter 6 about hydropathy and homeopathy.

78. Stebbins, *Address,* p. 11.

79. Colby paraphrased the Rush quote in *Guide to Health* (1844), t.p. John A. Brown used the same quotation, as cited in the text, in *Quackery Exposed!!! Or a Few Remarks on the Thomsonian System of Medicine, Consisting of Testimonies and Extracts from Various Writers. With Introductory Remarks* (Boston:

n.p., 1833), p. 3. Another version of the same quote is in Abbott, *Southern Botanic Physician*, p. v. For publishing information about Brown, see *NUC* 79: 181.

80. Robinson, *Fifteen Lectures*, p. iv. Most of these authors copiously cite orthodox medical authorities, particularly when giving descriptions of diseases. The range is wide, extending back as far as the ancients and forward to their contemporaries.

81. John A. Brown, *The Family Guide to Health, Containing a Description of the Botanic Thomsonian System of Medicine. With a Biographical Sketch of the Author* (Providence: B. T. Albro, Printer, 1827), p. v. For a description of the side effects of nineteenth-century heroic treatment, see Rothstein, *American Physicians*, pp. 41–62.

82. Doctor L. Sperry, *The Botanic Family Physician, or the Secret of Curing Diseases, with Vegetable Proportions. Also Containing Divers Formulas or Recipes, for the Cure of Almost Every Disease Incidental to Human Nature, Taken from the Best and Most Approved Botanical Publications, Together with the Most Approved Indian Methods of Using Roots and Herbs, by which Every One May Truly Be Said to Be His Own Physician, and Enjoy a Sound Mind in a Sound Body at a Cheap Rate* (Cornwall, Vt.: Published by the author, 1843), p. v.

83. Elias Smith's books were often reprinted, including his autobiography, *The Life, Conversion, Preaching, Travels and Sufferings of Elias Smith. Written by Himself. Vol. 1* [vol. 2 was never published] (Portsmouth, N.H.: Beck and Foster, 1816; reprint ed., New York: Arno Press, 1980). These remarks are from Smith's *The American Physician, and Family Assistant: In Five Parts. Containing: I. A General Description of Vegetable Medicines. II. The Manner of Preparing Them for Use. III. Description of Diseases, and Manner of Curing Them. IV. A Description of Mineral and Vegetable Poisons Given by Those Called Regular Doctors, under the Name of Medicines. V. Health Variously Illustrated,* 4th ed. (Boston: B. True, Printer, 1837), p. 211. Though Smith defended most Thomsonian practices, he criticized Thomson at length in some of his books. See, for example, Elias Smith, *The Medical Pocket-Book, Family Physician, and Sick Man's Guide to Health; Containing a Short Description of Vegitable Medicines; Manner of Preparing and Using Them; with a Description of Diseases which Attack the Human Frame, and the Mode of Cure, with Vegitables Only. Being an Extensive Improvement Beyond any Before Published* (Boston: Printed by Henry Bowen, 1822), pp. viii, 88, and passim. For publishing information, see *NUC* 550: 651–54.

84. This episode comes from Samuel B. Emmons, *'Every Man His Own Physician.' The Vegetable Family Physician: Containing a Description of the Roots and Herbs Common to This Country, With Their Medicinal Properties and Uses: Also Directions for the Treatment of the Diseases Incident to Human Nature, by Vegetables Alone; Embracing Many Valuable Indian Recipes* (Boston: George P. Oakes, 1836), pp. 167–69. For publishing information, see *NUC* 159: 483.

85. Abbott, *Southern Botanic Physician*, p. ix.

86. Daniel H. Whitney, *The Family Physician, or Every Man His Own Doctor: In Three Parts. Part I. Contains the Theory and Practice of Physic. Part II. Diseases of Women and Children, and the Botanic Practice. Part III. Dispensatory, Anatomy, and the Practice of Surgery: Together with the History, Causes, Symptoms and Treatment of Asiatic Cholera: A Glossary, Explaining the Most Difficult Words*

That Occur in Medical Science, and a Copious Index and Appendix (New York: Sold by N. and J. White, etc., 1834), p. 179. For publishing information, see *NUC* 661: 13.

87. Elias Smith, *American Physician,* pp. 275–306; quotes on pp. 304, 306.
88. Ibid., p. xvi.
89. Cited in Rothstein, *American Physicians,* p. 145.
90. Elias Smith, *American Physician,* p. xvi.
91. This 1838 editorial is quoted in Berman, "Thomsonian Movement," p. 535.
92. Abbott, *Southern Botanic Physician,* p. 17.
93. J. E. Carter [Written by A. H. Mathes], *The Botanic Physician, or Family Medical Advisor: Being an Improved System, Founded on Correct Physiological Principles. Comprising a Brief View of Anatomy, Physiology, Pathology, Hygiene, or the Art of Preserving Health: A Materia Medica, Exclusively Botanical, Containing a Description of More Than Two Hundred and Thirty of the Most Valuable Vegetable Remedies: To Which Is Added A Dispensatory, Embracing More Than Two Hundred Recipes for Preparing and Administering Medicine. The Diseases of the United States, with Their Symptoms, Causes, Cures, and Means of Prevention. Likewise, a Treatise on the Diseases Peculiar to Women and Children* (Madisonville, Tenn.: B. Parker and Co., 1837), pp. [13]–29 (anatomy), [30]–62 (physiology); quote on p. [13]. For publishing information, see *NUC* 97: 179.
94. M[orris] Mattson, *The American Vegetable Practice, or a New and Improved Guide to Health, Designed for the Use of Families. In Six Parts. Part I. Concise View of the Human Body, with Engraved and Wood-cut Illustrations. Part II. Glance at the Old School Practice of Physic. Part III. Vegetable Materia Medica, with Colored Illustrations. Part IV. Compounds. Part V. Practice of Medicine. Part VI. Guide for Women, Containing a Simplified Treatise on Childbirth, with a Description of the Diseases Peculiar to Females and Infants,* 2 vols., 2nd ed. (Boston: William Johnson, 1845), pp. 1–42 (anatomy); Whitney, *Family Physician,* pp. 339–97, quote on p. 396. For publishing information on Mattson, see *NUC* 370: 132.
95. See, for example, J. E. Carter, *Botanic Physician,* pp. 13–14; Mattson, *American Vegetable Practice,* pp. 3–4; and Sperry, *Botanic Family Physician,* pp. 54–55.
96. J. E. Carter, *Botanic Physician,* pp. [63]–112. Examples of writers whose preventive suggestions are found throughout their volumes are: Reuben Chambers, *The Thomsonian Practice of Medicine; Containing the Names, and a Description of the Virtues and Uses of the Medicines Belonging to this System of Practice; Also, Directions for Giving the Proper Quantity of Each Article for a Dose; Together with the Names and Symptoms of the Different Forms of Disease, and Ample Directions for Curing the Same, with Those Excellent Remedies* (Bethania, Pa.: n.p., 1842); George K. Bagley, *The Family Instructor, or Guide to Health: Containing the Names and Description of the Most Useful Herbs and Plants That Are Now in Use, with Their Medicinal Qualities Annexed. Also, A Treatise on Many of the Lingering Diseases to Which Mankind Are Subject, with New and Plain Directions Respecting the Management of the Same; with a Large List of Recipes, Which Have Been Carefully Selected from Indian Prescriptions, and from Those Who Were Cured by the Same After Every Other Remedy Had Failed. Designed for the Use of Families* ([Montpelier, Vt.]: Published for the Author, 1848);

Whitney, *Family Physician;* and Abbott, *Southern Botanic Physician.* For publishing information, see *NUC* 102: 629 (Chambers), 30: 306 (Bagley).

97. Benjamin Colby, *A Guide to Health; Being an Exposition of the Principles of the Thomsonian System of Practice, and Their Mode of Application in the Cure of Every Form of Disease; Embracing a Concise View of the Various Theories of Ancient and Modern Practice,* 3rd ed., enl. and rev. (Milford, N.H.: John Burns, 1846), p. 49.
98. Stebbins, *Address,* pp. 39–40.
99. "Medical Improvement—No. X," *BMSJ* 9(August 1833–February 1834): 253–56, at p. 253.

4. Toward a Literature of Prevention

1. Joseph F. Kett, *The Formation of the American Medical Profession: The Role of Institutions, 1780–1860* (New Haven: Yale University Press, 1968), pp. 12–13; William G. Rothstein, *American Physicians in the Nineteenth Century: From Sects to Science* (Baltimore: Johns Hopkins University Press, 1972), pp. 63–84. Their books also document the institutional and organizational efforts of orthodox physicians. See also Richard H. Shryock, *Medical Licensing in America, 1650–1965* (Baltimore: Johns Hopkins University Press, 1967).
2. Several scholars have pointed out the socialization value that this advice material had for a modernizing nation. See, for example: Daniel T. Rodgers, "Socializing Middle-Class Children: Institutions, Fables, and Work Values in Nineteenth-Century America," in N. Ray Hiner and Joseph M. Hawes, eds., *Growing Up in America: Children in Historical Perspective* (Urbana: University of Illinois Press, 1985), pp. 119–32; Regina Markell Morantz, "Nineteenth Century Health Reform and Women: A Program of Self-Help," in Guenter B. Risse, Ronald L. Numbers, and Judith Walzer Leavitt, eds., *Medicine Without Doctors: Home Health Care in American History* (New York: Science History Publications, 1977), pp. 73–93; and Regina Markell Morantz, "Making Women Modern: Middle Class Women and Health Reform in Nineteenth-Century America," *J. Soc. Hist.* 10(June 1977): 113–20.
3. Ronald L. Numbers, "The Rise and Fall of the American Medical Profession," in Judith Walzer Leavitt and Ronald L. Numbers, eds., *Sickness and Health in America: Readings in the History of Medicine and Public Health,* 2nd ed., rev. (Madison: University of Wisconsin Press, 1985), pp. 185–96.
4. Quoted in Kenneth M. Ludmerer, *Learning to Heal: The Development of American Medical Education* (New York: Basic Books, 1985), p. 13.
5. Quoted in Numbers, "Rise and Fall," p. 186.
6. Quoted in Regina Markell Morantz-Sanchez, *Sympathy and Science: Women Physicians in American Medicine* (New York: Oxford University Press, 1987 [1985]), p. 69.
7. Quoted in James Harvey Young, *The Toadstool Millionaires: A Social History of Patent Medicines in America Before Federal Regulation* (Princeton: Princeton University Press, 1961), p. 71. In a different context, Neil Harris has argued that nineteenth-century citizens actually enjoyed being hoodwinked: *Humbug: The Art of P. T. Barnum* (Boston: Little, Brown and Co., 1973).
8. Worthington Hooker, *Physician and Patient; or, A Practical View of the Mutual*

Duties, Relations and Interests of the Medical Profession and the Community (New York: Baker and Scribner, 1849), pp. vii–ix.

9. *Addresses Delivered by Professors Charles K. Winston and Paul Eve, at the Opening of the Medical Department of the University of Nashville* (Nashville, 1851), pp. 9–10. Quoted in Young, *Toadstool Millionaires*, p. 71. See also Caleb Ticknor, *Quacks and Quackery; Or, A Popular Treatise on Medical Philosophy and Imposture in Medicine by a Physician of New York* (New York: Mark H. Newman, 1844), pp. 219–66.

10. "Medical Ethics," *American Medical Recorder* 15(1829): 203–206, at p. 203.

11. "Report of the New Haven County Medical Society," *BMSJ* 16(February–August 1837): 341–47, 405–409; quotes at pp. 344, 346.

12. Lunsford P. Yandell, "An Address on the Improvement of the Medical Profession; Delivered before the Medical Society of Tennessee, at Its Twelfth Annual Meeting, in Nashville, in May, 1841," *Western Journal of Medicine and Surgery* 4(July–December 1841): 81–97; quotes at pp. 82–83. The Monroe County (New York) Medical Society saw the situation in much the same terms, as reported in "Medical Legislation," *BMSJ* 28(February–August 1843): 323–24.

13. "State Legislation Respecting Medical Practice," *BMSJ* 30(February–July 1844): 469–75. Quotes in this paragraph and the next two are from pp. 470–75.

14. These ideas provided much of the driving force to upgrade medical education. See, for example, Martin Kaufman, *American Medical Education: The Formative Years, 1765–1910* (Westport, Conn.: Greenwood Press, 1976).

15. Quoted in Rothstein, *American Physicians*, pp. 78–79.

16. "Importance of Punctuality to Medical Men," *BMSJ* 25(August 1841–February 1842): 228–29, at p. 228.

17. Stephen J. W. Tabor, "The Necessity of Urbanity in a Physician," *BMSJ* 30(February–July 1844): 294–97, at p. 294.

18. See, for example, John Harley Warner, *The Therapeutic Perspective: Medical Practice, Knowledge, and Identity in America, 1820–1885* (Cambridge: Harvard University Press, 1986), pp. 11–36.

19. Silas Holmes, "On the Means of Elevating the Medical Profession," *BMSJ* 16(February–August 1837): 152–55, 183–87. Quotes are from p. 154.

20. "Dr. Coventry's Valedictory Address," *American Medical Intelligencer*, n.s., 1(1841–42): 218.

21. John S. Wilson, "Remarks on the Use of Empirical Remedies; With Some Suggestions as to the Best Means of Abating the Evil," *Southern Medical and Surgical Journal*, n.s., 9(1853): 76–81. Quotes in this paragraph are from pp. 77–80.

22. Thus, in addition to articles published in *Godey's Lady's Magazine*, Wilson wrote books for women, including *Woman's Home Book of Health. A Work for Mothers and for Families. On a Plan, New, Safe, and Efficient. Showing, in Plain Language, How Disease May Be Prevented and Cured Without the Use of Dangerous Remedies* (Philadelphia: J. B. Lippincott and Co., 1860).

23. These conclusions are based on my comparisons of editions of Buchan from the first in 1769 through the twenty-ninth American edition in 1852. The younger Buchan signed his emendations A. P. B. The most notable alterations reflected A. P. Buchan's own experiences with consumption and the

widespread introduction of vaccination for smallpox. Other changes included the addition of substantial sections on diet and cold bathing, part of American editions from around 1809.

24. William Buchan, *Domestic Medicine, Or, a Treatise on the Prevention and Cure of Diseases, By Regimen and Simple Medicines: With Observations on Sea-Bathing, and the Use of the Mineral Waters. To Which Is Annexed, A Dispensatory for the Use of Private Practitioners,* 22nd ed., with considerable additions, and notes (London: T. Cadell, etc., 1826), pp. 102–103; William Buchan, *Domestic Medicine, Or, a Treatise on the Prevention and Cure of Diseases, by Regimen and Simple Medicines. Containing a Dispensatory for the Use of Private Practitioners. With Considerable Additions, and Various Notes, by A. P. Buchan, M.D. To Which Is Added, A Family Herbal. New Edition, Revised and Amended, by John G. Coffin, M.D.* (Boston: Phelps and Farnham, and Nathaniel S. Simpkins, 1825), p. 141. The 1826 volume was published in the United States under the same title and with the same text by J. and B. Williams in Exeter, New Hampshire, in 1828.

25. *New-England Journal of Medicine* 10(1821): 166–73; quotes in this paragraph and the next are from pp. 167–68, 172–73. See also Seebert J. Goldowsky, *Yankee Surgeon: The Life and Times of Usher Parsons, 1788–1868* (Boston: Francis A. Countway Library of Medicine in cooperation with Rhode Island Publications Society; Canton, Mass.: Sole distributor, Science History Publications/USA, 1988), pp. 150–52, 311, 167–68, n. 25.

26. *New-England Journal of Medicine* 11(1822): 321.

27. Ibid., 12(1823): 33–39; quotes in this paragraph and the next two are from pp. 35, 37, 38.

28. "Of the Medical Profession, and Of Its Preparation. An Introductory Lecture Read Before the Medical Class of Harvard University, Nov. 5, 1845, by Walter Channing, M.D.," *BMSJ* 33(August 1845–January 1846): 309–17; "Dr. Channing's Introductory Lecture," *BMSJ* 33(August 1845–January 1846): 329–37, 349–57. Quotes in this paragraph and the next three are from pp. 332–37.

29. "Coates's Popular Medicine," *BMSJ* 18(February–August 1838): 191–92. The "billing" is the substance of the title page of Reynell Coates's *Popular Medicine; or, Family Adviser; Consisting of Outlines of Anatomy, Physiology, and Hygiene, With Such Hints on the Practice of Physic, Surgery, and the Diseases of Women and Children, as May Prove Useful in Families when Regular Physicians Cannot Be Procured: Being a Companion and Guide for Intelligent Principals of Manufactories, Plantations, and Boarding-Schools, Heads of Families, Masters of Vessels, Missionaries, or Travellers; and a Useful Sketch for Young Men about Commencing the Study of Medicine* (Philadelphia: Carey, Lea and Blanchard, 1838). The other quotes are from the *BMSJ* review, p. 191.

30. Quotes in this paragraph and the previous one are from Coates, *Popular Medicine,* pp. 387, 290, 311, 319, 355, 487–88. Biographical information is from Howard A. Kelly and Walter L. Burrage, eds., *American Medical Biographies* (Baltimore: Norman Remington Co., 1920), pp. 328–29.

31. For many years the most accessible and comprehensive sources on unorthodox health-care options were: E. Douglas Branch, *The Sentimental Years: 1836–1860* (New York: D. Appleton-Century Co., 1934); Gilbert Seldes, *The Stammering Century* (New York: John Day Co., 1928); Grace Adams and

Edward Hutter, *The Mad Forties* (New York and London: Harper and Brothers, [1942]); and Gerald Carson, *Cornflake Crusade* (New York: Rinehart, 1957).

32. Richard H. Shryock, "Sylvester Graham and the Popular Health Movement, 1830–1870," *MVHR* 18(1931–32): 172–83. William B. Walker also placed Graham squarely within an ongoing health tradition: "The Health Reform Movement in the United States, 1830–1870" (unpublished Ph.D. dissertation, Johns Hopkins University, June 1955).

33. The most thorough discussion of Graham is Stephen Nissenbaum, *Sex, Diet, and Debility in Jacksonian America: Sylvester Graham and Health Reform* (Westport, Conn.: Greenwood Press, 1980). Though I stress dietary ideas here, it should be noted that Graham was equally famous—or infamous—for his teachings about sexuality. See also Nissenbaum's "Careful Love: Sylvester Graham and the Emergence of Victorian Sexual Theory in America, 1830–1840" (unpublished Ph.D. dissertation, University of Wisconsin, 1968). James C. Whorton's work is also useful: "Patient, Heal Thyself: Popular Health Reform Movements as Unorthodox Medicine," in Norman Gevitz, ed., *Other Healers: Unorthodox Medicine in America* (Baltimore: Johns Hopkins University Press, 1988), pp. 52–81; and "'Tempest in a Fleshpot': The Formation of a Physiological Rationale for Vegetarianism," *JHMAS* 32(1977): 115–39. I have used the revised version printed in Whorton's *Crusaders for Fitness: The History of American Health Reformers* (Princeton: Princeton University Press, 1982), pp. 62–91. Graham is also discussed in Whorton's "Christian Physiology," pp. 38–61 of the same volume. Two authors provide overviews for a more popular audience: Harvey Green, *Fit for America: Health, Fitness, Sport, and American Society* (New York: Pantheon Books, 1986), pp. 30–53; and Hillel Schwartz, *Never Satisfied: A Cultural History of Diets, Fantasies and Fat* (New York: Free Press, 1986), pp. 21–46.

34. Biographical details are taken from Nissenbaum, *Sex, Diet, and Debility*, pp. 3–24; quote at p. 79.

35. Ibid., pp. 13–21. See also Whorton, *Crusaders*, pp. 40–44.

36. Nissenbaum, *Sex, Diet, and Debility*, p. 14; "Health," *BMSJ* 5(August 1831–February 1832): 196.

37. "The Science of Life," *BMSJ* 13(August 1835–February 1836): 178–79.

38. Reprinted in *BMSJ* 13(August 1835–February 1836) were the following: S. Graham, "The Science of Life. Extracts from a Proem to a Course of Lectures at Boylston Hall," pp. 238–41; "The Science of Human Life: Extract from Mr. Graham's Introductory Lecture," pp. 317–19; and [S. Graham], "Vitality of the Blood," pp. 383–86.

39. Quotes in this and the following paragraph are from "Science of Life," p. 238; "Science of Human Life," pp. 318–19.

40. Luther V. Bell, "Boylston Prize Dissertation for 1835," *BMSJ* 13(August 1835–February 1836): 229–36, 247–56, 261–68, 280–86, 298–303. The editors used a more revealing title for all excerpts except the first: "Dr. Bell's Prize Dissertation on Diet."

41. Ibid., pp. 229, 303.

42. S. Graham, "Remarks on Dr. Bell's Prize Essay," *BMSJ* 13(August 1835–February 1836): 328–32, 347–52. Quotes are from pp. 332, 330, 351.

43. Luther V. Bell, "Cases in Pathological Anatomy," *BMSJ* 13(August

1835–February 1836): 405–409. Bell's remarks about Graham are on the final two pages, and the quotes are from p. 408.

44. Beta, "Dr. Bell's Prize Dissertation and Mr. Graham's Strictures," *BMSJ* 13(August 1835–February 1836): 379–82; quotes are from pp. 380–81.

45. A, "Beta *Versus* Mr. Graham," *BMSJ* 13(August 1835–February 1836): 396–98; quotes are from pp. 396, 397.

46. S. Graham, "Mr. Graham's Reply to Dr. Bell," *BMSJ* 14(February–August 1836): 22–28; quotes are from pp. 24–26.

47. Ibid., pp. 23, 27.

48. Quotes in this paragraph and the next are from W.★W.★, "Mr. Graham, Tea and Coffee, etc.," *BMSJ* 14(February–August 1836): 29–31.

49. R, "W.★W.★ and Mr. Graham," *BMSJ* 14(February–August 1836): 59–61.

50. M. L. North, "Dietetics," *BMSJ* 14(February–August 1836): 135–36.

51. S. Graham, "Grahamism NOT a Cause of Insanity," *BMSJ* 14(February–August 1836): 87–96, 103–108, 266–71, 319–22; quote at p. 93.

52. W.★W.★, "Some Facts and Logic Respecting Dietetics," *BMSJ* 14(February–August 1836): 166–72, at p. 166.

53. "Grahamism a Cause of Insanity," *BMSJ* 14(February–August 1836): 38–46.

54. S. Graham, "Dr. Pierson's Criticism on Mr. Graham," *BMSJ* 14(February–August 1836): 333–34, at p. 334. The editors' stifling of the Graham controversy was announced in the same issue under the title, "Difference of Opinion," p. 338.

55. The most useful sources for Alcott are Whorton's "Christian Physiology," cited above, and his "Physical Education," also in his *Crusaders for Fitness*, pp. 92–131.

56. Biographical details are culled from sources cited above as well as from William A. Alcott's fascinating autobiography, *Forty Years in the Wilderness of Pills and Powders: or, the Cogitations and Confessions of an Aged Physician* (Boston: John P. Jewett and Co., 1859). Quotes are from *Forty Years*, pp. 75, 77.

57. "Vegetable Diet as Sanctioned by Medical Men," *BMSJ* 18(February–August 1838): 352–53.

58. The article was continued in five issues of *BMSJ* 19(August 1838–February 1839): "Dr. Alcott's Work on Vegetable Diet," pp. 186–89; "Dietetics—Dr. Alcott's Work—No. II," pp. 220–23; "Dr. Alcott's Work on Vegetable Diet—No. III," pp. 252–55; "Dr. Alcott's Work on Vegetable Diet—No. IV," pp. 267–69; "Dr. Alcott's Work on Vegetable Diet—No. V," pp. 281–83. Quotes are from pp. 186, 220, 221.

59. "Dietetics—Dr. Alcott's Work—No. II," pp. 221–23.

60. W. A. Alcott, "Vegetable Diet," *BMSJ* 19(August 1838–February 1839): 316–20; quotes are from p. 317.

61. W. A. Alcott, "Temperance in All Things," *BMSJ* 21(August 1839–February 1840): 267–70; quotes are from p. 269.

62. For a discussion of "Christian physiology," consult sources listed above. See also John C. Burnham, *How Superstition Won and Science Lost: Popularizing Science and Health in the United States* (New Brunswick and London: Rutgers University Press, 1987), pp. 45–84; and Herbert Hovenkamp, *Science and Religion in America, 1800–1860* ([Philadelphia]: University of Pennsylvania Press, 1978).

63. Though it is beyond the scope of this book, it is important to note that while many scholars have agreed that physicians exerted enormous cultural authority through the publication of advice books, several studies have been more specific, arguing that this literature revealed and shaped a more rigid demarcation of sex roles. See, for instance, Carroll Smith-Rosenberg and Charles E. Rosenberg, "The Female Animal: Medical and Biological Views of Woman and Her Role in Nineteenth-Century America," *JAH* 60(1973): 332–56. Three articles by Smith-Rosenberg are also valuable: "Beauty, the Beast and the Militant Woman: A Study in Sex Roles and Social Stress in Jacksonian America," *AQ* 22(1971): 562–84; "The Hysterical Woman: Sex Roles and Role Conflict in Nineteenth-Century America," *Social Research* 39(1972): 652–78; and "Puberty to Menopause: The Cycle of Femininity in Nineteenth-Century America," *Feminist Studies* 1(1973): 58–72.
64. Publishing information is from *NUC* 7: 572–79. I have used William A. Alcott, *The Young Wife, Or Duties of Women in the Marriage Relation,* stereotype ed. (Boston: George W. Light, 1837; reprint ed., New York: Arno Press and the New York Times, 1972).
65. Ibid., pp. 21, 319.
66. Ibid., pp. 238–39, 254, 255.
67. Ibid., pp. 314–15. All of the books Alcott recommended were widely circulated and emphasized "that science and religion went hand in hand." William Paley's *Natural Theology: or Evidences of the Existence of the Attributes of the Deity, Collected from the Appearances of Nature,* for instance, "was imported by shiploads and endlessly adapted and revised for the American market" (Russel Blaine Nye, *Society and Culture in America, 1830–1860,* Harper Torchbooks ed. [New York: Harper and Row, 1974], p. 237).
68. I have used William A. Alcott, *The Young Mother; or Management of Children in Regard to Health,* 7th stereotype ed. (Boston: George W. Light, 1839).
69. Publishing information is from the *NUC* (cited above) and N, "The Young Mother," *BMSJ* 14(February–August 1836): 381–82. All quotes are from p. 381.
70. Alcott, *Young Mother,* pp. 19–20, 200–202, 25–26, 265.
71. Ibid., pp. 14, 97–98.
72. Ibid., pp. 30, 218.
73. I have used two identical editions: William A. Alcott, *The Young Woman's Guide to Excellence,* 6th stereotype ed. (Boston: George W. Light, 1841); and William A. Alcott, *The Young Woman's Guide to Excellence,* 13th ed. (Boston: Charles H. Pierce, etc., 1849). Publishing information is in *NUC* (see note above). Alcott published another book for this audience, but with a slightly different aim, as the title indicates: *Gift Book for Young Ladies; Or Familiar Letters on Their Acquaintances, Male and Female, Employments, Friendships, etc.* (Buffalo: George H. Derby and Co., 1852).
74. Alcott, *Young Woman's Guide* (1841), pp. 63–68. Most of these books, like the ones Alcott recommended elsewhere, were widely circulated, standard texts (Nye, *Society and Culture in America, 1830–1860,* pp. 324–27, 392–97; and *NUC* entries for each author). Alcott's inclusion of works by Catharine Maria Sedgwick, one of the mid-century female writers that Nathaniel Hawthorne so contemptuously dubbed "scribbling women," appears contradictory. But, as Ann Douglas has shown, in addition to their incredible pop-

ularity, Sedgwick's books helped define and popularize the ideal of domesticity. Also, Sedgwick's works had such strong religious overtones that a writer for the *Christian Examiner* likened her novels to "sermon[s]" (Ann Douglas, *The Femininization of American Culture,* Discus ed. [New York: Avon Books, 1978 (1977)], pp. 65, 129–30).

75. Alcott, *Young Woman's Guide* (1841), p. 227.
76. Ibid., pp. 78, 84, 85, 89.
77. Ibid., pp. 349, 262–63, 215–16.
78. W. A. Alcott, *The Young House-Keeper, or Thoughts on Food and Cookery,* 6th stereotype ed. (Boston: Waite, Peirce and Co., 1846), pp. 17–20.
79. I have used two editions: William A. Alcott, *The Young Man's Guide,* 2nd ed. (Boston: Lilly, Wait, Colman, and Holden, 1834); and the 14th edition of the same title (Boston: Perkins and Marvin, 1841). They are the same except that the later edition includes an "additional chapter" not found in the first. For the review, see "The Young Man's Guide," *BMSJ* 10(February–August 1834): 191.
80. William A. Alcott, *Familiar Letters to Young Men on Various Subjects. Designed as a Companion to the Young Man's Guide* (Buffalo: George H. Derby and Co., 1850), pp. 125–30. This volume was reissued in 1856 under a different title, reminiscent of the one Alcott had published for women: *Gift Book for Young Men; Or Familiar Letters on Self-Knowledge, Self-Education, Female Society, Marriage, etc.* (New York and Auburn: Miller, Orton and Mulligan, 1856).
81. Alcott, *Familiar Letters to Young Men,* p. 133. Allan S. Horlick has suggested that phrenology may have functioned as just the sort of practical tool Alcott was promoting: "Phrenology and the Social Education of Young Men," *History of Education Quarterly* 11(Spring 1971): 23–38.
82. I have used William A. Alcott, *The Young Husband, or Duties of Man in the Marriage Relation,* 20th stereotype ed. (New York: J. C. Derby, etc., 1855). All quotes in this paragraph and the next are from pp. 358–64.
83. Frank Ferguson, *The Young Man; Or Guide to Knowledge, Virtue, and Happiness* (Boston: G. W. Cottrell and Co.; New York: T. W. Strong, [1848], pp. 43–46 (regular hours), 46–50 (temperance).
84. Peter Parley [Samuel G. Goodrich], *The Every Day Book for Youth,* illustrated with numerous engravings (Philadelphia: Alexander Towar, 1836), pp. 76, 95, 173–74, 156–57; and Parley's *What To Do and How to Do It; or Morals and Manners Taught by Examples* (New York: Sheldon and Co., 1865 [1843]). Quotes are from *What To Do,* pp. 4–5.
85. I have used T. S. Arthur, *Advice to Young Men on Their Duties and Conduct in Life* (Philadelphia: John E. Potter and Co., [1860]); quotes are from pp. 214–17.
86. E. H. Chapin, *Duties of Young Men,* 9th ed., rev. (Boston: Putnam and Brother, 1856), pp. 7–38; quote at p. 11.
87. *The Well-Bred Boy and Girl; or, New School of Good Manners,* 2 vols. in 1 (Boston: B. B. Mussey and Co., 1850), pp. [59]–71.
88. Nearly a century earlier, at least one child did behave in a similar fashion. She was four-year-old Mary Noyes, only daughter of Mary Fish Noyes, who wrote in 1770 that "although so young, would take anything that was given her, if ever so bad to take. She would first taste it, and then would say, it is not good, Mama. I told her the Dr. said she must take it to make her better.

She would then open her little mouth and take anything." This passage also highlights the change in professional and nonprofessional roles in treating disease. In Alfred's case, the doctor's presence and authority were expected; seventy years earlier the doctor's presence signified an illness of some seriousness, and indeed little Mary died after ten days. See Joy Day Buel and Richard Buel, Jr., *The Way of Duty: A Woman and Her Family in Revolutionary America* (New York and London: W. W. Norton and Co., 1984), p. 61.

89. This statement is based on my survey of the magazines listed: *DeBow's Review* from its beginning in 1846 to vol. 20(January–June 1856); *North American Review* from the second to the sixth decade of the nineteenth century; *Southern Literary Messenger* 1(1835) through 22(1856); and *Peterson's Magazine* from inception in 1842 to the end of 1856.

90. Nissenbaum, *Sex, Diet, and Debility,* pp. 1–38.

91. Carl Degler, *At Odds: Women and the Family in America from the Revolution to the Present* (New York: Oxford University Press, 1980), p. 269.

92. Carroll Smith-Rosenberg, "Sex as Symbol in Victorian Purity: An Ethnohistorical Analysis of Jacksonian America," in John Demos and Sarane Spence Boocock, eds., *Turning Points: Historical and Sociological Essays on the Family, American Journal of Sociology,* vol. 84, Supplement (1978): S212–S247. For a later reference to one popular sexual physiology text, see Bernard J. Stern, ed., *Young Ward's Diary: A Human and Eager Record of the Years Between 1860 and 1870 as They Were Lived in the Vicinity of the Little Town of Towanda, Pennsylvania; in the Field as a Rank and File Soldier in the Union Army; and Later in the Nation's Capital* (New York: G. P. Putnam's Sons, 1935), pp. 41, 44, 45, 47, 56. I am indebted to Kathleen Neils Conzen for this reference. The best source on the literature of sexual physiology during this period is Janet Farrell Brodie, "Family Limitation in American Culture: 1830–1900" (unpublished Ph.D. dissertation, University of Chicago, 1982).

93. Sarah Josepha Hale, *The Good Housekeeper, or the Way to Live Well and To Be Well While We Live,* 2nd ed. (Boston: Weeks, Jordan and Co., 1839), t.p. The review is in *Godey's* 20(January–June 1840): 282–84.

94. Publishing information is from Ernest Earnest, *The American Eve in Fact and Fiction, 1775–1914* (Urbana: University of Illinois Press, 1974), pp. 93–98; see also the entry on Hale in Edward T. James et al., eds., *Notable American Women: A Biographical Dictionary* (Cambridge: Belknap Press of Harvard University Press, 1971), vol. 1, pp. 110–14. The statement about the magazine's contents is also based on my reading of it from the inception of the *Ladies' Magazine* through the late 1850s.

95. *Ladies' Indispensable Assistant, Being a Companion for the Sister, Mother, and Wife. Containing More Information for the Price than any Other Work Upon the Subject. Here Are the Very Best Directions for the Behavior and Etiquette of Ladies and Gentlemen, Ladies' Toilette Table, Directions for Managing Canary Birds, Also, Safe Directions for the Management of Children; Instructions for Ladies Under Various Circumstances; a Great Variety of Valuable Recipes, Forming a Complete System of Family Medicine. Thus Enabling Each Person to Become His or Her Own Physician: To Which Is Added One of the Best Systems of Cookery Ever Published; Many of These Recipes are Entirely New and Should Be in the Possession of Every Person in the Land* (New York: Published at 128 Nassau-Street, 1853), t.p.

96. Catharine Beecher, *A Treatise on Domestic Economy, for the Use of Young Ladies*

at Home, and at School, rev. ed., with numerous additions and illustrative engravings (New York: Harper and Brothers, 1845). This summary is based on Katherine Kish Sklar, *Catharine Beecher: A Study in American Domesticity* (New Haven: Yale University Press, 1973), pp. 151–67.

97. William A. Alcott, *Lectures on Life and Health; Or, The Laws and Means of Physical Culture* (Boston: Phillips, Sampson, and Co., 1853), p. 44.

5. The Pedagogical Crusade

1. Quoted in Lawrence A. Cremin, *American Education: The National Experience, 1783–1876* (New York: Harper and Row, 1980), p. 107.
2. Ibid., pp. 137–38; John H. Griscom, *Memoir of John Griscom, LL.D. With an Account of the New York High School; Society for the Prevention of Pauperism; the House of Refuge; and Other Institutions. Compiled from an Autobiography, and Other Sources* (New York: Robert Carter and Brothers, 1859), p. 346.
3. Cremin, *American Education,* pp. 107–47; quote on p. 138.
4. James C. Whorton, *Crusaders for Fitness: The History of American Health Reformers* (Princeton: Princeton University Press, 1982), pp. 112–14; quotes on p. 113.
5. There is no adequate study of American physiology, anatomy, and hygiene texts. The most convenient overview is Charles Carpenter, *History of American Schoolbooks* (Philadelphia: University of Pennsylvania Press, 1963); chapter 17 on "Physiologies and Mental Science Texts" is on pp. 233–44. Carpenter's essay, as he acknowledges, summarizes the major points in Helen Margaret Barton, "A Study of the Development of Textbooks in Physiology and Hygiene in the United States" (unpublished Ph.D. dissertation, University of Pittsburgh, 1942). Barton's coverage extends into the twentieth century, but it seldom advances beyond comparison of fact and feature to offer analysis or interpretation. Another survey is chapter 9 of John A. Nietz, *Old Textbooks. Spelling, Grammar, Reading, Arithmetic, Geography, American History, Civil Government, Physiology, Penmanship, Art, Music—As Taught in the Common Schools from Colonial Days to 1900* (Pittsburgh: University of Pittsburgh Press, 1961), pp. 290–318.
6. Frederick Rudolph, *Curriculum: A History of the American Undergraduate Course of Study Since 1636* (San Francisco: Jossey-Bass Publishers, 1977); C. I. Reed, "The Maturation of Physiology in America after 1830," *The Physiologist* 5(February 1962): 35–41.
7. On the perfectionistic impulse, see John L. Thomas, "Romantic Reform in America, 1815–1865," *AQ* 17(1965): 656–81. On pietism and public health, see Carroll Smith-Rosenberg and Charles E. Rosenberg, "Pietism and the Origins of the American Public Health Movement: A Note on John H. Griscom and Robert M. Hartley," *JHMAS* 23(1968): 16–35.
8. The best discussion of foreign influences and American attitudes is John Harley Warner, *The Therapeutic Perspective: Medical Practice, Knowledge, and Identity in America, 1820–1885* (Cambridge: Harvard University Press, 1986), pp. 13–14, 185–283. See also Warner's "'The Nature-Trusting Heresy': American Physicians and the Concept of the Healing Power of Nature in the 1850's and 1860's," *Perspectives in American History* 11(1977–78): 291–324; Kenneth M. Ludmerer, *Learning to Heal: The Development of American Medical*

Education (New York: Basic Books, 1985), pp. 11–38; and Robert G. Frank, Jr., "American Physiologists in German Laboratories, 1865–1914," in Gerald L. Geison, ed., *Physiology in the American Context, 1850–1914* (Bethesda, Md.: American Physiological Society, 1987), pp. 11–46.

9. The most comprehensive history of American physiology does not even treat events prior to mid-century: W. Bruce Fye, *The Development of American Physiology: Scientific Medicine in the Nineteenth Century* (Baltimore: Johns Hopkins University Press, 1987). Despite its title, Geison's volume of essays, cited above, also shortchanges the antebellum period. Edward C. Atwater mentions these writers, but does not discuss their works or influence in "'Squeezing Mother Nature': Experimental Physiology in the United States Before 1870," *BHM* 52(1978): 313–35. Martha H. Verbrugge briefly treats the reactions of orthodox physicians to popular lecturers on physiology in *Able-Bodied Womanhood: Personal Health and Social Change in Nineteenth-Century Boston* (New York: Oxford University Press, 1988), pp. 58–62, 214–16.

10. Warner mentions this link but does not develop the idea in his *Therapeutic Perspective*, pp. 236–37, 240–41. Despite the increasing importance of this point through the century, Anita Clair Fellman and Michael Fellman do not discuss it in *Making Sense of Self: Medical Advice Literature in Late Nineteenth-Century America* (Philadelphia: University of Pennsylvania Press, 1981).

11. James E. Cronin, ed., *The Diary of Elihu Hubbard Smith (1771–1798)* (Philadelphia: American Philosophical Society, 1973), pp. 306, 95.

12. I have used B[ernhard] C[hristoph] Faust, *Catechism of Health: For the Use of Schools and for Domestic Instruction,* trans. from last improved German ed. by J. H. Basse (London: Printed for C. Dilly, 1794). This edition is identical to the 1795 American one.

13. Ibid., pp. iii–viii, 14.

14. Ibid. In a book of 186 pages, the section on health was 104 pages (pp. 9–113). Quotes are from pp. 47, 86–87.

15. Ibid. This paragraph and the next are based on pp. 114–25, 134–58, 172–79, 182–83.

16. [Bernhard Christoph Faust], *A New Guide to Health. Compiled from the Catechism of Dr. Faust: With Additions and Improvements, Selected from the Writings of Medical Men of Eminence. Designed for the Use of Schools, and Private Families* (Newburyport, Mass.: W. and J. Gilman, 1810), t.p., pp. iii–iv.

17. Ibid., pp. 7–16; quotes on pp. 7, 13.

18. Ibid. The discussion of smallpox is updated to reflect Jenner's epochal 1796 experiment with the cowpox virus, pp. 113–15. The author's pronouncements about medicine and disease were quite familiar from the 1795 edition. See, for example, pp. 120–21, 123–24.

19. William [Fordyce] Mavor, *The Catechism of Health; Containing Simple and Easy Rules and Directions for the Management of Children, and Observations on the Conduct of Health in General. For the Use of Schools and Families,* with alterations and improvements (New York: Samuel Wood and Sons; Baltimore: Samuel S. Wood and Co., 1819), pp. 5, 54–55. Biographical material about Mavor is from *DNB* 13: 108–109.

20. Mavor, *Catechism of Health.* For instance, the fourth chapter of Mavor's text, "Of Air and Cleanliness—of Food and Drink," was six pages long, but it

covered the same topics treated in the 1810 volume in five chapters and four times as many pages.

21. Ibid., pp. 16, 62. The conclusion (pp. 64–68), a poetic tribute to the eradication of smallpox, also testifies to the intended readership. Entitled "Address to a Mother," it emphasizes the triumph of reason over superstition.

22. [Henry H. Porter], *The Catechism of Health* (Philadelphia: Offices of the *Journal of Health*, the *Journal of Law*, and the *Family Library of Health*, 1831), t.p.

23. Ibid., pp. 12–13, 66–67.

24. Ibid., pp. 125–94; quote on p. 125.

25. Review article, *Western Medical and Physical Journal* 5(April 1831–March 1832): 100–18; all quotes in this paragraph and the next two are from pp. 100–10.

26. Amariah Brigham, *Remarks on the Influence of Mental Cultivation and Mental Excitement Upon Health*, 2nd ed. (Boston: Marsh, Capen and Lyon, 1833; reprint ed., Delmar, N.Y.: Scholars' Facsimiles and Reprints, 1973), pp. iv–vi. Publishing history is from Ernest Harms's "Introduction" to the Brigham reprint, pp. v–xvi.

27. "Physical Education," *Western Medical and Surgical Journal* 7(1833–34): 226–56; quote on p. 227.

28. Brigham, *Remarks*, p. x; see also p. 52.

29. Roger Cooter, *The Cultural Meaning of Popular Science: Phrenology and the Organization of Consent in Nineteenth-Century Britain* (New York: Cambridge University Press, 1984).

30. Allan S. Horlick, "Phrenology and the Social Education of Young Men," *History of Education Quarterly* 11(Spring 1971): 23–38.

31. John D. Davies, *Phrenology, Fad and Science: A 19th-Century American Crusade* (New Haven: Yale University Press, 1955); Madeleine B. Stern, *Heads and Headliners: The Phrenological Fowlers* (Norman: University of Oklahoma Press, 1971).

32. Andrew Combe, *The Principles of Physiology Applied to the Preservation of Health, and to the Improvement of Physical and Mental Education*, stereotype ed. (New York: Harper and Brothers, 1836), t.p., pp. 15–16. The indefatigable Fowlers—Orson, Lorenzo, and Lydia—also published anatomy, physiology, and hygiene texts, as listed in *NUC* 179: 487–503. Since the orientation and audiences for these books were so different from the ones covered in this chapter, I have not included them in my discussion.

33. Combe, *Principles of Physiology*, p. [13], [1].

34. Ibid., pp. 43, 61, 160–61.

35. Ibid., pp. 88, 142–45.

36. As many scholars have shown, there was a close relationship between science and religion in antebellum America. See, for example, Herbert Hovenkamp, *Science and Religion in America, 1800–1860* ([Philadelphia]: University of Pennsylvania Press, 1978); Theodore Dwight Bozeman, *Protestants in an Age of Science: The Baconian Ideal and Antebellum American Religious Thought* (Chapel Hill: University of North Carolina Press, 1977); and John C. Burnham, *How Superstition Won and Science Lost: Popularizing Science and Health in the United States* (New Brunswick and London: Rutgers University Press, 1987), pp. 45–84.

37. Combe, *Principles of Physiology,* pp. 31–32.
38. Ibid., pp. 25–28. Charles Rosenberg places these ideas within a larger context in his "The Therapeutic Revolution: Medicine, Meaning, and Social Change in Nineteenth-Century America," in Morris J. Vogel and Charles E. Rosenberg, eds., *The Therapeutic Revolution: Essays in the Social History of American Medicine* (Philadelphia: University of Pennsylvania Press, 1979), pp. 3–25.
39. Combe, *Principles of Physiology,* pp. 24–28, 265–68, and passim. For discussions of changing concepts of health and sickness, see Verbrugge, *Able-Bodied Womanhood,* pp. 3–48; and Regina Markell Morantz, "Making Women Modern: Middle Class Women and Health Reform in Nineteenth-Century America," *J. Soc. Hist.* 10(June 1977): 113–20.
40. "Combe's Physiology," *American Medical Intelligencer* 1(1837): 50; Harriet Martineau, *Society in America,* 2 vols., 4th ed. (New York: Saunders and Otley, 1837), vol. 2, p. 151.
41. See two articles in *BMSJ* 43(August 1850–January 1851): William W. Finch, "Popular Physiology," pp. 133–34; and Medicus, "Popular Physiology," pp. 151–53. Verbrugge makes this point in *Able-Bodied Womanhood,* pp. 58–62, 214–16. On lecturing, see Donald M. Scott's suggestive "The Popular Lecture and the Creation of a Public in Mid-Nineteenth-Century America," *JAH* 66(1980): 791–809. Female health lecturers will be considered at greater length in chapter 6.
42. "Travelling Manakins," *BMSJ* 30(February–July 1844): 124–25; "American Manakins," *BMSJ* 30(February–July 1844): 407; "The Popular Study of Anatomy and Physiology," *BMSJ* 21(August 1839–February 1840): 188–93; and "Popular Anatomy," *BMSJ* 34(February–July 1846): 285–86.
43. Quoted in John B. Blake, "Health Reform," in Edwin S. Gaustad, ed., *The Rise of Adventism: Religion and Society in Mid-Nineteenth-Century America* (New York: Harper and Row, 1974), pp. 30–49, at pp. 43–44. See also I. F. Galloupe, "Popular Physiology," *BMSJ* 43(August 1850–January 1851): 59–62. Hyman Kuritz briefly discusses the entertainment aspect of popular science lectures in "The Popularization of Science in Nineteenth-Century America," *History of Education Quarterly* 21(Fall 1981): 259–74.
44. William A. Alcott, *The House I Live In. Part First. The Frame. For the Use of Families and Schools* (Boston: Lilly, Wait, Colman, and Holden, 1834); "The House I Live In," *BMSJ* 11(August 1834–February 1835): 18. For biographical and bibliographical information on Alcott, see sources listed in the previous chapter.
45. Alcott, *House I Live In,* pp. [13]–27, 41, 47, 112, 119, 106.
46. Ibid., pp. 62–63, 81, 127–28.
47. The only biographical data on Jane Taylor I have found is Charles Carpenter's statement that she was not the Jane Taylor who wrote children's books and the familiar nursery rhyme, "Twinkle, Twinkle Little Star" (*History of American Schoolbooks,* p. 236).
48. I have used the earlier title: Jane Taylor, *Physiology for Children,* rev. and corrected, twenty-ninth thousand (New York: Saxton and Miles, 1844). Publishing information is from *NUC* 584: 535–36.
49. Taylor, *Physiology for Children,* pp. 9, 16, [17], 25, 54, [59].
50. Jane Taylor, *Wouldst Know Thyself, or The Outlines of Human Physiology: De-*

signed for the Youth of Both Sexes, illustrated with numerous anatomical engravings (New York: George F. Cooledge and Brother, 1858), t.p., p. [5].

51. Ibid., pp. 9–13, 29–30.
52. Ibid. Quotes in this paragraph and the next are from pp. 62–64.
53. Worthington Hooker, *The Child's Book of Nature. Three Parts in One. Part I. Plants. Part II. Animals. Part III. Air, Water, Heat, Light, etc.,* illustrated by numerous engravings (New York: Harper and Brothers, 1874 [1857]), part 2, p. 11. For biographical information on Hooker, see sources listed in chapter 3.
54. Ibid., part 2, pp. 27, 35.
55. Ibid., part 2, pp. 77, 79, 70, 87, 47–48.
56. Ibid., pp. 51, 69–70. Chapters 19–32 of part 2 focus on animals and are profusely illustrated.
57. Publishing information is from *NUC* 236: 612–13 (Hayward) and *NUC* 118: 323–32 (Comstock). Aside from the anatomy and physiology textbooks discussed in this chapter, I know of only a few others published during this time period: Jerome V. C. Smith, *Class-Book of Anatomy* (Boston, 1834); Charles A. Lee, *Human Physiology* (New York, 1838); Edward Reynolds, *Importance of Knowledge of Physiology to Students* (1833); John C. Warren, *Physical Education and the Preservation of Health* (1846); John A. Tarbell, *Sources of Health and the Prevention of Disease* (1850); and LaRoy Sunderland, *Book of Health for the Million* (1847).
58. George Hayward, *Outlines of Human Physiology; Designed for the Use of the Higher Classes in Common Schools* (Boston: Marsh, Capen and Lyon, 1834), pp. 4, 60, 215 (God); 29–31, 67, 105, 111 (common language); and 172–73 (ear), 181–93 (eye). Biographical information is from Howard A. Kelly and Walter L. Burrage, eds., *American Medical Biographies* (Baltimore: Norman Remington Co., 1920), p. 547.
59. D. F. C., review of Hayward text, *American Journal of the Medical Sciences* 15(1834): 463–64, quote on p. 464.
60. The story of this controversy may be traced in: "School Physiology," *BMSJ* 29(August 1843–January 1844): 224; "Human Anatomy and Physiology for Schools," *BMSJ* 29(August 1843–January 1844): 523–24; "Popular Physiology," *BMSJ* 30(February–July 1844): 47; Alpha, "Lane's Physiology," *BMSJ* 30(February–July 1844): 139–40; Omega, "Lane's Anatomy and Physiology," *BMSJ* 30(February–July 1844): 178–80.
61. Hayward, *Outlines of Human Physiology,* for example, pp. 57, 179 (imperfect knowledge).
62. J. L. Comstock, *Outlines of Physiology, Both Comparative and Human; In Which Are Described the Mechanical, Animal, Vital, and Sensorial Organs, and Functions; Including Those of Respiration, Circulation, Digestion, Audition and Vision, as They Exist in the Different Orders of Animals, from the Sponge to Man. Also, The Application of These Principles to Muscular Exercise, and Female Fashions, and Deformities,* illustrated by numerous engravings, intended for the use of schools and heads of families (New York: Robinson, Pratt and Co., 1836). See, for example, pp. [iii]–iv, viii (scientific lineage); 85 (spine); 87 (collarbone); 166–78 (vision). Comstock wrote textbooks on a handful of other subjects; among the most popular were those in geology, botany, and es-

pecially chemistry. See *NUC* 118: 323–32; Nietz, *Old Textbooks,* pp. 303–305; and Carpenter, *History of American Schoolbooks,* pp. 234–35.

63. Comstock, *Outlines of Physiology,* pp. 88 (quote); 207–314 (exercise and fashion).

64. I have used a slightly later edition: Reynell Coates, *Physiology for Schools,* 4th ed., rev. (Philadelphia: Butler and Williams, 1845), pp. vi, 158 (quotes); 184–85, 244–45 (simple language); 36–39, 108, 226–27 (experiments); 140, 154, 175 (God). For publishing information, see *NUC* 113: 238–39.

65. Coates, *Physiology for Schools,* pp. 214–15, 230–31, 265–67 (behavior); 177 (quote). For biographical information, see sources listed in the previous chapter.

66. Biographical information is from: James H. Cassedy's entry in Martin Kaufman, Stuart Galishoff, and Todd L. Savitt, eds., *Dictionary of American Medical Biography,* 2 vols. (Westport, Conn.: Greenwood Press, 1984), vol. 1, pp. 308–309; and William F Norwood, *Medical Education in the United States Before the Civil War* (Philadelphia: University of Pennsylvania Press, 1944), pp. 130–31. See also Smith-Rosenberg and Rosenberg, "Pietism and the Origins of the American Public Health Movement," pp. 16–35.

67. John H. Griscom, *Animal Mechanism and Physiology; Being a Plain and Familiar Exposition of the Structure and Functions of the Human System. Designed for the Use of Families and Schools,* illustrated by numerous woodcuts by Butler (New York: Harper and Brothers, 1839), t.p., pp. i, 13–42. See also *NUC* 219: 289–91.

68. Ibid., pp. 319–42.

69. Ibid., pp. 88–90, 114, 137–39, 143; see also pp. 174–76.

70. Ibid., pp. 69–70, 62–63, 64–69, 162–73. The crusade against tight lacing spanned the nineteenth century. For an overview, see John S. Haller and Robin M. Haller, *The Physician and Sexuality in Victorian America* (Urbana: University of Illinois Press, 1974), pp. 146–74; Hillel Schwartz, *Never Satisfied: A Cultural History of Diets, Fantasies and Fat* (New York: Free Press, 1986), pp. 47–58; and Lois Banner, *American Beauty* (New York: Knopf, 1983).

71. I have used B[enjamin] N. Comings, *Class-Book of Physiology; For the Use of Schools and Families. Comprising the Structures and Functions of the Organs of Man, Illustrated by Comparative References to Those of Inferior Animals,* with twenty-four plates, and numerous engravings on wood, comprising in all above two hundred figures, 2nd ed., with appendix (New York: D. Appleton and Co., 1854), pp. 4, t.p. Biographical information is from Lisabeth M. Holloway, ed., *Medical Obituaries: American Physicians' Biographical Notices in Selected Medical Journals Before 1907* (New York: Garland Publishing, 1981), p. 94b. Bibliographical information is in *NUC* 117: 302–303; and Nietz, *Old Textbooks,* p. 309.

72. Comings, *Class-Book of Physiology,* t.p., 132–33 (quotes); 33, 51, 62 (experiments); 3, 184 (God).

73. Ibid., pp. 4 (quote); 59–61, 73, 92 (behavior); [240]–[249] (the human form); [251]–304 (appendix).

74. An excellent source on Jarvis's life and times is Gerald N. Grob, *Edward Jarvis and the Medical World of Nineteenth-Century America* (Knoxville: University of Tennessee Press, 1978). Grob summarizes in Kaufman, Galishoff, and Savitt,

eds., *Dictionary of American Medical Biography*, vol. 1, p. 392. See also Carpenter, *American Schoolbooks*, p. 236.

75. Edward Jarvis, *Primary Physiology, for Schools* (Philadelphia: Thomas, Cowperthwait, and Co., etc., 1848). For publishing details, see Grob, *Jarvis*, p. 77.

76. "Primary Physiology for Schools," *BMSJ* 39(August 1848–February 1849): 125; *NUC* 278: 247–50.

77. Jarvis, *Primary Physiology*, pp. [7]–8, 13, 28, 34.

78. Ibid., pp. [3], 87–89, 107–12, 132–41, 124–27.

79. Ibid., pp. 142–43, 14, 66, 15, 17–19, 44–45, 60, 85.

80. Ibid., p. 156.

81. Grob, *Jarvis*, p. 79.

82. Carpenter, *American Schoolbooks*, pp. 236–37; Nietz, *Old Textbooks*, pp. 305–307; Kelly and Burrage, eds., *American Medical Biographies*, pp. 283–84; *NUC* 130: 381–84.

83. Calvin Cutter, *First Book on Anatomy, Physiology, and Hygiene, for Grammar Schools and Families*, with eighty-three engravings, rev. stereotype ed. (New York: Clark and Maynard, etc., [1852]), p. 10.

84. Ibid., pp. 13, 14, 90 (everyday language); 17, 29 (Divine agency); 14, 20, 30–42, 97, 98 (experiments).

85. Ibid., pp. [v]–vi, 143–51. The opposite positions Jarvis and Cutter took on the use of slang words in many ways paralleled larger cultural concerns, as demonstrated in Kenneth Cmiel, "Democratic Eloquence: Language, Education and Authority in Nineteenth-Century America" (unpublished Ph.D. dissertation, University of Chicago, 1986), pp. 70–144, 210–60.

86. Cutter, *First Book*, pp. 158–75.

87. Calvin Cutter, *A Treatise on Anatomy, Physiology, and Hygiene: Designed for Colleges, Academies, and Families*, with one hundred and fifty engravings, stereotype ed. (Boston: Benjamin Mussey and Co., etc., 1850), pp. 6–8, 425–42.

88. Ibid., pp. 49–50 (quotes), 77 (experiment).

89. Lambert and his publishers had a proclivity for using variations of the same title over and over, which makes it extremely difficult to trace publishing details. This paragraph is based on *NUC* 313: 99–100; Nietz, *Old Textbooks*, pp. 308–309; and T[homas] S. Lambert, *Hygienic Physiology*, illustrated by numerous wood-cuts and colored engravings (Hartford: Brockett, Hutchinson and Co., etc., 1854), publishers' advertising supplement, pp. 1–2. Limited biographical details are available in Kelly and Burrage, eds., *American Medical Biographies*, p. 718.

90. "First, Second and Third Books of Anatomy," *BMSJ* 45(August 1851–January 1852): 437; J. D. Mansfield, "Dr. Lambert's Second Book on Anatomy and Physiology," *BMSJ* 44(February–August 1851): 35–37; "Dr. Lambert's Course of Lectures on Physiology," *BMSJ* 44(February–August 1851): 106.

91. J. D. Mansfield, "Dr. Lambert's Popular Anatomy and Physiology—Quackery, etc.," *BMSJ* 42(February–August 1850): 249–50; "Anatomy and Physiology," *BMSJ* 44(February–July 1851): 22–23.

92. T[homas] S. Lambert, *Popular Anatomy and Physiology, Adapted to the Use of Students and General Readers* (New York: Leavitt and Co., 1851), t.p., pp. 28n–29n, 32n, 218n. This book provides an excellent example of how dif-

ficult it is to establish publishing details for these texts. For the edition I have used, the title page gives one date (1851), the *NUC* lists a second (1850), and the copyright page records a third (1849).

93. Ibid., pp. 45–46, 89–90, 266–67, 315–16, 380, 324–25.

94. Ibid., pp. 142–82. Lambert condensed this material in his *Practical Anatomy, Physiology, and Pathology; Hygiene and Therapeutics,* illustrated by five hundred plates and over one hundred wood engravings (New York: Leavitt and Co., 1850), pp. 169–81. On p. 181 he referred readers who wanted additional information to *Popular Anatomy.*

95. Lambert, *Popular Anatomy,* pp. 155, 158, 167. One of the few who did also mention these parts was Hayward, *Outlines of Human Physiology,* pp. 184–86.

96. Lambert, *Hygienic Physiology,* pp. [15]–16, 136–43; quotes on p. 138.

97. Ibid., pp. 73, 56, 84, 87. In *Practical Anatomy, Physiology, and Pathology,* Lambert went further and highlighted the behavioral inferences that could be drawn from structure and function; see, for instance, p. 158, where eight inferences are specified. In addition, he peppered the text with descriptions of situations designed to convey proper and improper behavior; see pp. 127–28, where Lambert provides nine illustrations and four inferences.

98. Lambert, *Hygienic Physiology,* p. 135; *Popular Anatomy,* p. 408 (quote).

99. Worthington Hooker, *Human Physiology: Designed for Colleges and the Higher Classes in Schools, and for General Reading,* illustrated by nearly two hundred engravings (New York: Pratt, Oakley and Co., 1859), t.p. See, for example, pp. 56–57, 85, 145–46, 290. Nietz discusses this book briefly in *Old Textbooks,* pp. 307–308.

100. Hooker, *Human Physiology,* pp. 94–97.

101. Ibid., pp. 390–410; "Human Physiology," *BMSJ* 51(August 1854–January 1855): 244–45.

102. William A. Alcott, *Lectures on Life and Health; Or, The Laws and Means of Physical Culture* (Boston: Phillips, Sampson, and Co., 1853), pp. [iii]–iv.

103. Ibid., pp. 19–27.

104. Ibid., pp. 45, 452.

105. Ibid., pp. 47, 55, 317, 290, 220.

106. Catharine E. Beecher, *Physiology and Calisthenics. For Schools and Families* (New York: Harper and Brothers, 1856). Intended primarily for women readers, *Letters to the People on Health and Happiness* (New York: Harper and Brothers, 1855) was remarkably similar. Biographical information is drawn from Kathryn Kish Sklar's fine *Catharine Beecher: A Study in American Domesticity* (New Haven: Yale University Press, 1973) and the entries on Beecher in James et al., eds., *Notable American Women,* vol. 1, pp. 121–24, and *DAB* 2: 125–26. Bibliographical information may also be found in *NUC* 43: 46–50.

107. Beecher, *Physiology and Calisthenics,* p. [iii].

108. Ibid., pp. v–vi, 10–14.

109. Ibid., pp. 15, 18.

110. Ibid., pp. 74–77.

111. Ibid., pp. 21–25, [78].

112. Ibid., pp. [85]–87

113. Ibid., pp. [96]–102, [172]; quotes on pp. 102, [172].

114. Cremin, *American Education,* pp. 107–47; Reed, "Maturation of Phys-

iology," p. 36; William A. Link, *A Hard Country and A Lonely Place: Schooling, Society, and Reform in Rural Virginia, 1870–1920* (Chapel Hill: University of North Carolina Press, 1986), pp. 64–68, 149–60; John Kent Folmar, '*This State of Wonders*': *The Letters of an Iowa Frontier Family, 1858–1861* (Iowa City: University of Iowa Press, 1986), pp. xxv–xxvi, 62.

115. "Physiology and Animal Magnetism," *Western Journal of Medicine and Surgery*, n.s., 4(1841): 371.

116. Lack of delicacy and refinement were, however, cited as problems with another physiology text: Alpha, "Lane's Physiology" and Omega, "Lane's Anatomy and Physiology." However, even in the South, where these ideas were especially powerful and pervasive, there is evidence that some schools had incorporated anatomy and physiology into their curricula for women by the late 1850s. See, for example, Christie Farnham Pope, "Preparation for Pedestals: North Carolina Antebellum Female Seminaries" (unpublished Ph.D. dissertation, University of Chicago, 1977), pp. 140–70.

117. John B. Blake, "Anatomy," in Ronald L. Numbers, ed., *The Education of American Physicians: Historical Essays* (Berkeley and Los Angeles: University of California Press, 1980), pp. 29–47.

118. For information on general health reform, consult notes for the previous chapter. Good summaries of the mid-century exercise and dress crusades are: Harvey Green, *Fit for America: Health, Fitness, Sport, and American Society* (New York: Pantheon Books, 1986), pp. 77–100; and Whorton, *Crusaders*, pp. 92–131, 270–303. On changing concepts of health, see Verbrugge, *Able-Bodied Womanhood*, and Bruce Haley, *The Healthy Body and Victorian Culture* (Cambridge: Harvard University Press, 1978).

119. Quoted in Whorton, *Crusaders*, p. 272.

120. Edward Everett Hale, *A New England Boyhood and Other Bits of Autobiography* (Boston: Little, Brown, and Co., 1905), pp. 29–31, 40–42.

121. Edward Warren, *The Life of John Collins Warren, M.D.*, 2 vols. (Boston: Ticknor and Fields, 1860), vol. 1, pp. 223–26.

122. Whorton, *Crusaders*, pp. 270–303.

123. Edward Hitchcock, *Reminiscences of Amherst College, Historical, Scientific, Biographical, and Autobiographical: Also, of Other and Wider Life Experiences* (Northampton, Mass.: Bridgman and Childs, 1863), pp. 293–94; George F. Whicher, ed., *Remembrance of Amherst: An Undergraduate's Diary, 1846–1848* (New York: Columbia University Press, 1946), p. 192.

124. Young woman quoted in Elizabeth Alden Green, *Mary Lyon and Mount Holyoke: Opening the Gates* (Hanover, N.H.: University Press of New England, 1979), pp. 239–40; Whicher, ed., *Diary*, p. 142.

125. Ernest Earnest, *The American Eve in Fact and Fiction, 1775–1914* (Urbana: University of Illinois Press, 1974), pp. 90–92; Elizabeth A. Green, *Mary Lyon and Mount Holyoke*, pp. 64–65, 220–40; and Barbara Miller Solomon, *In the Company of Educated Women: A History of Women and Higher Education in America* (New Haven and London: Yale University Press, 1985), pp. 14–42.

126. Earnest, *American Eve*, pp. 93–98. The *Godey's* references are as follows: for Griscom, 19(July–December 1839): 192; for Coates, 22(January–June 1841): 190 and 24(January–June 1842): 239; for Hayward, 27(July–December 1843): 286–88.

6. The Unorthodox Physician

1. The most comprehensive study of homeopathy is Martin Kaufman, *Homeopathy in America: The Rise and Fall of a Medical Heresy* (Baltimore: Johns Hopkins University Press, 1971). A useful summary is Ronald L. Numbers, "Do-It-Yourself the Sectarian Way," in Guenter B. Risse, Ronald L. Numbers, and Judith Walzer Leavitt, eds., *Medicine Without Doctors: Home Health Care in American History* (New York: Science History Publications, 1977), pp. 58–62. Two other helpful discussions are William G. Rothstein, *American Physicians in the Nineteenth Century: From Sects to Science* (Baltimore: Johns Hopkins University Press, 1972); and Joseph F. Kett, *The Formation of the American Medical Profession: The Role of Institutions, 1780–1860* (New Haven: Yale University Press, 1968).

2. Until very recently, the only full-length study of hydropathy was Harry B. Weiss and Howard R. Kemble, *The Great American Water Cure Craze: A History of Hydropathy in America* (Trenton, N.J.: Past Times Press, 1967). This has now been supplemented by two substantial works, both of which focus on hydropathy's appeal to and impact on women: Susan E. Cayleff, *Wash and Be Healed: The Water-Cure Movement and Women's Health* (Philadelphia: Temple University Press, 1987); and Jane B. Donegan, *"Hydropathic Highway to Health": Women and Water-Cure in Antebellum America* (Westport, Conn.: Greenwood Press, 1986). Brief accounts are in Numbers, "Do-It-Yourself," pp. 62–68; Marshall Scott Kegan, "Hydropathy in America: A Nineteenth Century Panacea," *BHM* 45(1971): 267–80; and Kathryn Kish Sklar, "'All Hail to Pure Cold Water!'" *American Heritage* 26(December 1974): 64–69, 100–101. Sklar also describes one woman's water-cure experiences in *Catharine Beecher: A Study in American Domesticity* (New York: W. W. Norton and Co., 1973).

3. Though Rothstein's previously cited book is not the most representative of current scholarship, his title sums up the prevalent orientation: *American Physicians in the Nineteenth Century: From Sects to Science.*

4. Each of the most recent studies of hydropathy makes this general point in different ways, but neither elaborates on the meaning. In her synopsis of health-reform history, Cayleff highlights commonalities rather than divergences (*Wash and Be Healed*, pp. 11–16). Donegan asserts that scholarship is making it increasingly clear that regulars and sectarians embraced doctrines that "were not substantially at variance" (*"Hydropathic Highway to Health,"* pp. xii, xviin.8).

5. Cayleff discusses this point most clearly and at greatest length in *Wash and Be Healed*, pp. 44–74.

6. Allan Nevins and Milton Halsey Thomas, eds., *The Diary of George Templeton Strong*, 4 vols. (New York: Macmillan Co., 1952). Quotes are from vol. 1, pp. 238–39. Pike's establishment is not more precisely identified.

7. Ibid., vol. 1, p. 257 (16 March 1845).

8. Ibid., vol. 1, pp. 257 (16–23 March 1845), 261 (22 March 1845).

9. Ibid., vol. 1, p. 305 (26 October 1847).

10. Ibid., vol. 2, p. 289.

11. Edward C. Atwater, "The Lifelong Sickness of Francis Parkman (1823–93)," *BHM* 41(1967): 413–39, quote on p. 429.

12. Joanna L. Stratton, *Pioneer Women: Voices from the Kansas Frontier* (New York: Simon and Schuster, 1981), p. 73.

13. Curtis Carroll Davis, ed., "Chronicler of the Cavaliers: Some Letters from and to William Alexander Caruthers, M.D. (1802–1846)," *Virginia Magazine of History and Biography* 55(July 1947): 213–32. All of the quotes from Caruthers's letter are on pp. 227–29 (10 May 1846).
14. Ibid., p. 232 (18 May 1846).
15. "Law and Medicine," *Western Lancet* 2(1843): 47–48; all quotes in this paragraph are on p. 48.
16. "Empiricism: Quackery," *Western Lancet* 7(1848): 52–53; quotes on p. 53.
17. Worthington Hooker, *Physician and Patient; or, A Practical View of the Mutual Duties, Relations and Interests of the Medical Profession and the Community* (New York: Baker and Scribner, 1849), p. 55.
18. Dan King, *Quackery Unmasked: Or, a Consideration of the Most Prominent Empirical Schemes of the Present Time, With an Enumeration of Some of the Causes Which Contribute to Their Support* (Boston: Printed by David Clapp, 1858), t.p.
19. For discussion of this subject, see, for example, John Harley Warner, " 'The Nature-Trusting Heresy': American Physicians and the Concept of the Healing Power of Nature in the 1850's and 1860's," *Perspectives in American History* 11(1977–78): 289–324.
20. King, *Quackery Unmasked*, p. 120.
21. H, review of Samuel Henry Dickson's "A Lecture, Introductory to the Course on the Theory and Practice of Medicine, in the University of New York. Session 1847–1848," *Western Lancet* 7(1848): 153–57; quotes on p. 154.
22. Ibid., pp. 156–57.
23. Hooker, *Physician and Patient*, pp. 177–78.
24. See sources listed in note 2 of this chapter.
25. For these estimates, see Weiss and Kemble, *Water Cure Craze*, esp. pp. 24–41.
26. Sklar, *Beecher*, pp. 207–209; Cayleff, *Wash and Be Healed*, pp. 75–108. On hydropathy's appeal to men, see Donegan, *"Hydropathic Highway to Health,"* p. xv; and Ronald L. Numbers, *Prophetess of Health: A Study of Ellen G. White* (New York: Harper and Row, 1976), p. 228. Hydropaths wrote a great deal about pregnancy and childbirth. See, for instance, Joel Shew, *The Water-Cure in Pregnancy and Childbirth. Illustrated with Cases, Showing the Remarkable Effects of Water in Mitigating the Pains and Perils of the Parturient State*, stereotype ed. (New York: Fowlers and Wells, 1850). An example of a woman who praised hydropathy's effects after the birth of her third child is related in Claudia L. Bushman, *"A Good Poor Man's Wife": Being a Chronicle of Harriet Hanson Robinson and Her Family in Nineteenth-Century New England* (Hanover, N.H.: University Press of New England, 1981), p. 90.
27. Quoted in Numbers, "Do-It-Yourself," p. 64. The same kind of material was collected in books, such as *The Water Cure in America: Two Hundred and Twenty Cases of Various Diseases Treated with Water, by Drs. Wesselhoeft, Shew, Bedortha, Shieferdecker, and Others; with Cases of Domestic Practice; Notices of the Water Cure Establishments; Descriptive Catalogue of Hydropathic Publications, etc. Designed for Popular as well as Professional Reading. Edited by a Water Patient* (New York and London: Wiley and Putnam, 1848). The New York phrenological publishing house, Fowlers and Wells, produced an enlarged edition of the volume in 1852.
28. Numbers, "Do-It-Yourself," p. 67. On Austin, Jackson, and their work, see

Donegan, *"Hydropathic Highway to Health,"* pp. 54–59; and Numbers, *Prophetess of Health,* pp. 72–101, 202–207.

29. Weiss and Kemble, *Water Cure Craze,* p. 33; Donegan, *"Hydropathic Highway to Health,"* pp. 169–77; Cayleff, *Wash and Be Healed,* pp. 100–102.

30. Cayleff, *Wash and Be Healed,* pp. 100–102; Weiss and Kemble, *Water Cure Craze,* p. 38.

31. Though our perspectives are quite different, Cayleff's discussion of these issues is provocative: *Wash and Be Healed,* pp. 15–53 and passim.

32. Weiss and Kemble, *Water Cure Craze,* p. 69; Madeleine B. Stern, *Heads and Headliners: The Phrenological Fowlers* (Norman: University of Oklahoma Press, 1971), p. 51.

33. I have used Joel Shew, *Hydropathy; or, The Water-Cure: Its Principles, Processes, and Modes of Treatment. Compiled in Part from the Most Eminent Authors, Ancient and Modern, on the Subject. Together with an Account of the Latest Methods Adopted by Priessnitz. Illustrated by Numerous Cases of Cure* (New York: J. Wiley, 1849); and Joel Shew, *Hand-Book of Hydropathy: Or, A Popular Account of the Treatment and Prevention of Diseases, by Means of Water* (New York: Wiley and Putnam, 1844). Quotes are from *Hand-Book of Hydropathy,* p. iv. For publishing information, see *NUC* 543: 533–36.

34. Shew, *Hydropathy,* pp. [iii]–viii; quotes in this paragraph and the next are from p. iv. A convenient summary of the tractoration craze is Kett, *American Medical Profession,* pp. 97–99. See also Shew, *Hand-Book of Hydropathy,* pp. v–vi.

35. Quotes in this paragraph and the next are from Shew, *Hydropathy,* pp. 65–69.

36. Ibid., pp. ix–x.

37. I have used Joel Shew, *The Water-Cure Manual: A Popular Work, Embracing Descriptions of the Various Modes of Bathing, the Hygienic and Curative Effects of Air, Exercise, Clothing, Occupation, Diet, Water-Drinking, etc. Together with Descriptions of Diseases, and the Hydropathic Means To Be Employed Therein. Illustrated with Cases of Treatment and Cure. Containing, Also, a Fine Engraving of Priessnitz,* ninth thousand, improved (New York: Fowlers and Wells, 1849). Quotes in this paragraph and the next two are from pp. 12–18.

38. Cayleff notes the paradoxical nature of the hydropathic doctor-patient relationship. As she points out, water-cure rhetoric encouraged patients to achieve medical independence and self-sufficiency, but they were also advised to look to physicians for advice and inspiration (*Wash and Be Healed,* pp. 52–53).

39. Shew, *Water-Cure Manual,* pp. 258, 97, 136–38.

40. Joel Shew, *The Hydropathic Family Physician, A Ready Prescriber and Hygienic Adviser. With Reference to the Nature, Causes, Prevention, and Treatment of Diseases, Accidents, and Casualties of Every Kind,* illustrated with nearly 300 engravings (New York: Fowlers and Wells, 1854), pp. [iii], [9].

41. Russell Trall went well beyond Shew in this area; he devoted nearly half of his thousand-page *Hydropathic Encyclopedia* to these subjects, a level of detail probably better suited to the doctors and students among his readers than the average citizen. See R[ussell] T. Trall, *The Hydropathic Encyclopedia: A System of Hydropathy and Hygiene. In Eight Parts: I. Outlines of Anatomy, Illustrated. II. Physiology of the Human Body. III. Hygienic Agencies, and the Preservation of Health. IV. Dietetics and Hydropathic Cookery. V. Theory and Practice of Water*

Treatment. VI. Special Pathology and Hydro-Therapeutics, Including the Nature, Causes, Symptoms, and Treatment of All Known Diseases. VII. Application to Surgical Diseases. VIII. Application of Hydropathy to Midwifery and the Nursery. Designed as a Guide to Families and Students, and a Text-book for Physicians, with numerous engraved illustrations, 2 vols. (New York: Fowlers and Wells, 1851–52), vol. 1. For publishing information, see *NUC* 599: 591–95.

42. Shew, *Hydropathic Family Physician;* quotes in this paragraph and the next are from pp. 42–43.

43. Ibid., pp. 30–43, 402. Shew reiterated these points in *Children, Their Hydropathic Management in Health and Disease* (New York: Fowler and Wells, 1857), pp. 290–99.

44. Quotes in this paragraph and the next are from Shew, *Hydropathic Family Physician,* pp. 45, 122–23, 396.

45. Ibid., pp. 403, 464–66 (scarlet fever).

46. Ibid., pp. 403–404. Three years later Shew was still denouncing laryngotomies: *Children,* pp. 298–99.

47. Shew, *Hydropathic Family Physician,* pp. 522, 455. Shew had a strong interest in consumption and devoted an entire volume to it: *Consumption: Its Prevention and Cure by the Water Treatment, With Advice Concerning Haemorrhage from the Lungs, Coughs, Colds, Asthma, Bronchitis, and Sore Throat* (New York: Fowlers and Wells, 1850).

48. Shew, *Hydropathic Family Physician,* p. 690.

49. Estimates about female practitioners are from Numbers, "Do-It-Yourself," p. 64. See also Cayleff, *Wash and Be Healed,* pp. 68–74.

50. Mary S. Gove Nichols tells the story of her life in *Experience in Water-Cure: A Familiar Exposition of the Principles and Results of Water Treatment, in the Cure of Acute and Chronic Diseases, Illustrated by Numerous Cases in the Practice of the Author; With an Explanation of Water-Cure Processes, Advice on Diet and Regimen, and Particular Directions to Women in the Treatment of Female Disease, Water Treatment in Childbirth, and the Diseases of Infancy,* stereotype ed. (New York: Fowlers and Wells, 1852). For additional biographical information I have relied especially on John Blake, "Mary Gove Nichols, Prophetess of Health," in Judith Walzer Leavitt, ed., *Women and Health in America: Historical Readings* (Madison: University of Wisconsin Press, 1984), pp. 359–75. Blake offers a brief account in Edward T. James et al., eds., *Notable American Women: A Biographical Dictionary,* 3 vols. (Cambridge: Belknap Press of Harvard University Press, 1971), at vol. 2, pp. 627–29. For publishing information, see *NUC* 418: 193–94.

51. Mary S. Gove, *Lectures to Ladies on Anatomy and Physiology* (Boston: Saxton and Peirce, 1842), p. [iii]; Blake, "Prophetess of Health," p. 359.

52. Gove, *Lectures to Ladies,* p. iv.

53. Ibid., p. iv.

54. In addition to Blake, "Prophetess of Health," see Hillel Schwartz, *Never Satisfied: A Cultural History of Diets, Fantasies and Fat* (New York: Free Press, 1986), pp. 47–65.

55. Gove's book is cited above. The brief notice of it appeared in "Lectures to Ladies on Anatomy and Physiology, by Mary S. Gove," *BMSJ* 25(August 1841–February 1842): 374.

56. "Lectures to Ladies on Anatomy and Physiology," *BMSJ* 26(February–August 1842): 97–98.

57. Gove Nichols, *Experience in Water-Cure,* pp. 24–29; Gove, *Lectures to Ladies,* pp. [9]–11, 18, 57.

58. Gove Nichols, *Experience in Water-Cure,* pp. 17–21; Cayleff, *Wash and Be Healed,* pp. 49–74; Regina Morantz-Sanchez, *Sympathy and Science: Women Physicians in American Medicine* (New York: Oxford University Press, 1987 [1985]), pp. 28–46.

59. Mary S. Gove, *Lectures to Women on Anatomy and Physiology. With an Appendix on Water-Cure* (New York: Harper and Brothers, 1846), pp. [iii]–iv, 245.

60. Ibid., pp. 274, 242, 239, 289. In *Experience in Water-Cure,* however, she emphasized that water-cure, if "skilfully directed," would nearly always cure (pp. 7–12).

61. Quotes are from Gove, *Lectures to Women,* p. 275. One clear expression of her stance on lay versus professional healers is in Gove Nichols, *Experience in Water-Cure,* pp. [v]–[vi]. See also Cayleff's discussion of this point in *Wash and Be Healed,* pp. 52–53.

62. Gove, *Lectures to Women,* pp. 257–58, 263. She reiterates these sentiments in *Experience in Water-Cure,* pp. 60–79.

63. M[arie] L[ouise] Shew, *Water-Cure for Ladies; A Popular Work on the Health, Diet, and Regimen of Females and Children, and the Prevention and Cure of Diseases, With a Full Account of the Processes of Water-Cure; Illustrated with Various Cases. Revised by Joel Shew, M.D.* (New York: Wiley and Putnam, 1844), pp. [iii], 29–30, vi. For publishing information, see *NUC* 543: 536–37.

64. M. L. Shew, *Water-Cure for Ladies,* pp. 20–21.

65. Ibid., pp. 25–28, iv, 21–22, 15.

66. Historians have largely neglected the study of private preventive medicine. For an excellent representative sample of the existing literature, see Judith Walzer Leavitt and Ronald L. Numbers, eds., *Sickness and Health in America: Readings in the History of Medicine and Public Health* (Madison: University of Wisconsin Press, 1978) and the revised edition of the same title, published in 1985.

67. Sally Gregory Kohlstedt, "Physiological Lectures for Women: Sarah Coates in Ohio, 1850," *JHMAS* 33(1978): 75–81; all quotes are from p. 79.

68. This information has been culled from the biographical entries in James et al., eds., *Notable American Women:* vol. 1, pp. 444–45 (Davis); vol. 2, pp. 285–86 (Jones); and vol. 1, pp. 654–55 (Fowler). On Fowler, see also Madeleine B. Stern, "Lydia Folger Fowler, M.D.: First American Woman Professor of Medicine," *New York State Journal of Medicine* 77(June 1977): 1137–40.

69. Mary Roth Walsh emphasizes Hunt's historical importance in *"Doctors Wanted. No Women Need Apply": Sexual Barriers in the Medical Profession* (New Haven: Yale University Press, 1978).

70. Harriot K. Hunt, *Glances and Glimpses; Or Fifty Years Social, Including Twenty Years Professional Life* (Boston: John P. Jewett and Co., etc., 1856; reprint ed., New York: Source Book Press, 1970). Unless otherwise noted, her comments about this experience are drawn from pp. 81–88. The entry in James et al., eds., *Notable American Women,* consists almost entirely of excerpts from this work: vol. 2, pp. 235–37.

71. The seton—a thread, horsehair, piece of lint, or some other foreign matter—worked much like a blister. Placed on an open wound or a surgical incision, it

promoted infection and produced "laudable pus," which orthodox physicians thought a certain sign of healing.

72. Hunt, *Glances and Glimpses,* pp. 110–15.
73. Ibid., pp. 120–27, 171–72.
74. Ibid., pp. 140–44.
75. Ibid., pp. 156–57.
76. Ibid., pp. 86–91.
77. Ibid., pp. 88–89.
78. Ibid., pp. 151–56, 170–71.
79. Ibid., pp. 192–93.
80. Ibid., pp. 175, 185, 407.
81. For sources on homeopathy, see the first note of this chapter.
82. Estimates of homeopathic strength are drawn from Kett, *American Medical Profession,* pp. 137–39, and Numbers, "Do-It-Yourself," p. 58.
83. Oliver Wendell Holmes, "Some More Recent Views on Homoeopathy," *Atlantic Monthly* 1(December 1857): 187. The other quote is cited in Numbers, "Do-It-Yourself," p. 58.
84. Constantin Hering, *The Homoeopathist, or Domestic Physician. Two Parts* (Philadelphia: J. G. Wesselhoeft, 1835, 1838). I have also used: [Constantin Hering], *C. Hering's Domestic Physician. Third American Edition, Comprising the Former Edition of the Homoeopathist, or Domestic Physician, Revised, with Additions from the Author's Manuscript of the Fifth German Edition, Together with the Additions of Drs Goullon, Gross, and Stapf, To Which Is Added a Chapter on the Diseases of Women* (Philadelphia: For sale at C. L. Rademacher's Homoeopathic Book and Medicine Store, 1845). For publishing information, see *NUC* 242: 106–109.
85. Hering, *The Homoeopathist,* part 1, pp. 2–3; part 2, p. 241; and Constantin Hering, *The Homoeopathic Domestic Physician,* 7th Am. ed. (Philadelphia: F. E. Boericke, Hahnemann Publishing House, 1883), p. 15. For similar phrasing, see also Hering, *C. Hering's Domestic Physician,* pp. [vi]–vii. Edward C. Chepmell's title encapsulates the idea: *A Domestic Homoeopathy, Restricted to Its Legitimate Sphere of Practice; Together with Rules for Diet and Regimen,* 1st Am. ed. with additions and improvements, by Samuel B. Barlow (New York: William Radde, 1849), pp. 50–51, 179–80.
86. Quotes are from Hering, *Homoeopathic Domestic Physician,* pp. 15–31. Except for the instructions on diagnosis, the wording is very similar to that used in Hering, *C. Hering's Domestic Physician,* pp. [vi]–viii.
87. Egbert Guernsey, *The Gentleman's Hand-Book of Homoeopathy; Especially for Travelers, and for Domestic Practice* (Boston: Otis Clapp; New York: William Radde, 1855), p. v; Egbert Guernsey, *Homoeopathic Domestic Practice, Containing Also Chapters on Anatomy, Physiology, Hygiene, and an Abridged Materia Medica* (New York: William Radde, 1853), p. [iii]. For publishing information, see *NUC* 222: 19–22.
88. Guernsey, *Homoeopathic Domestic Practice,* pp. [iii]–v.
89. George E. Shipman, *The Homoeopathic Family Guide, For the Use of Twenty-Five Principal Remedies in the Treatment of the More Simple Forms of Disease. Together with Directions for the Treatment of Dengue and Yellow Fever, by W. H. Holcombe, M.D.,* 2nd ed. (Chicago: C. S. Halsey, 1865), pp. ix, 32–38, 72–77. At least one author showed no concern about lay treatment, perhaps because he addressed his book to students, doctors, and families: M. Freligh, *Homoeopathic*

Practice of Medicine: Embracing the History, Diagnosis and Treatment of Diseases in General, Including Those Peculiar to Females: and the Management of Children. Designed as a Text-book for the Student, as a Concise Book of Reference for the Profession, and Simplified and Arranged for Domestic Use, new ed., rev. and enl. (New York: Sheldon, Lamport and Blakeman, etc., 1855). For publishing information, see *NUC* 544: 114–15 (Shipman).

90. J[oseph] H[ipplyt] Pulte, *Homoeopathic Domestic Physician; Containing the Treatment of Diseases; with Popular Explanations of Anatomy, Physiology, Hygiene and Hydropathy: Also an Abridged Materia Medica,* enl. with special hydropathic directions, and illustrated with anatomical plates, eighth thousand (Cincinnati: Moore and Anderson, etc., 1852), p. [v]; J[oseph] H[ipplyt] Pulte, *Homoeopathic Domestic Physician; Containing the Treatment of Diseases; with Popular Explanations of Anatomy, Physiology, Hygiene and Hydropathy: Also an Abridged Materia Medica. With Important Additions, Especially in Surgery and the Diseases of Women and Children,* illustrated in anatomy and surgery, 7th ed., enl. and rev., twenty-seventh thousand (Cincinnati: Moore, Wilstach, Keys and Co., etc., 1859), p. vi. It was especially important, argued Pulte, that women, the primary victims of prevailing canons of propriety, be provided with the means to diagnose and treat themselves: *Woman's Medical Guide; Containing Essays on the Physical, Moral and Educational Development of Females, and the Homoeopathic Treatment of Their Diseases in All Periods of Life, Together with Directions for the Remedial Use of Water and Gymnastics,* 2nd ed., rev. (Cincinnati: Moore, Wilstach, Keys and Co., 1859), pp. [iv], [xiii]–xviii. For publishing information, see *NUC* 475: 298–99.

91. Quoted in Numbers, "Do-It-Yourself," p. 61.

92. Hering, *The Homoeopathist,* part 1, p. 7; John Epps, *Domestic Homoeopathy: Or Rules for the Domestic Treatment of the Maladies of Infants, Children, and Adults, And for the Conduct and the Treatment During Pregnancy, Confinement, and Suckling,* 3rd Am. from the 4th London ed., edited and enl. by George W. Cook, M.D. (Boston: Otis Clapp, etc., 1849), p. 8; Holmes, "Recent Views," p. 187. For biographical and bibliographical information about Epps, see *DNB* 6: 800–801; and *NUC* 161: 28–29.

93. Carol Bleser, ed., *The Hammonds of Redcliffe* (New York: Oxford University Press, 1981), pp. 101–102; Drew Gilpin Faust, *James Henry Hammond and the Old South: A Design for Mastery* (Baton Rouge: Louisiana State University Press, 1982), pp. 76–83. George Templeton Strong's remarks, cited earlier in this chapter, are also eloquent testimony to the perceived safety of homeopathic remedies.

94. Gayle Thornbrough et al., eds., *The Diary of Calvin Fletcher,* 6 vols. (Indianapolis: Indiana Historical Society, 1972–78), vol. 6, pp. 46–50 (9–18 April 1857).

95. Numbers, "Do-It-Yourself," p. 61.

96. King, *Quackery Unmasked,* pp. 112–78, esp. pp. 132–33.

97. Hooker, *Physician and Patient,* p. 145.

98. Kett, *American Medical Profession,* pp. 185–86; Paul Starr, *The Social Transformation of American Medicine* (New York: Basic Books, 1982), p. 99. See also Rothstein, *American Physicians,* pp. 234–36.

99. One example is osteopathy: Norman Gevitz, *The D.O.'s: Osteopathic Medicine in America* (Baltimore: Johns Hopkins University Press, 1982).

100. Starr, *Social Transformation*, p. 135; Rothstein, *American Physicians*, p. 266.
101. Quoted in Starr, *Social Transformation*, p. 141.
102. See, for example, Thomas McKeown, *The Modern Rise of Population* (New York: Academic Press, 1976). The provision of modern services was also extremely important, as highlighted in Jean-Pierre Goubert, *The Conquest of Water: The Advent of Health in the Industrial Age* (Princeton: Princeton University Press, 1986), and Ann Durkin Keating, *Building Chicago: Suburban Developers and the Creation of a Divided Metropolis* (Columbus: Ohio State University Press, 1988).
103. René DuBois, "Introduction," in Norman Cousins, *Anatomy of an Illness as Perceived by the Patient: Reflections on Healing and Regeneration* (New York: Bantam Books, 1981 [1979]), p. 11.
104. Cousins, *Anatomy of an Illness*, p. 48.
105. John C. Burnham has drawn more pessimistic conclusions about the long-term impact of the health popularization efforts begun in the mid-eighteenth century in his *How Superstition Won and Science Lost: Popularizing Science and Health in the United States* (New Brunswick and London: Rutgers University Press, 1987).

Bibliographic Essay: A Note on Sources and Method

Primary Sources

This study draws on a range of late eighteenth- and nineteenth-century sources: popular periodical literature; autobiographies, letters, and diaries of physicians and lay people, both male and female; and medical journals. However, it relies most heavily on the advice literature that appeared during the same period; much of it ephemeral and most of it now obscure, its selection depended on occasional serendipitous discovery but primarily on diligent, creative searching.

The most important criterion in choosing books for this project was that their principal aim be to impart systematically arranged information about the management of health and disease. This operational definition quickly excluded several types of literature that conveyed treatment information in a more random or subsidiary fashion: almanacs (though the existence of health almanacs should be noted); patent medicine circulars and advertisements; cookbooks; and beauty books. Two other categories have been purposely omitted. The first, phrenological books, have been excluded because, like the health guides discussed in the concluding section of chapter 4, they sought mainly to inculcate general principles of good living. Concerned more with the practical affairs of life, they seldom directly addressed questions of disease management. The other genre of health advice that is not represented in this study is sexual hygiene literature. Though there was a proliferation of written sexual advice during the antebellum period, much of it, as scholars have noted, remained semi-licit, unlike the popular literature here discussed. Equally important, sexual advice—except as related to pregnancy, childbirth, and occasionally conception—remained beyond the scope of the domestic health guide, whatever its sectarian origin.

Because medical advice literature remains largely untapped by researchers, locating the publications required both ingenuity and luck. The first step in this task was to comb secondary literature for any mention of household guides. This process yielded roughly two-thirds of the material included here. That list was supplemented by reading library shelf lists, bibliographic checklists, and published catalogs of other collections. The existence of a large number of these works in the general, science, and rare collections of the University of Chicago Library was enormously beneficial. Also helpful were contemporary medical journal notices, diaries and letters, and publishers' advertisements found in books, magazines, and newspapers. The goal has been to make the search as exhaustive as possible, and the resulting body of materials probably represents roughly seventy-five to ninety percent of the total pool.

Book classification normally presented no problems, since eighteenth- and nineteenth-century medical authors displayed a useful penchant for clearly identifying their works with particular genres. Thus a household or domestic health guide is a volume intended for general family use that presents comprehensive information on disease causation and treatment, often boasting a materia medica section as well. Frequently, they also contain discussions of women's diseases, which include pregnancy, childbirth, and children's complaints. However, only those volumes weighted toward the afflictions of women and children, almost always so billed, are treated in this study as "maternal physicians." Homeopathic and hydropathic authors without exception identify their works with their respective sects. Thomsonians sometimes did not, but the therapeutic advice they gave unequivocally signaled their affiliations. On the other hand, some authors— John Gunn is a good example—not only recommend remedies drawn from different therapeutic traditions, but also fail to associate themselves with any particular one. In those rare cases, classification has proceeded according to the therapeutic emphasis, which is usually, as in the case of Gunn, fairly distinct. Finally, this study also examines schoolbooks on anatomy, physiology, and hygiene. Gathering these titles proved to be more difficult than anticipated, since scholars have largely ignored the subject. Moreover, Helen Barton's frequently cited 1944 dissertation is a poor guide to the textbook literature, because her criteria for inclusion are unreliable and arbitrary. The books themselves, once located through secondary literature and contemporary popular and medical periodicals, are straightforwardly promoted as textbooks; all display increasingly sophisticated efforts to convey information about anatomy, physiology, and hygiene.

Secondary Sources

Before the 1960s historians of American medicine concentrated on documenting advances in medical knowledge, which, they argued, hastened medical professionalization and encouraged expanded public health responsibilities. Downplaying social and cultural factors, they emphasized instead biographical, institutional, and intellectual elements in medical development. Many of the resulting studies were infused with a misleading sense of straightforward progress from an unenlightened, misguided past to a rational, scientific present and future. Three historiographical essays discuss this point from different perspectives: Gerald Grob, "The Social History of Medicine and Disease in America: Problems and Possibilities," *J. Soc. Hist.* 10(1977): 391–409; Charles E. Rosenberg, "The Medical Profession, Medical Practice, and the History of Medicine," in Edwin Clarke, ed., *Modern Methods in the History of Medicine* (London: Althone Press, 1971), 22–35; and Ronald L. Numbers, "The History of American Medicine: A Field in Ferment," *Reviews in American History* 10(1982): 245–63.

The scholarship of the past three decades has followed a different path, highlighting the fact that the "triumph of scientific medicine" was not a foreordained conclusion. This revisionist literature has stressed the extent to which nonmedical factors have influenced both medical developments and life expectancy. Richard H. Shryock was the pioneer here, and at least two of his books remain standard, if somewhat outmoded, references: *The Development of Modern Medicine: An Interpretation of the Social and Scientific Factors Involved* (New York: Alfred A. Knopf, 1947); and *Medicine and Society in America, 1660–1860* (New York: New York University Press, 1960). Several of Shryock's medically trained contemporaries expressed similar themes, among them George Rosen, Edwin Ackerknecht, Owsei Temkin, and Henry Sigerist.

Building on this legacy, many researchers have broadened the study of medical history. Good overviews include Joseph Kett, *The Formation of the American Medical Profession: The Role of Institutions, 1780–1860* (New Haven: Yale University Press, 1968); William G. Rothstein, *American Physicians in the Nineteenth Century: From Sects to Science* (Baltimore: Johns Hopkins University Press, 1972); Martin Kaufman, *American Medical Education: The Formative Years, 1765–1910* (Westport, Conn.: Greenwood Press, 1976); Paul Starr, *The Social Transformation of American Medicine* (New York: Basic Books, 1982); Martin S. Pernick, *A Calculus of Suffering: Pain, Professionalism, and Anesthesia in Nineteenth-Century America* (New York: Columbia University Press, 1985); Charles E. Rosenberg, *The Cholera Years: The United States in 1832, 1849, and 1866,* Phoenix paperback ed. (Chicago: University of Chicago Press, 1962); and Charles E. Rosenberg, "The Therapeutic Revolution: Medicine, Meaning, and Social Change in Nineteenth-Century America," in Morris J. Vogel and Charles E. Rosenberg, eds., *The Therapeutic Revolution: Essays in the Social History of American Medicine* (Philadelphia: University of Pennsylvania Press, 1979), 3–25. Two excellent essay collections exemplify current trends in the writing of medical history: Judith Walzer Leavitt and Ronald L. Numbers, eds., *Sickness and Health in America: Readings in the History of Medicine and Public Health* (Madison: University of Wisconsin Press, 1978), and the second, revised edition that appeared in 1985; and Judith Walzer Leavitt, ed., *Women and Health in America* (Madison: University of Wisconsin Press, 1984).

Of course, many older studies are also indispensable aids. The medical histories of particular states or cities are often filled with valuable information. Among the most useful for this study were: Eugene F. Cordell, *The Medical Annals of Maryland, 1799–1899* (Baltimore: Press of Williams and Wilkins Co., 1903); John R. Quinan, *Medical Annals of Baltimore. From 1608 to 1880, Including Events, Men and Literature* (Baltimore: Press of Isaac Friedenwald, 1884); and two books by Wyndham B. Blanton, *Medicine in Virginia in the Eighteenth Century* (Richmond: Garrett and Massie, 1931) and *Medicine in Virginia in the Nineteenth Century* (Richmond: Garrett and Massie, 1933).

Institutional histories were less helpful, but published biographies, autobiographies, and diaries should not be overlooked. The most valuable for this project were Whitfield J. Bell, Jr., *John Morgan, Continental Doctor* (Philadelphia: University of Pennsylvania Press, 1965); Cecil K. Drinker, *Not So Long Ago: A Chronicle of Medicine and Doctors in Colonial Philadelphia* (New York: Oxford University Press, 1937); and Jack P. Greene, ed., *The Diary of Colonel Landon Carter of Sabine Hall, 1752–1778,* 2 vols. (Charlottesville: Published for the Virginia Historical Society by the University Press of Virginia, 1965). Epidemics were a near-constant trial to our forebears, but few histories match the caliber of Rosenberg's work on cholera. John Duffy's *Sword of Pestilence: The New Orleans Yellow Fever Epidemic of 1853* (Baton Rouge: Louisiana State University Press, 1966) is disappointing; John H. Powell, on the other hand, paints an evocative picture in his *Bring Out Your Dead: The Great Plague of Yellow Fever in Philadelphia in 1793* (Philadelphia: University of Pennsylvania Press, 1949).

The history of public and private disease management reveals a great deal about changing concepts of public health and hygiene. Among the most useful references on these subjects are: James H. Cassedy, *Demography in Early America: The Beginnings of the Statistical Mind, 1600–1800* (Cambridge: Harvard University Press, 1969); James H. Cassedy, *Charles V. Chapin and the Public Health Movement* (Cambridge: Harvard University Press, 1962); Judith Walzer Leavitt, *The Healthiest City: Milwaukee and the Politics of Health Reform* (Princeton: Princeton University Press, 1982); Barbara Gutmann Rosenkrantz, *Public Health and the State: Changing Views in Massachusetts, 1842–1936* (Cambridge: Harvard University Press, 1972); Carroll Smith-Rosenberg and Charles E. Rosenberg, "Pietism and the Origins of the American Public Health Movement: A Note on John H. Griscom and Robert M. Hartley," *JHMAS* 23(1968): 16–35; Thomas McKeown, *The Modern Rise of Population* (New York: Academic Press, 1976); and John Duffy, *Epidemics in Colonial America* (Baton Rouge: Louisiana State University Press, 1959). The history of urban services is also pertinent, as demonstrated in Jean-Pierre Goubert, *The Conquest of Water: The Advent of Health in the Industrial Age* (Princeton: Princeton University Press, 1986); Ann Durkin Keating, *Building Chicago: Suburban Developers and the Creation of a Divided Metropolis* (Columbus: Ohio State University Press, 1988); and Nelson Blake, *Water for the Cities* (Syracuse: Syracuse University Press, 1956).

Colonial medicine cannot be understood without reference to the Old World context, and Lester S. King provides a detailed introduction in *The Medical World of the Eighteenth Century* (Chicago: University of Chicago Press, 1958). Whitfield J. Bell, Jr., has written a great deal about colonial medical practices, much of which is reprinted in *The Colonial Physician & Other Essays* (New York: Science History Publications, 1975). Bell's work should be supplemented by the fine essays in Philip Cash, Eric H. Christianson, and J. Worth Estes, eds., *Medicine in Colonial Massachusetts, 1620–1820*, vol. 57 of the *Publications* of The Colonial Society of Massachusetts (Boston: The Colonial Society of Massachusetts, 1980). For a comparative perspective, see Ronald L. Numbers, ed., *Medicine in the New World: New Spain, New France, and New England* (Knoxville: University of Tennessee Press, 1987).

Until very recently, medical historians focused primarily on the doctor's role in providing health care. The research focus is now shifting to include the patient, his or her caregivers, and other participants. Judith Walzer Leavitt stresses the central importance of lay women in the development of obstetrics and gynecology in *Brought to Bed: Childbearing in America, 1750 to 1950* (New York: Oxford University Press, 1986). In *Alice James: A Biography* (Boston: Houghton Mifflin, 1980), Jean Strouse does justice to the nuances of the invalid-doctor relationship and its larger familial and social contexts. Several British researchers provide fascinating insights into early medical care: Dorothy Porter, *Patient's Progress: Doctors and Doctoring in Eighteenth-Century England* (Cambridge: Polity Press, 1989); Roy Porter, ed., *Patients and Practitioners: Lay Perceptions of Medicine in Pre-Industrial Society* (Cambridge: Cambridge University Press, 1985); and Roy Por-

ter and Dorothy Porter, *In Sickness and In Health: The British Experience,
1650–1850* (New York: Basil Blackwell, 1989 [1988]).

Greater sensitivity to the wide range of health-care roles in the premodern
world has led to an increased awareness of the complex structure of medical care
in those times. Roy Porter offers a brief typology in "The Language of Quackery
in England, 1660–1800," in Peter Burke and Roy Porter, eds., *The Social History
of Language* (Cambridge: Cambridge University Press, 1987), 73–103. A more
ambitious effort is Matthew Ramsey's *Professional and Popular Medicine in France,
1770–1830: The Social World of Medical Practice* (Cambridge and New York:
Cambridge University Press, 1988). Using popular health literature, William
Coleman has also explored the French medical landscape: "Health and Hygiene in
the *Encyclopédie:* A Medical Doctrine for the Bourgeoisie," *JHMAS* 29(1974):
399–421; and "The People's Health: Medical Themes in 18th-Century French
Popular Literature," *BHM* 51(1977): 55–74.

Students of nineteenth-century American medical history have likewise delved
into popular literature. Of particular value is Guenter B. Risse, Ronald L. Numbers, and Judith Walzer Leavitt, eds., *Medicine Without Doctors: Home Health Care
in American History* (New York: Science History Publications, 1977). Thus far the
tendency has been to depict professional and domestic practice in antagonistic
terms, but a few scholars see the relationship as having been more fluid:
Charles E. Rosenberg, "Medical Text and Social Context: Explaining William
Buchan's *Domestic Medicine,*" *BHM* 57(1983): 22–42; Charles E. Rosenberg,
"Introduction to the New Edition," *Gunn's Domestic Medicine, or, Poor Man's
Friend* (Knoxville, Tenn.: Printed under the immediate superintendance of the
author, a physician of Knoxville, 1830; facsimile ed., Tennesseana Editions,
Knoxville: University of Tennessee Press, 1986), [v]–xxi; Judith Walzer Leavitt,
Brought to Bed: Childbearing in America, 1750–1950 (New York: Oxford Univer-
sity Press, 1986); and Richard D. Brown, "The Healing Arts in Colonial and
Revolutionary Massachusetts: The Context for Scientific Medicine," in Philip
Cash, Eric H. Christianson, and J. Worth Estes, eds., *Medicine in Colonial Massachusetts, 1620–1820,* vol. 57 of the *Publications* of The Colonial Society of Mas-
sachusetts (Boston: The Colonial Society of Massachusetts, 1980), 35–47.

As James Harvey Young has documented, domestic practitioners had ready
access to an exploding patent medicine industry: "American Medical Quackery
in the Age of the Common Man," *MVHR* 47(1961): 579–93; *The Toadstool Millionaires: A Social History of Patent Medicines in America Before Federal Regulation*
(Princeton: Princeton University Press, 1961); *American Self-Dosage Medicines: An
Historical Perspective* (Lawrence, Kansas: Coronado Press, 1974). Sarah Stage extended Young's work with a fascinating case study, *Female Complaints: Lydia
Pinkham and the Business of Women's Medicine* (New York: W. W. Norton, 1979).
Madge E. Pickard and R. Carlyle Buley examined both home remedies and un-
orthodox practitioners in their less scholarly but useful *The Midwest Pioneer: His
Ills, Cures, and Doctors* (Crawfordsville, Ind.: R. E. Banta, 1945).

Popular health movements, especially sectarian alternatives to regular medicine, have received a great deal of research attention since Richard Shryock's
"Sylvester Graham and the Popular Health Movement, 1830–1870," *MVHR*
18(1931–1932): 172–83. William B. Walker also placed Graham squarely within
an ongoing health tradition in "The Health Reform Movement in the United
States, 1830–1870" (Ph.D. dissertation, Johns Hopkins University, June 1955),

but the best source on Graham and his work is Stephen Nissenbaum's *Sex, Diet, and Debility in Jacksonian America: Sylvester Graham and Health Reform* (Westport, Conn.: Greenwood Press, 1980).

During the past twenty years, specialized studies of medical sects have appeared. For overviews, see the general medical histories listed above and Norman Gevitz, ed., *Other Healers: Unorthodox Medicine in America* (Baltimore: Johns Hopkins University Press, 1988). On Thomsonianism, Alex Berman's work provides the most exhaustive discussion: "The Impact of the Nineteenth Century Botanico-Medical Movement on American Pharmacy and Medicine" (Ph.D. dissertation, University of Wisconsin, 1954); "Neo-Thomsonianism in the United States," *JHMAS* 11(1956): 133–55; and "The Thomsonian Movement and Its Relation to American Pharmacy and Medicine," *BHM* 25(1971): 405–28. The most comprehensive study of homeopathy is Martin Kaufman, *Homeopathy in America: The Rise and Fall of a Medical Heresy* (Baltimore: Johns Hopkins University Press, 1971). Harry B. Weiss and Howard R. Kemble's *The Great American Water Cure Craze: A History of Hydropathy in America* (Trenton, N.J.: The Past Times Press, 1967) has been supplemented by two substantial works, both of which focus on hydropathy's appeal to and impact on women: Susan E. Cayleff, *Wash and Be Healed: The Water-Cure Movement and Women's Health* (Philadelphia: Temple University Press, 1987); and Jane B. Donegan, *"Hydropathic Highway to Health": Women and Water-Cure in Antebellum America* (Westport, Conn.: Greenwood Press, 1986). Kathryn Kish Sklar describes one woman's water-cure experiences in *Catharine Beecher: A Study in American Domesticity* (New York: W. W. Norton, 1973), and Ronald L. Numbers gives another intimate perspective in *Prophetess of Health: A Study of Ellen G. White* (New York: Harper and Row, 1976).

The story of nineteenth-century medical sectarianism cannot be told without reference to other contemporary reform movements. In the vast secondary literature on antebellum reform, some of the most useful works are: Alice Felt Tyler's classic *Freedom's Ferment: Phases of American Social History from the Colonial Period to the Outbreak of the Civil War,* Harper Torchbook ed. (New York: Harper and Row, 1962 [1944]); David Rothman's influential *The Discovery of the Asylum: Social Order and Disorder in the New Republic* (Boston: Little, Brown and Company, 1971); and John L. Thomas's succinct "Romantic Reform in America, 1815–1865," *AQ* 17(1965): 656–81.

That these larger reform currents affected matters of health and medicine has been well demonstrated. See James C. Whorton, *Crusaders for Fitness: The History of American Health Reformers* (Princeton: Princeton University Press, 1982); Martha H. Verbrugge, *Able-Bodied Womanhood: Personal Health and Social Change in Nineteenth-Century Boston* (New York: Oxford University Press, 1988); Ronald G. Walters, *American Reformers, 1815–1860* (New York: Hill and Wang, 1978); John C. Burnham, *How Superstition Won and Science Lost: Popularizing Science and Health in the United States* (New Brunswick and London: Rutgers University Press, 1987); and Bruce Haley, *The Healthy Body and Victorian Culture* (Cambridge: Harvard University Press, 1978). Two authors make similar points for a more popular audience: Harvey Green, *Fit for America: Health, Fitness, Sport, and American Society* (New York: Pantheon Books, 1986); and Hillel Schwartz, *Never Satisfied: A Cultural History of Diets, Fantasies and Fat* (New York: The Free Press, 1986).

Popular physiologists played an important role in educating Americans about health through lectures and books. Donald M. Scott makes some suggestive remarks in "The Popular Lecture and the Creation of a Public in Mid-Nineteenth-Century America," *JAH* 66(1980): 791–809. There is no adequate study of American physiology, anatomy, and hygiene textbooks. The standard references are Charles Carpenter, *History of American Schoolbooks* (Philadelphia: University of Pennsylvania Press, 1963), and John A. Nietz, *Old Textbooks. Spelling, Grammar, Reading, Arithmetic, Geography, American History, Civil Government, Physiology, Penmanship, Art, Music—As Taught in the Common Schools from Colonial Days to 1900* (Pittsburgh: University of Pittsburgh Press, 1961). Carpenter acknowledges his reliance on Helen Margaret Barton's superficial "A Study of the Development of Textbooks in Physiology and Hygiene in the United States" (Ph.D. dissertation, University of Pittsburgh, 1942).

It is difficult to place popular physiologists within the field of physiology, since histories of the discipline shortchange antebellum developments: W. Bruce Fye, *The Development of American Physiology: Scientific Medicine in the Nineteenth Century* (Baltimore: Johns Hopkins University Press, 1987); and Gerald L. Geison, ed., *Physiology in the American Context, 1850–1914* (Bethesda, Md.: American Physiological Society, 1987). Edward C. Atwater's "'Squeezing Mother Nature': Experimental Physiology in the United States Before 1870," *BHM* 52(1978): 313–35 is more helpful, as is Gerald N. Grob's biography of a leading textbook writer, *Edward Jarvis and the Medical World of Nineteenth-Century America* (Knoxville: University of Tennessee Press, 1978). John Harley Warner provides useful background information in "'The Nature-Trusting Heresy': American Physicians and the Concept of the Healing Power of Nature in the 1850's and 1860's," *Perspectives in American History* 11(1977–1978): 291–324. Despite the growing importance of the relationship between anatomy, physiology, and hygiene throughout the century, Anita Clair Fellman and Michael Fellman do not discuss it in *Making Sense of Self: Medical Advice Literature in Late Nineteenth-Century America* (Philadelphia: University of Pennsylvania Press, 1981).

In the private domain, burgeoning advice literature both reflected and assuaged widespread popular anxieties about suitable personal behavior and expectations. Studies of phrenology illustrate this theme: Roger Cooter, *The Cultural Meaning of Popular Science: Phrenology and the Organization of Consent in Nineteenth-Century Britain* (New York: Cambridge University Press, 1984); John D. Davies, *Phrenology, Fad and Science: A 19th-Century American Crusade* (New Haven: Yale University Press, 1955); Madeleine B. Stern, *Heads and Headliners: The Phrenological Fowlers* (Norman: University of Oklahoma Press, 1971); and especially Allan S. Horlick, "Phrenology and the Social Education of Young Men," *History of Education Quarterly* 11(Spring 1971): 23–38. Daniel T. Rodgers has argued more cogently that advice literature had great socialization value for a modernizing nation: "Socializing Middle-Class Children: Institutions, Fables, and Work Values in Nineteenth-Century America," in N. Ray Hiner and Joseph M. Hawes, eds., *Growing Up in America: Children in Historical Perspective* (Urbana: University of Illinois Press, 1985), 119–32.

Many scholars have used advice literature to chart a growing cultural investment in childhood after the American Revolution: Bernard Wishy, *The Child and the Republic: The Dawn of Modern American Child Nurture* (Philadelphia: University of Pennsylvania Press, 1968); Jacqueline S. Reiner, "Rearing the Republican

Child: Attitudes and Practices in Post-Revolutionary Philadelphia," *WMQ*, 3rd ser., 39(1982): 150–63. See also Ruth H. Bloch, "American Feminine Ideals in Transition: The Rise of the Moral Mother, 1785–1815," *Feminist Studies* 4(1978): 101–26; Anne L. Kuhn, *The Mother's Role in Childhood Education: New England Concepts, 1830–1860* (New Haven: Yale University Press, 1947).

Sparked by Barbara Welter's "The Cult of True Womanhood, 1820–1860," *AQ* 18(1966): 151–74, other researchers have investigated the concurrent and interrelated glorification of the domestic sphere. Among them are Laurel Thatcher Ulrich, *Good Wives: Image and Reality in the Lives of Women in Northern New England, 1650–1750* (New York: Alfred A. Knopf, 1982), and Nancy Cott, *The Bonds of Womanhood: "Women's Sphere" in New England, 1780–1835* (New Haven: Yale University Press, 1977). Citizens of the new nation extended the benefits of female domesticity to encompass the public realm as well, as Mary Beth Norton points out in *Liberty's Daughters: The Revolutionary Experience of American Women, 1750–1850* (Boston: Little, Brown and Company, 1980). Linda Kerber has convincingly corroborated and advanced this argument by linking it explicitly to republican ideology: "The Republican Mother: Women and the Enlightenment—An American Perspective," *AQ* 28(1976): 187–205; "Daughters of Columbia: Educating Women for the Republic, 1787–1805," in Stanley Elkins and Eric McKitrick, eds., *The Hofstadter Aegis: A Memorial* (New York: Alfred A. Knopf, 1974), 36–59; and *Women of the Republic: Intellect and Ideology in Revolutionary America* (Chapel Hill: University of North Carolina Press, 1980). Also helpful in understanding republicanism are Robert E. Shalhope, "Republicanism and Early American Historiography," *WMQ*, 3rd ser., 39(1982): 334–56; Gordon S. Wood, *The Creation of the American Republic, 1776–1787* (New York: W. W. Norton, 1972); Garry Wills, *Inventing America: Jefferson's Declaration of Independence* (Garden City, N.Y.: Doubleday and Co., 1978); and Rhys Isaac, *The Transformation of Virginia, 1740–1790* (Chapel Hill: Published for the Institute of Early American History and Culture by the University of North Carolina Press, 1982).

Given the increasing emphasis on childhood and family, it is not surprising that this period also saw the birth of pediatrics. Yet the subject has received little scholarly attention beyond compilations akin to Arthur F. Abt, ed., *Abt-Garrison History of Pediatrics* (Philadelphia: W. B. Saunders Co., 1965). Sydney A. Halpern mentions antebellum events only briefly in *American Pediatrics: The Social Dynamics of Professionalism, 1880–1980* (Berkeley and Los Angeles: University of California Press, 1988). Virginia A. Metaxas Quiroga supplies some facts in "Female Lay Managers and Scientific Pediatrics at Nursery and Child's Hospital, 1854–1910," *BHM* 60(1986): 194–208. Valerie A. Fildes offers more substantial coverage of pediatric developments in two books: *Breasts, Bottles and Babies: A History of Infant Feeding* (Edinburgh: Edinburgh University Press, 1986); and *Wet Nursing: A History from Antiquity to the Present* (Oxford: Basil Blackwell, 1988).

In sharp contrast to the paucity of our knowledge about the origins of pediatrics in America, our understanding of antebellum midwifery, obstetrics, and gynecology is growing rapidly. See especially Judith Walzer Leavitt, *Brought to Bed: Childbearing in America, 1750–1950* (New York: Oxford University Press, 1986); Judith Walzer Leavitt, "'Science' Enters the Birthing Room: Obstetrics in America since the Eighteenth Century," *JAH* 70(1983): 281–304; Jane B. Donegan, *Women and Men Midwives: Medicine, Morality and Misogyny in Early America* (Westport, Conn.: Greenwood Press, 1978); Richard W. Wertz and Dorothy C.

Wertz, *Lying-In: A History of Childbirth in America* (New York: The Free Press, 1977); Catherine M. Scholten, "'On the Importance of the Obstetrick Art': Changing Customs of Childbirth in America, 1760 to 1825," *WMQ*, 3rd ser., 34(1977): 426–45; Catherine M. Scholten, *Childbearing in American Society, 1650–1850* (New York: New York University Press, 1985); and Gerda Lerner, "The Lady and the Mill Girl," *American Studies (Midcontinent American Studies Journal)* 10(1969): 5–15.

Heightened interest in women's experiences has encouraged historical study of sexuality and sex roles. In this area, researchers argue, medical men and medical ideas have had significant impact, largely through the dissemination of advice literature. For a synthetic overview, see Carl Degler, *At Odds: Women and the Family in America from the Revolution to the Present* (New York: Oxford University Press, 1980). Relatively little work has been done on male sexuality, and the most useful discussions are: Carroll Smith-Rosenberg, "Sex as Symbol in Victorian Purity: An Ethnohistorical Analysis of Jacksonian America," in John Demos and Sarane Spence Boocock, eds., *Turning Points: Historical and Sociological Essays on the Family (American Journal of Sociology,* vol. 84, Supplement, 1978): S212–S247; and Charles E. Rosenberg, "Sexuality, Class, and Role," *AQ* 25(1973): 131–53. G. J. Barker-Benfield's work is laced with misogynism: *The Horrors of the Half-Known Life: Male Attitudes Toward Women and Sexuality in 19th Century America* (New York: Harper, 1976); and a summary version, "The Spermatic Economy: A Nineteenth-Century View of Sexuality," *Feminist Studies* 1(Summer 1972): 45–74.

But, as Carl Degler warned in 1974, one of the greatest dangers in tackling this type of research is the temptation to interpret prescriptive literature as directly reflective of past behavior (Carl Degler, "What Ought To Be and What Was: Women's Sexuality in the Nineteenth Century," *AHR* 79(1974): 1479–90). John S. Haller and Robin M. Haller inadequately heed Degler's warning in *The Physician and Sexuality in Victorian America* (Urbana: University of Illinois Press, 1974). Ann Douglas Wood's strident feminism greatly weakens her argument in "The 'Fashionable Diseases': Women's Complaints and Their Treatment in Nineteenth Century America," *JIH* 4(1973–1974): 25–52. Regina Markell Morantz offers sensible rejoinders in "The Perils of Feminist History," *JIH* 4(1973–1974): 649–60 and "The Lady and Her Physician," in Mary Hartmann and Lois Banner, eds., *Clio's Consciousness Raised: New Perspectives on the History of Women* (New York: Harper and Row, 1974), 38–53. Another pertinent study is Regina Markell Morantz and Sue Zschoche, "Professionalism, Feminism, and Gender Roles: A Comparative Study of Nineteenth-Century Medical Therapeutics," *JAH* 67(1980): 568–88.

Students of sexuality and female invalidism implicitly or explicitly accord physicians great cultural authority. But the means by which doctors attained and maintained this authority have seldom been well analyzed. This is true, for instance, of the stridently polemical works of Barbara Ehrenreich and Deirdre English: *Complaints and Disorders: The Sexual Politics of Sickness* (Old Westbury, N.Y.: Feminist Press, 1973) and *Witches, Midwives and Nurses* (Old Westbury, N.Y.: Feminist Press, 1973). Similarly biased is their later volume, *For Her Own Good: 150 Years of the Experts' Advice to Women* (New York: Anchor Press/Doubleday, 1978). Carroll Smith-Rosenberg and Charles E. Rosenberg have done more thoughtful work in this area: Rosenberg and Smith-Rosenberg, "The Female Animal: Medical and Biological Views of Woman and Her Role in Nineteenth-Century America," *JAH* 60(1973): 332–56; Smith-Rosenberg, "The Hysterical Woman: Sex Roles and Role Conflict in Nineteenth-Century America," *Social Research* 39(1972): 652–78; Smith-Rosenberg, "Puberty to Menopause: The Cycle of Femininity in Nineteenth-Century America," *Feminist Studies* 1(1973): 58–72; and Smith-Rosenberg, "Beauty, the Beast and the Militant Woman: A Study in Sex Roles and Social Stress in Jacksonian America," *AQ* 22(1971): 562–84.

The situation on both public and private fronts was enormously complicated by the precarious state of the medical profession. Strong public support for alternative medical practices undermined the regulars' claims to legitimacy just as the regulars felt buffeted by tremendous internal discord and fragmentation. As the general histories make clear, orthodox physicians tried to use legislation to strengthen the profession. See also Richard H. Shryock, *Medical Licensing in America, 1650–1965* (Baltimore: Johns Hopkins University Press, 1967); Donald E. Konold, *A History of American Medical Ethics, 1847–1912* (Madison: State Historical Society of Wisconsin, 1962); John Duffy, *The Healers: The Rise of the Medical Establishment* (New York: McGraw-Hill Book Co., 1976); George Rosen, *Fees and Fee Bills: Economic Aspects of Medical Practice in Nineteenth Century America* (Baltimore: Johns Hopkins University Press, 1947); and Paul Starr, "Medicine, Economy and Society in Nineteenth-Century America," *J. Soc. Hist.* 10(1976–1977): 588–607.

Regulars also tried to strengthen the profession by improving medical education. Still useful is William F. Norwood's exhaustive *Medical Education in the United States Before the Civil War* (Philadelphia: University of Pennsylvania Press, 1944). For more recent overviews, see Martin Kaufman, *American Medical Education: The Formative Years, 1765–1910* (Westport, Conn.: Greenwood Press, 1980); Ronald L. Numbers, ed., *The Education of American Physicians: Historical Essays* (Berkeley: University of California Press, 1979); Kenneth M. Ludmerer, *Learning to Heal: The Development of American Medical Education* (New York: Basic Books, 1985); and John Harley Warner, *The Therapeutic Perspective: Medical Practice, Knowledge, and Identity in America, 1820–1885* (Cambridge: Harvard University Press, 1986).

Women and blacks fared no better than sectarians in winning equal educational and associational opportunities. On women, see Regina Markell Morantz-Sanchez, *Sympathy and Science: Women Physicians in American Medicine* (New York: Oxford University Press, 1987 [1985]); Mary Roth Walsh, *"Doctors Wanted. No Women Need Apply": Sexual Barriers in the Medical Profession* (New Haven: Yale University Press, 1978); John B. Blake, "Women and Medicine in Antebellum America," *BHM* 39(1965): 99–123; and Regina Markell Morantz, "The 'Connecting Link': The Case for the Woman Doctor in 19th-Century America," in Judith Walzer Leavitt and Ronald L. Numbers, eds., *Sickness and Health in America: Readings in the History of Medicine and Public Health* (Madison: University of Wisconsin Press, 1978), 117–28.

On blacks, see Herbert M. Morais, *The History of the Negro in Medicine* (New York: Publishers Co., 1967). William D. Postell's *The Health of Slaves on Southern Plantations* (Baton Rouge: Louisiana State University Press, 1951) has been updated by Todd L. Savitt, *Medicine and Slavery: The Health Care and Diseases of Blacks in Antebellum Virginia* (Urbana: University of Illinois Press, 1978), and Todd L. Savitt, "Black Health on the Plantation: Masters, Slaves, and Physicians," in Judith Walzer Leavitt and Ronald L. Numbers, eds., *Sickness and Health in America: Readings in the History of Medicine and Public Health*, 2nd ed., revised (Madison: University of Wisconsin Press, 1985), 313–30.

To some extent these barriers worked for women by shunting them into nursing. A good overview is Richard H. Shryock, *The History of Nursing: An Interpretation of the Social and Medical Factors Involved* (Philadelphia: Saunders, 1959). Shryock summarizes the American situation in "Nursing Emerges as a Profession: The American Experience," *Clio Medica* 3(1968): 131–47. The charge of sexism is leveled crudely in JoAnn Ashley, *Hospitals, Paternalism, and the Role of the Nurse* (New York: Teachers College Press, 1976). Better treatments are Susan Reverby, *Ordered to Care: The Dilemma of American Nursing, 1850–1945* (Cambridge: Cambridge University Press, 1987); and Barbara Melosh, *"The Physician's Hand": Work Culture and Conflict in American Nursing* (Philadelphia: Temple University Press, 1982). On the history of hospitals, see especially Morris J. Vogel, *The Invention of the Modern Hospital: Boston, 1870–1930* (Chicago: University of Chicago Press, 1980), and Charles E. Rosenberg, *The Care of Strangers: The Rise of America's Hospital System* (New York: Basic Books, 1987). A useful source for the antebellum period is Charles E. Rosenberg, "And Heal the Sick: The Hospital and the Patient in 19th Century America," *J. Soc. Hist.* 10 (1976–1977): 428–47.

While it is true that women have had to struggle to be admitted to orthodox training programs and to accredited practice, there is another side to their historical relationship with professional medicine. Physicians, as scholars are beginning to realize, recognized that women were important providers and consumers of health care. It has been argued that medical debates over the role of women both revealed and encouraged slowly changing nineteenth-century attitudes toward sickness and death. See, for example, two articles by Regina Markell Morantz, "Nineteenth Century Health Reform and Women: A Program of Self-Help," in Guenter B. Risse, Ronald L. Numbers, and Judith Walzer Leavitt, eds., *Medicine Without Doctors: Home Health Care in American History* (New York: Science History Publications, 1977), 73–93; and "Making Women Modern: Middle Class Women and Health Reform in Nineteenth Century America," *J. Soc. Hist.* 10(1976–1977): 490–507. See also Martha H. Verbrugge, "The Social Meaning of Personal Health: The Ladies' Physiological Institute of Boston and Vicinity in the 1850s," in Susan Reverby and David Rosner, eds., *Health Care in America: Essays in Social History* (Philadelphia: Temple University Press, 1979), 45–66.

Some have extended this argument by pointing out that for many women health-reform activities became steppingstones to more aggressive feminism, both within the public sphere and within the more narrowly defined context of family and friends. Carroll Smith-Rosenberg has depicted "The Female World of Love and Ritual: Relations Between Women in Nineteenth-Century America," *Signs* 1(1975): 1–29. Others have explored issues of birth control, family limitation, and abortion: Daniel Scott Smith, "Family Limitation, Sexual Control, and Domestic Feminism in Victorian America," in Mary Hartmann and Lois Banner, eds., *Clio's Consciousness Raised: New Perspectives on the History of Women* (New York: Harper and Row, 1974), 119–36; David Kennedy, *Birth Control in America: The Career of Margaret Sanger* (New Haven: Yale University Press, 1970); James Reed, *From Private Vice to Public Virtue: The Birth Control Movement and American Society Since 1830* (New York: Basic Books, 1978); Linda Gordon, *Woman's Body,*

Woman's Right: A Social History of Birth Control in America (New York: Grossman Publishers, 1976); and James Mohr, *Abortion in America: The Origins and Evolution of National Policy* (New York: Oxford University Press, 1977). An excellent summary of the Reed book is James Reed, "Doctors, Birth Control, and Social Values, 1830–1970," in Morris J. Vogel and Charles E. Rosenberg, eds., *The Therapeutic Revolution: Essays in the Social History of American Medicine* (Philadelphia: University of Pennsylvania Press, 1979), 109–33.

Index

Abbott, Simon, 94, 97, 99
Account of Some of the Vegetable Productions Naturally Growing in This Part of America, An (Cutler), 72
Account of the Diseases Most Incident to Children, An (Armstrong), 45–46
Ackerknecht, Erwin, 226
Ackerley, G., 59–60
Adams, Abigail, 9
Advice books. *See* Domestic health manuals
Advice to Mothers (Buchan), 42–43
Advice to Young Men on Their Duties and Conduct in Life (Arthur), 134–36
Advice to Young Mothers on the Physical Education of Children (Moore), 65–66
Alcohol: Graham on use of, 116; temperance movement, 116
Alcott, William Andrus, 115, 141, 160, 162, 175, 202; on education, 123–25, 139; career and beliefs, 123–34; textbooks by, 154–55, 176–77; influence on later textbooks, 156, 159
Allentown Academy, 218
American Domestick Medicine (Jameson), 19–21, 28, 30

American Family Physician (Ewell), 19, 57
American Frugal Housewife (Child), 66, 138–39
American Herbal (Stearns), 72
American Hydropathic Society, 197
American Hygienic and Hydropathic Association of Physicians and Surgeons, 197
American Institute of Homeopathy, 218, 220
American Journal of the Medical Sciences, 161, 165
"American Matron" (author), 63–65
American Medical Association, 102, 218
American Medical Botany (Bigelow), 72–73
American Medical Intelligencer (journal), 152
American Museum (journal), 27
American Physician (Smith), 96–98
American Physiological Society, 206
American Revolution, 25–27, 97, 140–41
American Tract Society, 84
American Vegetable Practice (Mattson), 99
Ames, Fisher, 11–12
Ames, Nathaniel, Jr., 24
Amherst College, 184
Analytic Anatomy and Hygiene (Cutter), 168

303